LIFE AND DEATH ON THE NILE

UNIVERSITY PRESS OF FLORIDA

Florida A&M University, Tallahassee
Florida Atlantic University, Boca Raton
Florida Gulf Coast University, Ft. Myers
Florida International University, Miami
Florida State University, Tallahassee
New College of Florida, Sarasota
University of Central Florida, Orlando
University of Florida, Gainesville
University of North Florida, Jacksonville
University of South Florida, Tampa
University of West Florida, Pensacola

LIFE AND DEATH ON THE NILE

A Bioethnography of Three Ancient Nubian Communities

GEORGE J. ARMELAGOS
AND DENNIS P. VAN GERVEN

University Press of Florida
Gainesville · Tallahassee · Tampa · Boca Raton
Pensacola · Orlando · Miami · Jacksonville · Ft. Myers · Sarasota

Printed in the United States of America on acid-free paper

This book may be available in an electronic edition.

22 21 20 19 18 17 6 5 4 3 2 1

Library of Congress Cataloging-in-Publication Data
Names: Armelagos, George J., author. | Van Gerven, Dennis P., author.
Title: Life and death on the Nile : a bioethnography of three ancient Nubian communities / George J. Armelagos and Dennis P. Van Gerven.
Description: Gainesville : University Press of Florida, 2017. | Includes bibliographical references and index.
Identifiers: LCCN 2017016668 | ISBN 9780813054452 (cloth)
Subjects: LCSH: Nubia—History. | Nubia—Antiquities. | Excavations (Archaeology)—Nubia. | Excavations (Archaeology)—Sudan.
Classification: LCC DT159.6.N83 A76 2017 | DDC 939/.78—dc23
LC record available at https://lccn.loc.gov/2017016668

The University Press of Florida is the scholarly publishing agency for the State University System of Florida, comprising Florida A&M University, Florida Atlantic University, Florida Gulf Coast University, Florida International University, Florida State University, New College of Florida, University of Central Florida, University of Florida, University of North Florida, University of South Florida, and University of West Florida.

University Press of Florida
15 Northwest 15th Street
Gainesville, FL 32611-2079
http://upress.ufl.edu

In Memory of George John Armelagos

(1936–2014)

The Greatest Scholar and Funniest Man I Ever Knew

CONTENTS

FIGURES

TABLES

PREFACE

Perfect is the enemy of done.
Meg Seiler

This book is a tribute to George John Armelagos. He was a prolific writer authoring hundreds of articles and over a dozen books. His curriculum vita was some 85 pages long. He was one of the leaders of an intellectual movement in biological anthropology known today as bioarchaeology. It is impossible to identify his area of expertise. His contributions spanned the breath of biological anthropology, and he made important contributions to archaeology and cultural anthropology as well. His reputation was international. He was my friend and mentor. He was the funniest man I ever knew.

Our friendship and his mentorship go back to 1965. I was an undergraduate at the University of Utah, and George was an instructor in the Department of Anthropology while completing his Ph.D. in anthropology at the University of Colorado. I took his Introduction to Physical Anthropology course, and halfway through he invited me to visit his lab. That visit was the beginning of over a half century of collaboration and friendship. We published together in six decades. We were both shooting for a seventh. Most of the articles dealt with skeletal remains from Sudanese Nubia.

George's dissertation research was based on the study of Nubian remains excavated near the town of Wadi Halfa on the border between modern Egypt and Sudan. He and a team of other Colorado graduate students had excavated the material in 1959 as part of a program funded by the United Nations Educational, Scientific, and Cultural Organization (UNESCO) to save the monuments of Nubia. The Colorado expedition was one of some 36 mounted from across Europe and the United States.

The goal of the UNESCO Campaign was to salvage as much of the human and archaeological remains as possible before they were buried under a 340-mile-long, 22-mile-wide, and 100-foot-deep lake. The lake would extend from Aswan in Egypt across the Egyptian-Sudanese border for some 80 miles. The lake would entirely bury a region of the Nile known in antiquity as Nubia. The Sudanese portion of the lake is called Lake Nubia. The Egyptian portion is called Lake Nasser. Because of the dam and its lake, the Nubia you will be learning about in this book no longer exists.

While I collaborated with George on his Nubia work, I had no opportunity to conduct my own research until 1979. David Greene, William Adams, and I obtained a National Science Foundation grant to excavate two cemeteries at the site of Kulubnarti located at the very tip of the lake. The folk interred in the cemeteries were the Christian ancestors of the modern Muslim people living in the neighboring village of Kulb today.

Life and Death on the Nile: A Bioethnography of Three Ancient Nubian Communities represents a half century of collaboration between George, me, and our students studying the remains from Wadi Halfa and Kulubnarti. It was conceived during a casual conversation about nothing in particular. George mentioned that we had published articles together in six decades. That led us to thinking back about our Nubian research—about how many theses and articles had been published, and how creative our students' research had been.

George remarked on how we'd never had an organized plan as to how the research would proceed. Neither of us could recall a time when we had actually assigned a student a project. George always believed that students learned most—did their best—when he left them alone. George had a teaching mantra—the less you teach the more they learn.

While there wasn't a plan, there was an overarching principle: every aspect of the Nubians' lives—how they grew and developed, the diseases that afflicted them, and the diets that sustained them—was the result of a complex interaction between their biology and the physical-cultural environment in which they lived. The goal under George's leadership was to tease out and understand those relationships. So, while the work has most often been spontaneous, it has never been incoherent.

George's commitment to a biocultural approach and his faith in the creativity of his students—including me—have given our work an intellectually natural, organic quality. Viewed from early days to most recent times, the work has grown like a family tree of accomplishment with roots running deep into a biocultural perspective. Each branch represents a new line of inquiry grown from the work that preceded it. There are functional morphology and demography branches down near the roots, with the growth and development and paleopathology branches farther up. And there were always new branches sprouting at the top.

We of course knew there were connections among the projects, but we had never realized how natural those relationships were. We had never fully realized the unifying power of a biocultural approach until we reflected back on our half century together. We knew it, but we hadn't seen it because we had worked too close to the branches and hadn't stepped back to look at the tree. That realization gave rise to this book.

The book would have a monograph quality—that is, it would present a single body of work—but it wouldn't be a traditional monograph. Monographs are most often written in the present tense. They represent the culmination of research at that moment. Ours would be written largely in the past tense. It would be a retrospective on our five decades of work with our students. There would be an emphasis on the research process as well a product. The book would end with our view of the future. We would reflect on the future and how new discoveries, both biological and archaeological, promised a future as productive as the past.

We became convinced that a book such as ours would have value—certainly for us. We were anxious to set down in print what we had come to think of as our research family tree. We wanted others to appreciate the remarkable creativity of our students and the natural progression of their unfettered work.

We hoped it would be of interest to others as well. We believe that ours is an interesting story for students and nonprofessionals interested in the study of ancient human remains. Of course ancient Nubia is an interesting story in itself. And there is the story of how research like ours is done. In telling that story, we hoped to illustrate the natural synergy between teaching and research. In doing so, we hoped to dispel the myth of an inherent conflict between the two.

George's first love was teaching and sharing the excitement of learning with his students. Indeed, George working apart from students—graduate and undergraduate alike—was unthinkable. He believed that doing science without teaching was a lonely business, and a scientist who didn't teach was squandering an important opportunity. George never missed a teaching opportunity. His reputation as a world-class scientist sometimes obscured that.

We decided to write this book in a personal voice speaking to the audiences that attend our talks and lectures. They don't come to hear the technical analyses we publish in journals. They want to know about how we read the bones for clues and how we use the clues to bring to light "Life and Death on the Nile." They want us to take them behind the scenes and show them how we do what we do. That is what we hoped to do with this book. At the same time, we hoped to present the science in a way that the nonspecialist could understand and appreciate.

As for how the volume is organized, we followed the advice the king gave to the white rabbit in *Alice and Wonderland*. "Begin at the beginning," the king said, very gravely, "and go on till you come to the end: then stop."

George passed away on May 15, 2014, just as we completed the first draft of this book. He died the way he lived—surrounded by friends and his students. The world lost a great mind and a remarkable innovator. Many colleagues acknowledged George as the greatest biological anthropologist of his time. I believe we lost the best, most diverse and creative biological anthropologist of the twentieth century.

This volume is the last work that we did together. I hope that you will enjoy reading it as much as we did writing it.

ACKNOWLEDGMENTS

There is no question that our most sincere and heartfelt thanks must go to the many students—both undergraduate and graduate—who made this book possible. They brought the constant supply of new eyes and fresh legs that fueled our six decades of research. There is no aspect of our research that could have been accomplished without their energy and creativity. We would like to extend a special thanks to David Greene. David's analysis of the dental morphology of the Wadi Halfa and Kulubnarti remains provided a seminal role in our understanding of continuity and change in the Nubian populations. His integration of genetic and archaeological data helped lay the foundation for what would become our biocultural approach. On a more personal note, I would have never gotten to Nubia without his collaboration on the National Science Foundation grant that funded the Kulubnarti expedition. Bill Adams's collaboration on the Kulubnarti grant was equally critical, but we owe him a debt far greater than that. The force of his intellect and the body of his research on the culture history of Nubia touched every aspect of our work. David and Bill have also been wonderful friends. I personally would like to thank Ed Rowen, who worked alongside me in the cemeteries. We would also like to thank Kendra Sirak for the many hours she spent editing our prose. We would like to thank Clark Larsen, series editor, for the important influence he has had on our work. He is a true leader in biocultural analysis. Last but not least, we want to thank the staff at the University Press of Florida, most particularly Ali Sundook, acquisitions assistant, and Eleanor Deumens, project editor.

1

LIFE AND DEATH ON THE NILE

Bones are like old books in strange languages. Learn how to read them and they have wonderful tales to tell.

In the Beginning

This book is the story of life and death, health and disease of three ancient Nubian communities. The first community was Meinarti. It sat astride the Nile River on what is today the Egyptian-Sudanese border. The river was the economic artery connecting Egypt and interior Africa to the Mediterranean basin (Adams 1977). Meinarti was a town of merchants, tradesmen, bureaucrats, and farmers. The second community was Kulubnarti, a tiny hamlet of freehold farmers eking out a living on the west bank of the Nile some 80 miles to the south of Meinarti in the most isolated and hostile of Nubia's environments. Their descendants live there today in the village of Kulb.[1] The third was a shantytown of landless, itinerant laborers living on an island adjacent to the west bank little more than a mile from the Kulubnarti folk they served. The three villages together span some 1,500 years of Nubian history beginning 350 years before the Common Era (CE) (the birth of Christ) and extending to the middle of the twelfth century.

While our subjects have provided us little more than bones, teeth, and desiccated flesh, they tell a tale of wealth and poverty, chance, and opportunity universal to the human condition. It's a tale best told from anthropology's most time-honored perspective—ethnography or, in our case, bioethnography.

If anthropology had an origin story it could start with a simple sentence like this: *in the beginning there was ethnography*. All of the areas of the discipline—including archaeology and physical anthropology—go back to ethnography. Ethnography has been anthropology's window into other cultures and the home base from which anthropologists have unraveled the complexities of human culture, adaptation, and evolution. All anthropology has been built on the foundation laid by the early ethnographers.

The wonder of a great ethnography is its capacity to give us an intimate understanding of other people—their hopes and dreams, the values and beliefs that guide their lives; the setting in which they live; their patterns of subsistence, kinship, social organization, religion, and ideology that constitute *that complex whole* envisioned over a century ago by E. B. Tylor (1871).

We mention this because contemporary biological anthropologists, particularly those who study skeletal remains, have often moved away from their ethnographic roots. As a result, it has become increasingly difficult to find what we call a *bioethnographic* window on ancient cultures and the people who created them. It seems as though wide-ranging treatments comparable to *The Indians of Pecos* (Hooton 1930) or *The Stone Age of Mount Carmel* (Garrod et al. 1939) have become increasingly rare. This isn't to say skeletal analyses have fallen into a dark age—far from it. Modern analytical techniques combined with a new interest in population ecology have created a florescence of research in paleodemography, paleopathology, bone growth and development, and functional morphology (Armelagos 2013). While the technical quality of such research has never been higher, there have been consequences. Human and cultural remains are less often treated as integrated historical phenomena, but rather as material for a series of separate, highly sophisticated analyses.

The trend is not, however, inevitable. Indeed, the abundance of information available today has created a rich potential for what might be termed a new "bioethnographic" approach in which the biology and culture of ancient people are integrated into the cultural historical process. Synthetic treatments such as Clark and Brandt's *From Hunters to Farmers* (Clark and Brandt 1984), Cohen and Armelagos's *Paleopathology at the Origins of Agriculture* (Cohen and Armelagos 1984, 2013), Larsen and Milner's *In the Wake of Contact: Biological Responses to Conquest* (Larsen and Milner 1993), and Larsen's *Bioarchaeology of Spanish Florida* (Larsen 2001) are excellent examples. Our hope is to continue in that tradition by creating a bioethnography of three Nubian communities.

Nubia

Nubia is a land between the cataracts—what we call rapids. It begins in Egypt at the first cataract of the Nile (the town of Aswan) and extends

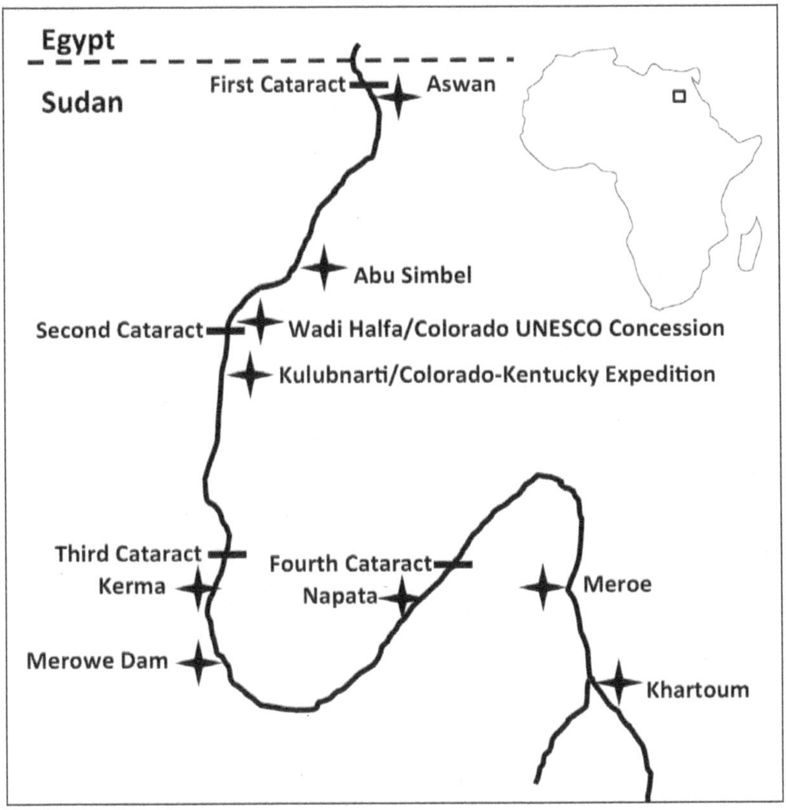

Figure 1.1. Map of Sudanese Nubia.

southward across the Egyptian-Sudanese border to the 4th cataract near the Sudanese capital of Khartoum. It is a region rich in history as well as archaeological treasures, and yet unlike Egypt, the archaeology of Nubia has never captured the imagination of the general public.

The problem has been Nubia's image. Appearance has always trumped importance. William Y. Adams, the world authority on ancient Nubia, describes Nubia as "a hot, dry and barren land of few resources and limited subsistence potential" (Adams 1977:19), but he goes on to tell us that "poor as it was and is, however, the Nile Valley between Aswan and Khartoum offered, for millennia on end, the only way across the great desert barrier of the Sahara."

Adams's definitive volume on ancient Nubia is titled *Nubia: Corridor to Africa* (Adams 1977), and the title is apt. Nubia was Egypt's land of gold as well as slaves, ivory, and other riches. The treasures of interior Africa

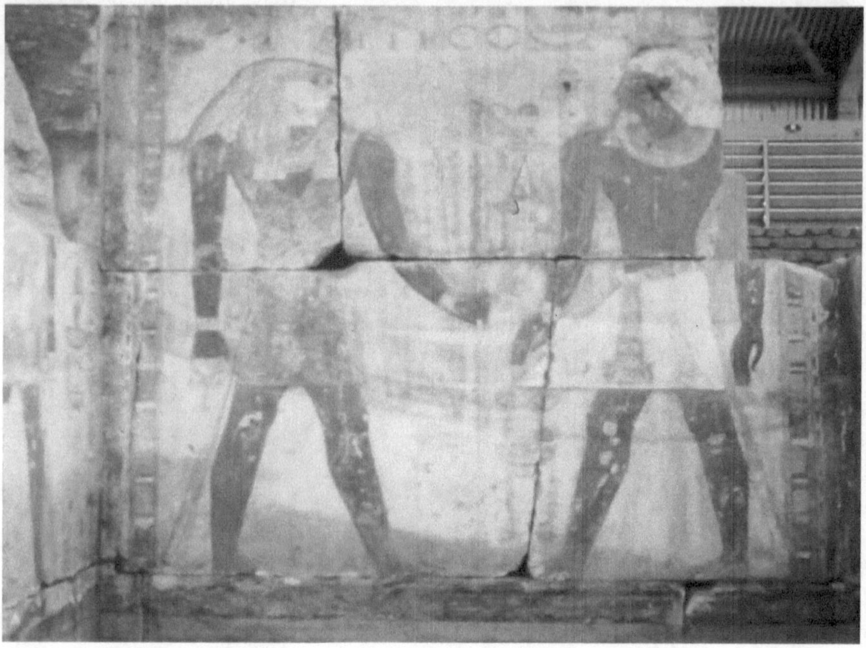

Figure 1.2. The Buhen temple.

moved northward down the Nile through the lands of Nubia. Nubia would remain a vital economic corridor until the advent of the great camel caravans in 300 CE. Nubia also provided legions of soldiers for Egypt's armies—soldiers famous for their deadly skill with the long bow.

It's not surprising that Egyptian pharaohs fought to extend control farther and farther southward into the lands of Nubia, and it's also not surprising that Nubia is today home to large numbers of pharaonic monuments, temples, and tombs proclaiming royal dominion.

Nubia could, in a sense, be thought of as two corridors laid end to end. Lower Nubia extends southward from Aswan to Wadi Halfa, with Upper Nubia extending southward from Wadi Halfa to near Khartoum. The Nile passing through Lower Nubia is broad, slow moving, and productive for the human population inhabiting its banks. As the Nile passes into Upper Nubia, it becomes increasingly wild and fast-flowing. Its channel becomes strewn with rocks, making navigation increasingly difficult. The populations of Upper Egypt have always remained huddled along the river, extending only as far as irrigation would permit (Adams 1977).

With the flow of goods through Nubia naturally came a flow of people and ideas. Roman legions passed into sub-Saharan Africa through Nubia, and indeed one can still see Roman ruins far into Sudan. There can be no doubt that Romans and others passing through Nubia left their genes along the Nubian corridor, and that should not be understood as their Levi pants! Given this continuous flow of peoples and cultures, it's not surprising that Nubian populations and cultures "are neither wholly Mediterranean nor wholly African: since earliest times they have presented a unique blend of the two" (Adams 1967:12). You need only look at Nubian villagers of today to appreciate that fact.

There is one final point that needs to be made. Nubians are often portrayed in ancient Egypt as servants and slaves. A servile position wasn't always the case. Egypt was ruled by a succession of Nubian pharaohs from 760 to 656 BCE. Their seat of power was Napata at the 4th cataract—far to the south of Egypt. Modern Nubians rightly consider themselves to be the descendants of pharaohs.

We should point out that the influence of population centers at Nubia's southern extreme has been poorly understood until recently (Edwards 2004). We are only now beginning to appreciate the importance of the ancient Kingdom of Kush with its capitals near the 4th cataract to the history of Nubia.

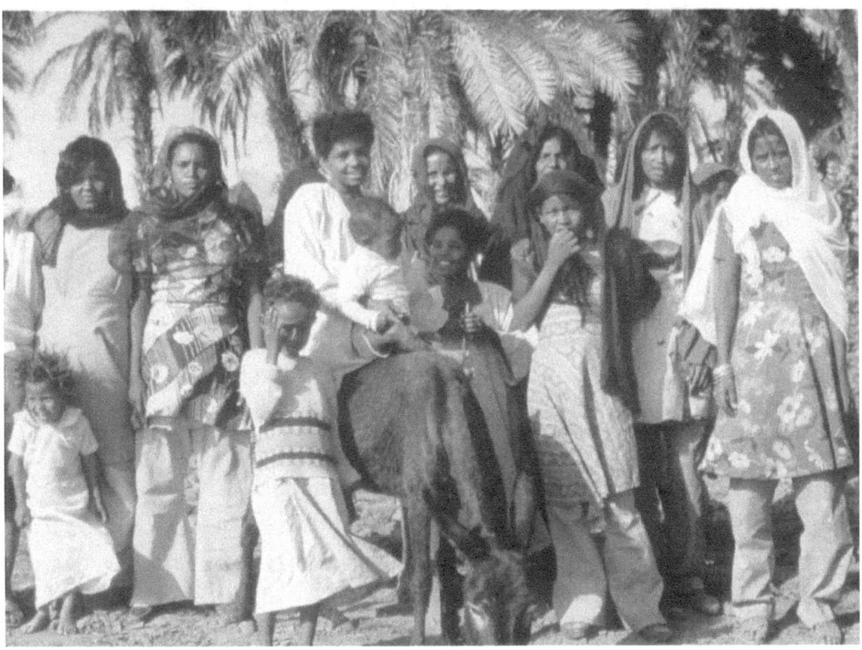

Figure 1.3. Kulb village women and children.

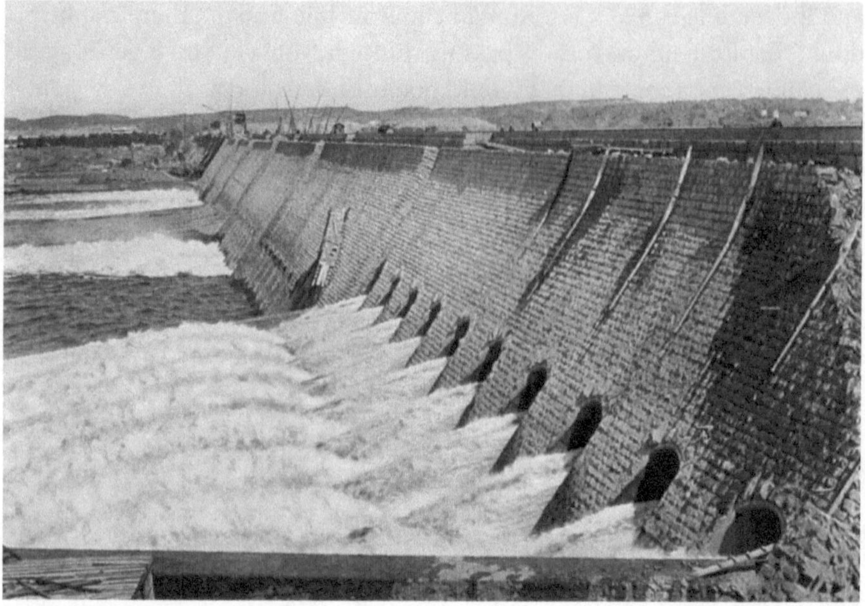

Figure 1.4. The Aswan Low Dam.

So why Nubia? William Flinders Petrie, a pioneer in scientific archaeology, made his first visit to Egypt in 1880. The Egypt Exploration Society was founded two years later. But it would be some 20 more years before a serious interest in Nubian archaeology developed. Even then, Nubian archaeology remained in the shadow of Egypt (Edwards 2004). Why did it take so long? It comes down to the old adage: "you only miss it when you lose it," or, in this case, are about to lose it. Archaeology in Lower Nubia has been the result of dam building at Aswan. Each dam has been larger than the one before it. Construction on the first began in 1899 and was completed in 1902. It was built in order to increase food production and generate electricity. Unfortunately, silt that had formerly renewed soil along the river now accumulated behind the dam—raising the level of the reservoir. The dam was enlarged twice to solve the problem—once in 1908 and again between 1929 and 1934.

In order to salvage as much of Nubia's archaeological and human remains as possible, two archaeological surveys were organized. Staffed by scientists from around the world, the surveys were the largest salvage programs of their day. Physical anthropology would play a vital role in both surveys. The first began in 1907 and was first directed by George A. Reisner and then by C. M. Firth (Reisner 1909; Firth 1912, 1915, 1927). The second

(1929–1934) was directed by W. B. Emery (Emery 1948, 1954) and L. P. Kirwan (Kirwan 1937). As with archaeology in Egypt, the work focused on cemeteries. The First Survey excavated more than 8,000 graves from 151 cemeteries (Adams 1977:72). The second excavated over 2,400 graves from 76 cemeteries (Adams 1977:76). Nubia rapidly became one of the world's great centers of archaeological research. Its desert climate (portions of Nubia receive less than 1 millimeter of rain per year) preserved a treasure trove of archaeological and human remains. It wasn't unusual for human remains to be partially or completely mummified. Nubia has also provided a wonderful combination of both historical (written) and archaeological materials. Adams has observed that Egypt at the lower end of the Nile has the longest recorded history on earth. Inner Africa, at the headwaters of the Nile, has one of the shortest. Consequently, Nubia has alternated between history and prehistory. In fact, its most recent "dark age" was the centuries before the coming of Islam (Adams 1967).

Everyone expected Nubian history to follow Egyptian history period for period and phase for phase. But that expectation failed to materialize. There appeared to be entire periods of Nubian history that had no counterpart in Egypt. Reisner used alphabetical designations such as A, B, and C in order to fit them into the Egyptian sequence (Reisner 1909). These unexpected periods created a serious problem, but the problem was not without

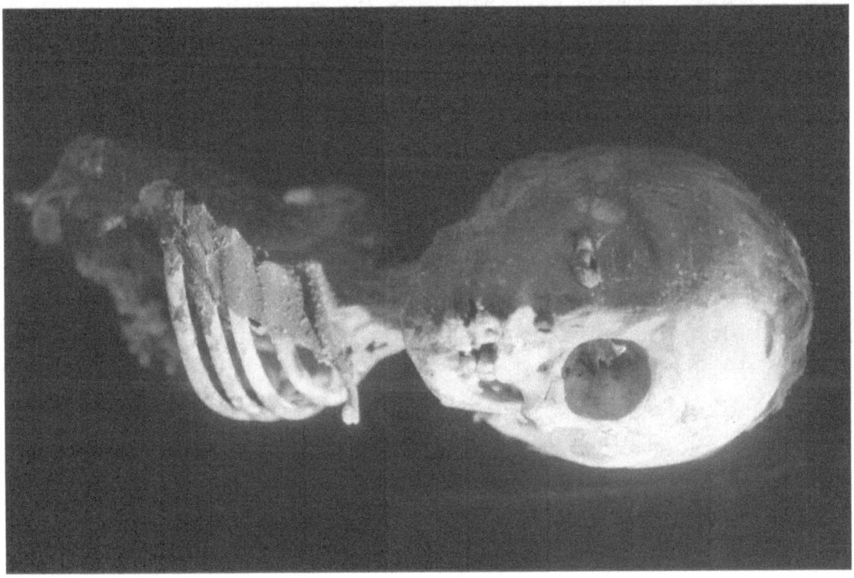

Figure 1.5. Partially mummified child from Kulubnarti.

Table 1.1. Nubian cultural sequences

Holocene Populations 10,500 BCE
Settled hunting, fishing, and gathering
First pottery 10,000 BCE
First domestic livestock 7600 BCE
Sorghum domesticated 6500 BCE
A-Group 3800–2800 BCE
Regional elites associated with pre-Dynastic Egyptian kings
First urban kingdom south of the Sahara consisting of three periods each associated with a political center
Kerma period 2500–1500 BCE (Lower Nubian C-Group)
Napatan period 1550–350 BCE
Meroitic period 350 BCE
X-Group (Ballana) 350 BCE–550 CE
Independent agrarian communities
Christian period 550–1400
Economic expansion and trade
Lower Nubia becomes a free trade zone with Egypt
Introduction of the saquia (water wheel) and multiple crop regimes
Islamic period 1323–present

its benefits. New research opportunities emerged—particularly for physical anthropology. Reisner and colleagues needed to know who—meaning what races—made these unexpected cultures.

You see, anthropology was dominated by a deeply held belief in racial determinism. It was accepted as a given that differences in intellectual capacity among races determined the nature of the cultures they created. Racial determinism held that cultures flourished and declined as races came, went, and mixed. Civilizations were made by civilized races; dark ages were produced by inferior, savage races. From that perspective, understanding Nubian history demanded the study of race, which in turn demanded the study of the anatomical remains.

It should come as no surprise then that the archaeological adviser to the First Archaeological Survey of Nubia (1909–1913) was an anatomist. His name was Grafton Elliot Smith.

Following the traditions of race science going back over a century (Blumenbach 1795; Morton 1844), Smith focused on the skull for his racial diagnoses. The approach is well exemplified by his comparison between the

Proto-Egyptian and Egyptian races. Referring to the Egyptian race, Smith tells us:

> The brain case often impresses me at a glance, not only by its greater capacity and lack of the meager, ill fitted character usually presented by the Proto-Egyptian skull. . . . The top of the head is now often flattened, and it becomes rare to find the bulged-out occiput, which is such a peculiarly distinctive feature of the Proto-Egyptian and their kinsmen of the Brown race. (Smith 1909b:110)

His racial determinism has a distinctly aquatic theme in keeping with the setting. According to Smith:

> Nubia has for long ages been the vessel in which the black and red races of Africa have been mixed and blended: in the course of the fluctuations of the human stream in the Nile Valley Nubia has been occupied at one time by the Egyptian, and another by the Negro: the dregs of one receding human tide mingled with the oncoming wave of population, and so, from time to time, produced racial mixtures in which now the Egyptian, or at another times the Negro element predominated. (Smith 1909b:23)

As for the consequences of this racial ebb and flow, Smith makes it clear that "the smallest infusion of Negro-blood immediacy manifests itself in a dulling of initiative and a 'drag' on the further development of the arts of civilization" (Smith 1909b:25).

The lead physical anthropologist for the Second Survey was also a physician and anatomist. His name was Ahmed Batrawi. Batrawi (1935, 1945, 1946, 1947) initially endorsed the determinist views of Smith and coworkers, but then changed his position considerably. He argued that

> failure to distinguish clearly between the achievements of populations and their inherent biological characteristics has caused much confusion in anthropological writing. The literature dealing with the racial history of Egypt [and Nubia] provides an outstanding example of the danger. (Batrawi 1946:131)

Batrawi's rejection of racial determinism notwithstanding, his racial typology didn't miss a beat. In his view, A-Group people appeared to be a hybrid race resulting from the mixture of pure Negroids and Caucasoids. The following C-Group people showed a continuation of A-Group features with an increase in Negroid characteristics among the women. He went on to argue that this mixing of Caucasoid men and Negroid women continued through Meroitic times but ended with the arrival of a new *alien* race at the beginning of the X-Group period. All of this interpretation was based on cranial features.

While Batrawi and others modified and remodified their racial categories—redefining this or that attribute—the view of Nubian history as a series of disconnected episodes continued to dominate theories of Nubian history. There was, however, one notable exception. Back in 1905, C. S. Myers challenged a racial approach that in many ways anticipated critiques of the post-1950s (Myers 1905, 1908). He pointed out significant statistical errors in all of the analyses as well as a total lack of any appreciation of human variation. He went on to expand his criticisms beyond Nubia to all racial analyses. Myers was a man ahead of his time, and as with most such persons, his criticisms largely fell on deaf ears.

The Colorado Expedition

Interest in ancient Nubia diminished until 1959 with the announcement of a new dam to be built 7 kilometers south of the old dam. The proposed High Dam would be orders of magnitude larger and more complex than the Low Dam. It would be 200 feet high, 3 miles long, and capable of impounding 4×10^{12} cubic feet of water. When complete, its reservoir would extend southward some 130 kilometers into Sudan. The consequences for Nubian antiquities and monuments would be catastrophic. Lower Nubia would be entirely inundated.

The old dam had a far smaller impact on the monuments. The reservoir behind the old dam was drained each summer. As a result, the monuments weren't entirely lost. They could at least be seen each year. The new reservoir would be permanent, leaving some of the greatest monuments in the Nile Valley submerged forever. If such a loss were to be avoided, thousands of sites would have to be excavated, and some 35 major monuments as well as smaller temples would have to be moved (Adams 1977). In some cases that would mean cutting them from the rock and rebuilding them on higher ground.

In response to the impending catastrophe, funds were provided by the United Nations Educational, Scientific, and Cultural Organization (UNESCO) for an international campaign to save the monuments of both Egypt and Nubia (Smith 1962). During the ten years of the campaign, some 18 foreign expeditions from around the world identified over 1,000

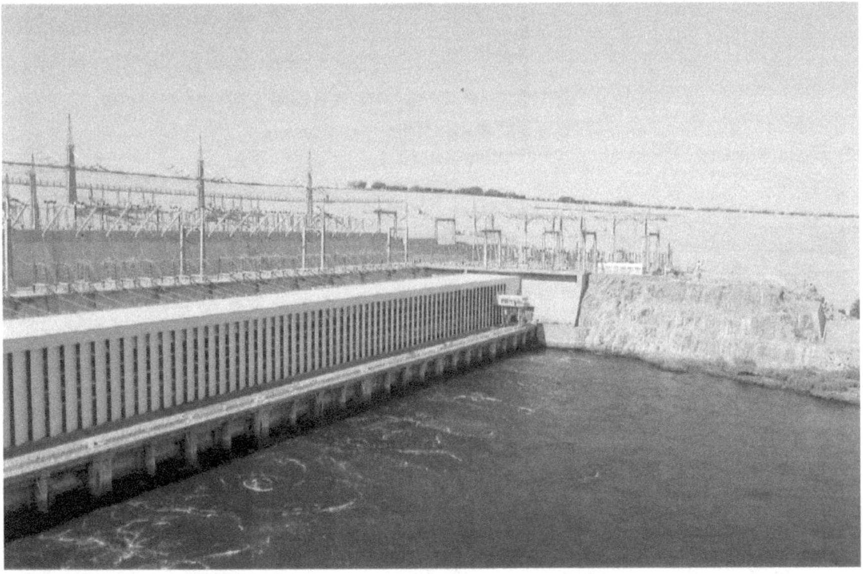

Figure 1.6. The Aswan High Dam.

archaeological sites and excavated over one-third of them (Adams 1977). The defining accomplishment of the entire Nubian campaign was the cutting and relocation of Abu Simbel (figure 1.7) (Save-Soderbergh 1987). The temple was constructed in 1257 BCE in honor of Ramses II (1279–1213 BCE).

Tragically, there was one problem that UNESCO couldn't solve. Some 50,000 Egyptian Nubians were forced to resettle some 10 kilometers from their homes on the Nile. Sudanese Nubians fared even worse. They were to be moved 700 kilometers south and then several hundred kilometers up the Atbara River—a tributary of the Nile (Fernea and Kennedy 1966). Forced into this new environment with its seasonal rains (never experienced by Nubians before), thousands died of malaria. Ethnic Nubians are still fighting for the right to return to the Nile Valley and reestablish their traditional villages and lifeways along the shores of the lake.

In the fall of 1961, the Nubian portion of the UNESCO Campaign was under way, and the University of Colorado was destined to play an important part. The late professor Gordon Hewes gained support from the National Science Foundation and the U.S. State Department to mount a two-year University of Colorado Nubia Expedition (Armelagos et al. 1968). The university was given a 14 square kilometer concession opposite Wadi Halfa. Fans of Agatha Christie's *Death on the Nile* (Christie 1937) will recognize

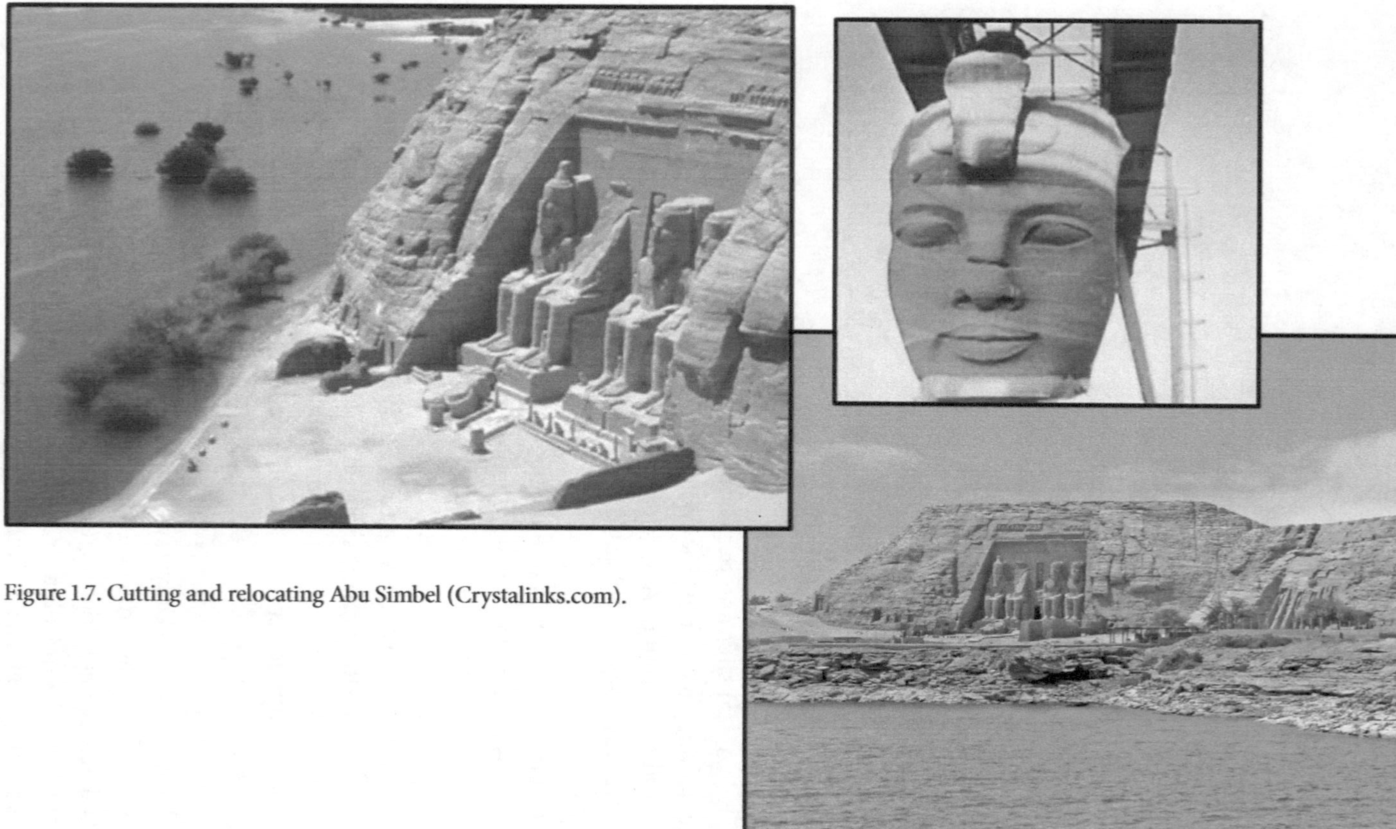

Figure 1.7. Cutting and relocating Abu Simbel (Crystalinks.com).

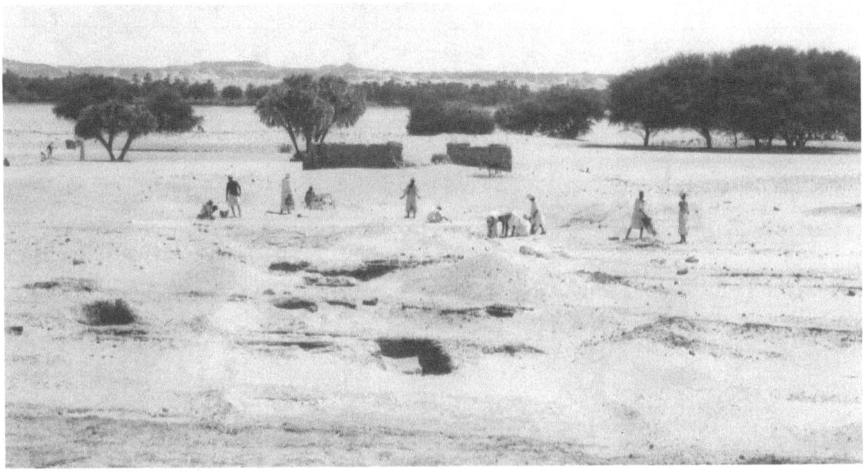

Figure 1.8. Excavation at the Colorado Wadi Halfa concession.

Wadi Halfa as the destination for tourist steamers traveling up the Nile from Aswan.

The plan for the first year was to investigate the relationship between Napatan-Meroitic (350 BCE–350 CE), X-Group (350 CE–550 CE), and Christian (550–1350 CE) periods; survey Paleolithic sites; and sample a number of cemeteries uncovered by previous investigators (Adams and Nordstrom 1963; Nordstrom 1962; Verwers 1962). In the course of the first year, the Colorado team discovered exceptionally preserved human remains. Many were mummified by a combination of sand, heat, and virtually no rainfall. A fossilized human mandible was also discovered (Armelagos 1964). By the end of the season it was clear that the next year's expedition would have to include a team of physical anthropologists. George remembers the year well, and it's a story best told in his own words.

George Ewing and I took the lead in developing plans for the next year. Our field season would last from November 1, 1963, until April 1, 1964. Excavations were always conducted in the winter when temperatures were tolerable. Summer temperatures often top 100°F and the sand can reach temperatures above 120°F. This makes walking uncomfortable even wearing sandals. Winter days were more commonly in the 70s, although any day could be miserably hot. There was a striking diurnal range in every season. It could be in the low 40s at 7 am and over 100°F at the end of the day.

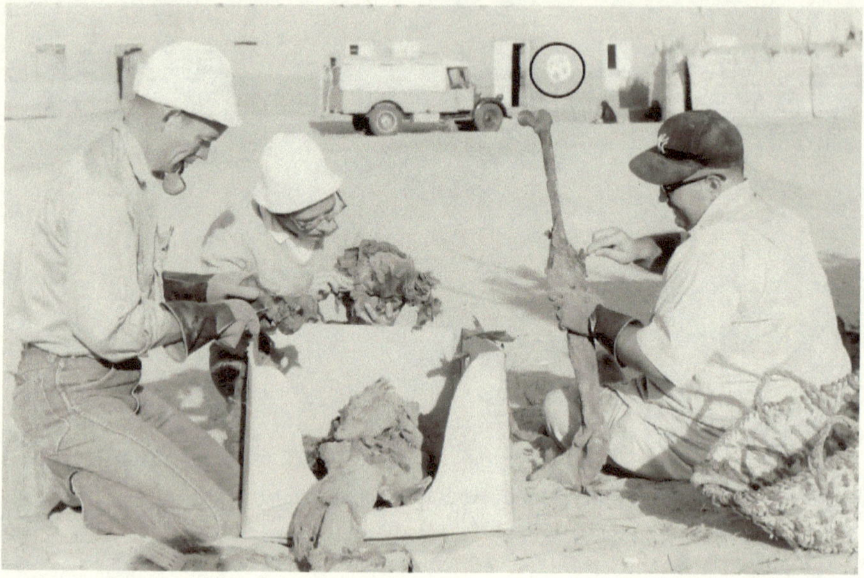

Figure 1.9. George Armelagos (*right*) processing a mummy.

Our research plan was vague (Armelagos et al. 1968). The previous expedition's discovery of a fossilized mandible gave us hope that we could study the relationships among Nubia's various cultural periods covering perhaps the last 10,000 years. We were particularly interested in the transition from the Meroitic period to the following X-Group period.

We had read the reports of the First and Second Surveys and understood the interpretations that resulted. According to the reports, the Meroitic period was one of civilization and cultural florescence created by an indigenous Caucasoid people. The X-Group period was one of cultural decline—a virtual dark-age resulting from the arrival of a Negroid race with some other unknown race mixed in. We planned to evaluate the question of population replacement, but without the racial-determinist element.

We had other objectives as well. We planned to conduct a thorough analysis of the various pathologies evidenced in the remains. We even planned to autopsy mummies in the hope of recovering diseases of internal organs. Since the mummies were natural (burial in the hot sand desiccated the bodies before they decayed) and not intentionally prepared, the internal organs would not have been removed as was the practice in Egypt.

There would be a morphology piece. The focus would be far broader than craniometrics. We planned to collect data on post-cranial and sub-adult remains as well. This would provide us with a wider range of research questions than would racial diagnosis. There would also be a genetic analysis. The genetics would be based on a thorough analysis of the dentition with an eye to various features—such as cusps and fissure patterns of the molars—known to have some genetic basis. We hoped that this would provide us with an additional means of assessing the genetic relationships between Meroitic, X-Group, and Christian populations. We would ultimately be disappointed in only one area of the proposed work. While many of the mummies were well preserved on the outside, insect infestations had made them virtually hollow torsos. Thus the hope to conduct autopsies vanished.

Our expedition was headquartered in Wadi Halfa within easy reach of the sites to be excavated. When we arrived, I was struck by two things—the stores had Pepsi Cola and the street signs were in Greek![2] There were two compounds sufficient to provide living quarters as well as laboratory space. As all but a few of the more interesting specimens were destined for reburial, proper data collection was vital. This made laboratory space far more important than the living space. I made my room by shoveling out a goat pen full of feces and whitewashing the walls.

Wadi Halfa was still a thriving city with several thousand residents. It was founded by the British in the 19th century as a headquarters for British forces during the re-conquest of Sudan. The military action, led by Herbert Kitchener, was provoked by an insurrection led by Muhammad Ahmad, the self-proclaimed Mahdi. We actually found spent shells that remained in the desert from Kitchener's campaign (Magnus 1968; Daly 2004). There was a very old man that the locals referred to as "Kitchener's son." I thought it was amusing until I returned to Colorado and read about the British campaign against the Mahdi. There was a picture of Kitchener and the old man was his spitting image.

Located as it was on the border between Egypt and Sudan, Wadi Halfa was a center of trade—both legitimate and illegitimate—between the two countries. I remember visiting a store whose owner I had befriended. On this particular day he was selling 10,000 razor blades to an Egyptian on his way home. I only had to walk around town to realize how much Wadi Halfa (and Nubia) remained a crossroads between cultures. A local shop had an Ann-Margret "Bye Bye Birdie" poster on the wall, and the shopkeeper wore part of an old Nazi uniform. Wadi Halfa had been a WWII

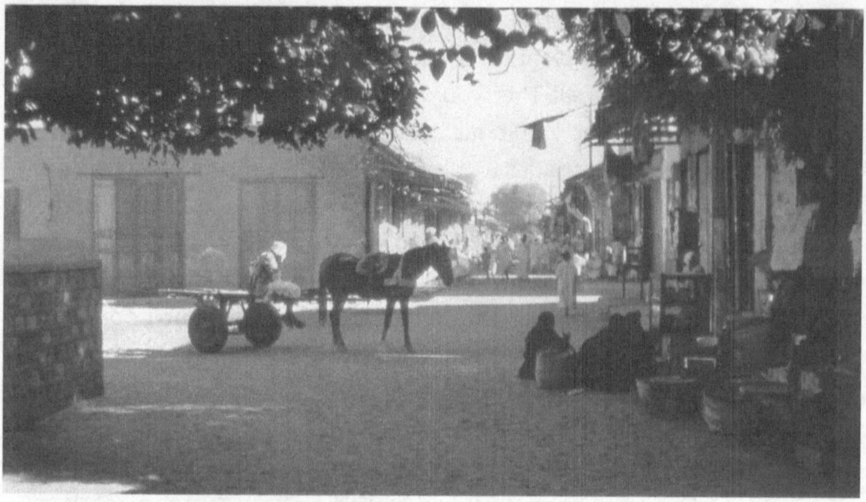

Figure 1.10. Wadi Halfa before the flood.

communications center during the Africa Campaign. The shopkeeper had no idea what the uniform meant. It was difficult to imagine that in a few years' time, Wadi Halfa would be buried forever under some 200 feet of water.

On a typical workday the others would be up by 6:00 am—I would wake up at 6:25. There was a half hour for breakfast—I had five minutes. I would make a sweep through the dining area picking up the liver—served every day—which no one else would eat. By 7:00 am we were off on our half-mile walk to the boat that would take us to the sites. We anticipated no problems excavating all of the remains necessary for the project. However, after the first month of excavation, it became clear that we wouldn't find an adequate sample of X-Group material. Fortunately we managed to obtain the permission of both W. Y. Adams (director of the UNESCO Survey in Nubia), and also from the Sudan Antiquities Service to excavate a portion of an additional X-Group cemetery (2413) within the Franco-Argentine Concession. An additional sample of some 140 skeletons was graciously made available to us by the Spanish. As it turned out, they didn't obtain funds for shipping the material back to Spain. That left the skeletons from their concession stranded in Wadi Halfa. The Colorado team owed the Spanish a great deal for their generosity.

The Meroitic and Christian remains presented less of a problem. One cemetery provided an excellent Meroitic sample and two additional cemeteries provided Christian remains. The Christian sample was expanded further when Adams requested help aging and sexing Christian-period skeletons from the Island of Meinarti. The archaeological context was extraordinary.

Unlike all of the other cemeteries, Meinarti was stratified. That is to say the graves occurred at different depths in chronological order. Furthermore, the village and cemetery were periodically whitewashed at the same time. As a result, the history of the cemetery (time of the interments) could be calibrated with historical events within the village. This produced an unprecedented opportunity to examine changing patterns of mortality and disease over a three-hundred year period. This kind of joint archaeological and biological record was unheard of in excavations elsewhere in Nubia.[3]

As important as Meinarti was, the most exciting remains didn't appear until the last month of the season. After excavations at the village sites were complete, we began looking for additional sites to excavate. Our chance of finding anything of importance was small but as it turned out, luck was with us. During one of our trips out into the desert, we noticed what appeared to be a human mandible protruding from a track left by a passing truck. It was fossilized! We immediately began a thorough

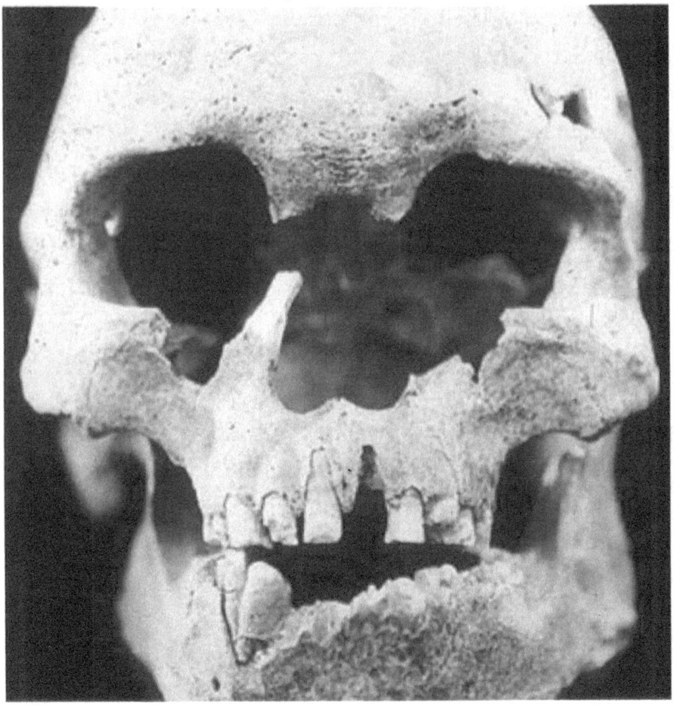

Figure 1.11. Mesolithic skull.

excavation of the area. The mandible led us to a 12,000-year-old Mesolithic cemetery containing 39 partially fossilized skeletons. We had discovered one of the most important fossil human sites in North Africa (Hewes et al. 1964)—all due to a passing truck.

The old saying was true—at least for us—it's better to be lucky than good. Raymond Dart would visit the University of Colorado some years after the expedition was concluded. Upon seeing the Mesolithic collection, he stated that that alone made the expedition worthwhile.

We had excellent samples of human remains by the end of the season. The most recent had died at the very doorstep of the Islamic era in the mid-14th century. The most ancient lived and died some 12,000 [years] earlier. We all knew exactly what we would be doing when we got back to Colorado. We would be working to answer two questions. Who were these Nubians, and what happened to them in the course of their lives?

There is the parable of the ant on the leaf that goes like this: The ant had made his home on a leaf. He spent every day cleaning his house, tending his garden, keeping everything just as it should be. He knew what he was doing, and he had a clear vision of his future. What the ant didn't know was that his leaf was flowing down a great river heading for rapids.

When we returned to Colorado to begin our work, we were like the ant. We had our data, we had our questions and we knew what we intended to do. We were in good shape and we had a clear vision of our future. But in reality we were floating on a river of old ideas about race heading for rapids. We were about to be taken to places none of us had anticipated. But unlike the ant merely floating along, we were about to help stir the rapids. We didn't know it at the time, but our analyses of the Wadi Halfa remains would be part of a scientific revolution.

Ideas, Theories, and Paradigms

Back in 1962, a physicist-philosopher by the name of Thomas Kuhn wrote a book on the history and philosophy of science titled *The Structure of Scientific Revolutions* (Kuhn 1962). The book challenged the way scientists thought about scientific progress. Traditionalists saw progress as incremental. In their view, scientists made observations, developed theories, and tested hypotheses. Theories competed for acceptance. Some were validated and others weren't. The successful theories added to the collective body of knowledge. Kuhn proposed a different view. Where traditionalists saw incremental changes, Kuhn saw long periods of normalcy followed by abrupt intellectual transformations. These, in Kuhn's view, were scientific revolutions.

Let's make an example using a simplified bit of history. By the second century CE an Alexandrian Greek named Ptolemy had a theory concerning the movements of celestial bodies. His theory proposed that all of the stars, planets, comets, and even the sun rotated around the earth. Over time, Ptolemy's theory became so widely accepted it became a kind of astronomical truth (Ellis 2004). Scholars and theologians believed it, taught it, and students learned it. Students needed to learn Ptolemy if they wanted to practice astronomy. At that point Ptolemy's celestial scheme had risen above the status of a theory; it had become what Kuhn called a paradigm.

Once the Ptolemaic theory reached paradigm status, other theories became irrelevant. Astronomers studied Ptolemy. But ironically that was the rub. With so many astronomers studying Ptolemy, small inconsistencies, puzzles, and problems were bound to be noticed. You see, the business of what Kuhn calls everyday "normal science" was trying out Ptolemy on new problems as they appeared. Astronomers such as Kepler and Copernicus conducted experiments that exposed inconsistencies and weak spots in the paradigm. Small cracks in the paradigm grew until they became chasms.

Copernicus finally proposed an alternative theory based on a sun-centered solar system (Lakatos and Zahar 1975). Why? He had lost confidence in Ptolemy. And there was worse to come for Ptolemy's beleaguered paradigm. Galileo looked through his telescope and discovered moons orbiting Jupiter. Not all celestial bodies orbited the earth! The Ptolemaic system finally collapsed under the sheer weight of the facts it couldn't explain. The fall of Ptolemy and the rise of Copernicus *revolutionized* how astronomers saw the universe. Over time, the Copernican system was elevated from a theory to the new paradigm.

When the Colorado team arrived in Nubia back in 1959, the race paradigm was coming apart at the seams, much like the last days of Ptolemy. The notion of a racial hierarchy had already collapsed. A generation of anthropologists such Franz Boas, Ruth Benedict, Robert Lowe, and Alfred Kroeber had gone out among the so-called savage races and found none. There were no primitive languages, systems of kinship, art, or religion. Race couldn't explain hierarchies of cultural capacity because there were no hierarchies to explain.

But the proponents of race were not going down without a fight. After all, they and generations of anthropologists before them had built their careers on race. They were invested in it. Astronomers invested in Ptolemy had proposed an absurd system of planetary loop-the-loops trying to save their view. That didn't work, but surely physical anthropologists could save the idea of racial categories if they remodeled them enough. Let's repeat Grafton Elliot Smith's view of race compared to Batrawi's:

> Nubia has been occupied at one time by the Egyptian, another by the Negro . . . the smallest infusion of Negro-blood immediately manifests itself in a dulling of initiative and a "drag" on the further development of the arts of civilization. (Smith 1909b:23)

> Failure to distinguish clearly between the achievements of populations and their inherent biological characteristics has caused much confusion in anthropological writing. The literature dealing with the racial history of Egypt [and Nubia] provides an outstanding example of the danger of assessing biological relationships from cultural evidence. (Batrawi 1946:131)

Batrawi's abandonment of racial determinism gave hope to traditionalists invested in race science. The study of race could be saved if the creation of racial hierarchies was abandoned and the categories reorganized. In reality, the race concept could no more be saved by abandoning racial ranking and fiddling with the categories than Ptolemy could be saved by adding one more loop to the loop-the-loop. Think about it this way. To this day, physical anthropologists can't agree on how many races there are (Armelagos 1994). The number ranges from five geographic races to an uncountable number of microraces, each based on the study at hand (Garn 1961; Garn and Coon 1955). It's loop-the-loops. Imagine a science of physics where mass could be any number of things! Imagine a science of chemistry where the number of elements in the periodic table depended on the study at hand!

As the Colorado Expedition began its work at Wadi Halfa the race paradigm had run out of loop-the-loops, and a new theory was on the ascent. While not yet a paradigm, it was a theory so elegant and simple in conception that it could be expressed in one simple sentence: "Race is an arbitrary category invented to fit a misunderstanding about how humans evolve" (Anonymous). I found that sentence on a greeting card of all places. What occasion the card was for is a mystery to this day.

The road to a demise of the race concept had two capstone moments. Both were just gaining traction at the outset of the Colorado Expedition.

The first was Sherwood Washburn's "The New Physical Anthropology" published in 1951 (Washburn 1951). The second was Frank Livingstone's "Anthropological Implications of the Sickle Gene Cell in West Africa" published in 1958 (Livingstone 1958). Washburn challenged physical anthropology to move away from the endless description of human attributes (races) toward a new physical anthropology grounded in the methods of modern science and informed by modern evolutionary theory. Livingstone's analysis of sickle cell demonstrated the explanatory power of a new biocultural approach to human adaptation and evolution. In many ways, Livingstone's work stands as one of the most significant applications of the "new physical anthropology" to a human genetic trait.

We are going to spend some time looking at Livingstone's analysis even though it may appear far removed from our work in Nubia. It's not. It is an exemplar of two principles that have guided our research for over 50 years. The principles are these:

- Human evolution is the result of an interaction between biological and cultural systems.
- Human evolution isolated from its cultural context is unintelligible.

These principles have not only informed our work, they are the foundation on which this volume is built. So let's look at the "Anthropological Implications of the Sickle Cell Gene in West Africa." As with all biocultural analyses, there is a biological baseline and a biocultural interaction.

The Biological Baseline

In 1910 a physician and professor of medicine, James Herrick, reported on a case of anemia in a dental student from the West Indies (Savitt and Goldberg 1989). The patient's red blood cells were distorted into a variety of unusual elongated forms, some of which had a peculiar sickle shape. The affected cells couldn't circulate properly and had a life span of only around 15 days compared to 120 days for normal cells—hence the anemia. Herrick's report provided the first description in the medical literature of sickle cell anemia.

Linus Pauling (Pauling et al. 1949) and James Neel (Neel 1949) worked out the genetics and biochemistry of sickle cell in 1949. The anemia was caused by a single gene mutation resulting in the production of a modified form of hemoglobin. Homozygotes (inheritors of the trait from both parents) produced large amounts of the modified hemoglobin. They were described as having sickle cell anemia. Heterozygotes (inheritors from one parent) produced a lesser amount and were described as having sickle cell trait.

Cell distortion (sickling) occurred when the modified hemoglobin was exposed to a low oxygen environment. Victims of sickle cell anemia were sensitive to even minor levels of oxygen depletion, resulting in frequent sickle cell "crises." Those with sickle cell trait were seldom affected and typically enjoyed normal life spans. In fact, they often never knew they had the trait. The sickle cell gene appeared to be African in origin. Almost all cases in the United States involved persons of African ancestry, and up to 40 percent of some African populations expressed sickle cell trait. It was not, however, entirely African. The gene was also present in parts of India and the Mediterranean.

Explanations of sickle cell were proposed from two points of view—one racial and one clinal (Trapper 1995, 1998). The racial view went like this: sickle cell was African and therefore a Negroid trait. It therefore must have originated in some Negroid population from which it spread across Africa and then onto India and the Mediterranean by way of migration and interbreeding between Africans and indigenous Indian and Mediterranean races. From a racial perspective, that was the only reasonable explanation.

Anthony Allison approached the sickle cell problem from a different perspective (Allison 1954). He observed that the distribution of sickle cell was clinal, not racial. A cline is a gradient across physical space. A lot of natural phenomena are clinal. Mean annual temperature, rainfall, and altitude all form gradients from one place to another. Gradients are often represented by bands of different colors. There are also genetic clines. The sickle cell gene formed a genetic cline that he could map. The contours crosscut racial boundaries. Allison next discovered that the distribution of sickle cell matched the distribution of malaria.

Malaria is a parasitic disease transmitted by a mosquito—primarily the *Anopheles* mosquito. The malaria parasite is a single-celled organism known as a plasmodium. Once injected into the blood stream by the mosquito's bite, the parasite invades red blood cells, consumes oxygen and hemoglobin, and multiplies until the cells are killed. Before the advent of modern medical treatment, malaria was the number one source of human mortality in the world (Piel et al. 2013). Today one child dies of malaria every 45 seconds in sub-Saharan Africa alone.

Allison discovered that individuals born with sickle cell trait survived malarial infection more frequently than those without the trait. Allison's

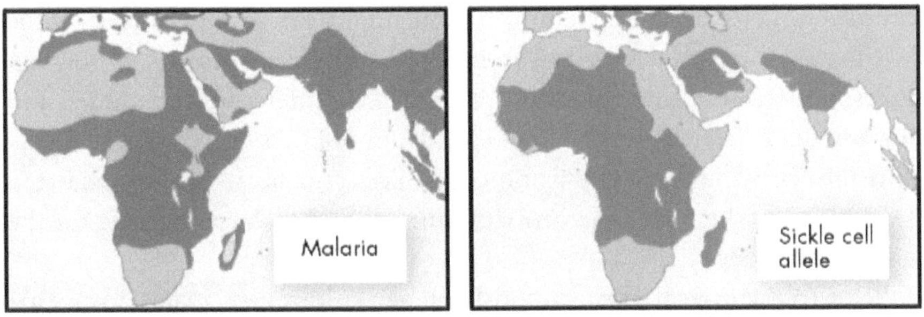

Figure 1.12. The distribution of malaria and the sickle cell allele.

statistical evidence was indisputable. Malaria-infected individuals with sickle cell trait maintained fewer parasites, developed fewer symptoms, and had higher survival rates compared to those who couldn't sickle. This is particularly important for infants and children. A child with sickle cell trait had a 40 percent greater chance of reaching his or her fifth birthday than a child who lacked the capacity to sickle.

The mechanism of resistance lies in the behavior of sickling hemoglobin. As we have already discussed, individuals with sickle cell trait only sickle under conditions of extreme oxygen deprivation, which seldom occurs under everyday conditions. Conditions change dramatically when a cell is attacked by parasites. Once attacked, the parasites rob the red cell of oxygen and induce it to sickle. This is catastrophic for the parasite. Unable to circulate properly, the sickled red cell is destroyed, and the parasite is destroyed along with it. This does not provide immunity to malaria; it provides resistance by keeping parasite numbers low.

The Biocultural Interaction

With the biological baseline established by Allison, Livingstone explained the evolution of sickle cell trait as a series of biological and cultural (biocultural) interactions (Livingstone 1958). The story began in West Africa some 2,500 years ago with the convergence of two cultural events—iron smelting introduced from the Near East, and the yam, taro, and banana introduced by Malayo-Polynesian explorers. Axes produced from iron made it possible to cut stands of tropical forest, and the new cultigens provided the first food crops capable of growing in the thin, acid soils of the forest floor.

Iron axes combined with the new cultigens gave birth to what is known as slash-and-burn agriculture. Slash-and-burn agriculture is predatory on forests. Gardens are cut by felling and burning trees. Ash produced by the burning provides nutrients to the exposed soil. Even so, tropical soil can only support about three plantings. Exhausted gardens are abandoned and new ones cut. The result is a relentless advance of people, villages, and gardens into pristine forest environments. Slash-and-burn gardens changed the ecology of the forest and brought humans and malaria together for the first time in history.

Prior to the arrival of slash-and-burn agriculturalists, malaria was primarily a disease of nonhuman primates—particularly chimpanzees (Harper and Armelagos 2013). Its distribution was limited to those areas where the *Anopheles* mosquito could reproduce. The mosquito requires pools of fresh standing water and sunlight—both rare under the forest canopy. Slash-and-burn agriculture created a whole new dynamic for humans and malaria. Gardens provided sunlight, and cut trees provided nooks, crannies, cracks, and crevices for small pools of standing water. Primates were hunted and driven from gardens, mosquito breeding grounds multiplied, and humans became a new host for malaria. In the beginning, the sickle cell gene was a rare random mutation. The frequency of villagers with sickle cell trait was probably little more than 0.1 percent. The evolutionary advantage of those with sickle cell trait increased the trait's frequency to over 40 percent in little more than 35 generations.

Allison demonstrated the biological link between sickle cell trait and malarial resistance. Livingstone demonstrated the biocultural link to slash-and-burn agriculture. He went on to demonstrate that the highest frequencies of sickle cell occurred in populations that had been practicing slash and burn the longest. Livingstone later wrote an article arguing that "there are no races, there are only clines" (Livingstone 1962:279). From the standpoint of sickle cell, race was nothing more than an arbitrary category invented to fit a misunderstanding about how humans evolve. A racial approach not only failed to explain sickle cell, racial boundaries imposed over the clinal gradients obscured the explanation. Livingstone's analysis of sickle cell was to race what Copernicus was to Ptolemy.

So why have we given so much space to Allison and Livingstone in a volume about long-dead Nubians? Allison's and Livingstone's analyses provided the intellectual foundation for our research agenda begun back in 1959. Our work has proceeded for some 60 years on the presumption that patterns of morphology, growth and development, and disease result from biocultural interactions, just as Livingstone observed in the case of sickle cell and agriculture.

Teasing out those interactions constitutes the intellectual thread that binds this volume together. The cases we present and the problems we address incorporate a biological baseline and a biocultural analysis. We do it in the spirit of a proposition made by V. Gordon Child some 80 years ago. It ran something like this: humankind is as much a product of culture as culture is a product of humankind (Child 1936).

The Kulubnarti Expedition

The Kulubnarti research is somewhat like the story of the Wadi Halfa Mesolithic. It is a story of coincidence, opportunity, and sheer dumb luck. I discovered Nubia in 1965 at the University of Utah in an Introduction to Anthropology class. George was the instructor. He had taken the instructorship in the Department of Anthropology while he finished writing his dissertation on the paleopathology and paleodemography of the Wadi Halfa remains.

While George knew nothing about Nubia before the UNESCO program, I knew nothing about either anthropology or Nubia before 1965. I hadn't heard the word "anthropology" or seen it in print. I'd enrolled in Introduction to Anthropology because it met Mondays, Wednesdays, and Fridays at 9:00 a.m. and filled a social science requirement. By the end of the term, I was an anthropology major fascinated by Nubia and hoping for an opportunity to do my own research there.

My opportunity didn't come until 1978. In the meantime, I finished my degree at Utah and followed George to the University of Massachusetts. I earned my master's in 1969 and my Ph.D. in 1971. George was my adviser and mentor for all three degrees. I took a position in the Department of Anthropology at the University of Kentucky in 1971. As it happened, Bill Adams, the former director of UNESCO's Nubia Campaign, was a senior professor in the department.

Bill introduced me to Kulubnarti one night over dinner at his house. He explained that it was a Christian site some 80 miles south of the Egyptian border in a stretch of the Nile known as the *Batn el Hajar* (Belly of Rock). The *Batn el Hajar* begins at the 2nd cataract (Wadi Halfa) and extends for approximately 100 miles. It is a region where the Nile passes through a geological feature known as the North African Basement Complex. Giant granite boulders dominate the landscape down to and into the river channel. Rapids make the river effectively unnavigable. The desert beyond the river is a moonscape of jebels (large outcroppings of rock) separated by sandy valleys known as wadis. The *Batn el Hajar* is, without a doubt, the most desolate and inhospitable of all Nubian environments. Adams once made the comment that while there isn't 300 feet of elevation, there isn't 3 square feet of level ground. While that is a bit of an exaggeration, it captures the nature of the *Batn el Hajar*. Although population densities in the region varied through time, the area was never heavily populated, and subsistence was always marginal:

> The tortured landscape of bare granite ridges and gullies which characterizes this part of Nubia begins at the bank of the river itself; alluvium exists not as a continuous floodplain, but only in protected pockets and coves. Fields and tiny hamlets hug the banks wherever such soil is available, but for long stretches neither natural nor cultivated vegetation is to be seen. The narrow channel and steep riverbanks make agriculture difficult even where alluvium is present, because of the extreme differential between high and low Nile levels. At the slack season the surface of a stream may be 50 feet or more below the neighboring fields; in these circumstances irrigation is a practical impossibility without the aid of modern pumps. (Adams 1977:26)

Kulubnarti takes its name from its location on a small island adjacent to the west bank village of Kulb. Kulb is a small village of perhaps a dozen households located on a high jebel overlooking the narrow strip of river

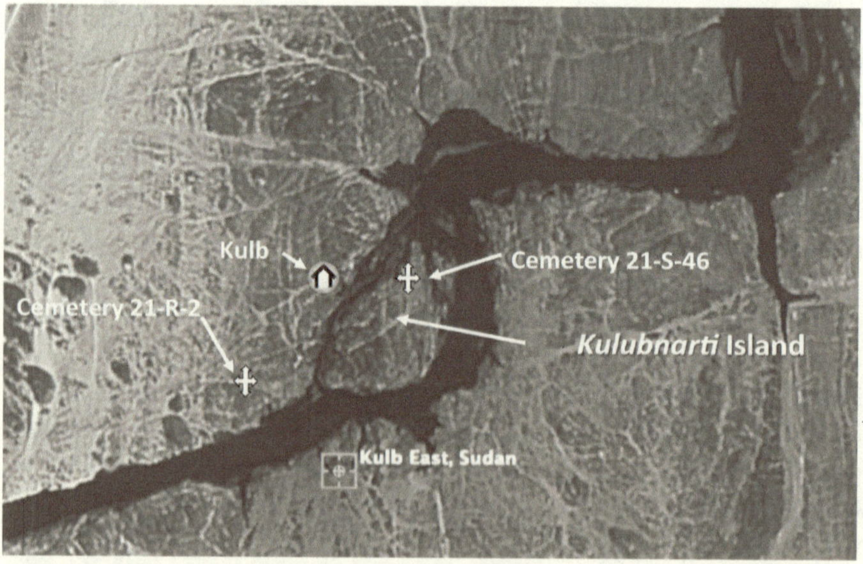

Figure 1.13. Satellite view of the Kulubnarti sites (adapted by author from Google Earth).

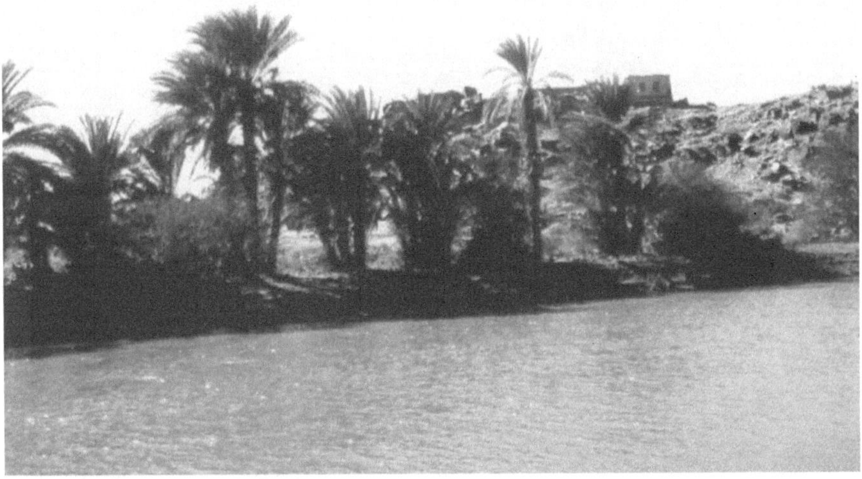

Figure 1.14. The modern village of Kulb.

separating the island from the west bank. It is typical of the villages dotting this stretch of the Nile.

Bill had surveyed Kulubnarti during the UNESCO Campaign, but it was south of the flooding and never excavated. Nevertheless, the site remained on his to-do list. It contained an abundance of architectural remains, including habitation sites, a large medieval castle, and several churches. There were also two cemeteries. One (21-S-46) was located on the island about a mile north of the castle. The second (21-R-2) was on the mainland west of the village.[4] Adams opened several graves and found preservation to be excellent. Many of the individuals were mummified as at Wadi Halfa. This, of course, drew my interest. It was clear to me that Kulubnarti's location in the *Batn el Hajar*, combined with mummified human remains, made it more than just another Christian site. It provided an opportunity to explore life and death in ancient Nubia in a setting never studied before. What was life like in the harshest of Nubian environments?

Bill and I hoped to mount an expedition to excavate the cemeteries, but I left Kentucky in 1974 for a position at the University of Colorado where of course George, David, and Kathy had discovered Nubia in the first place. Again, coincidentally, David was on the faculty. David had done his dissertation on the dentition of the Wadi Halfa remains (Greene 1965). Like stars, the coincidences were aligned, and in 1978 Bill at Kentucky and David and

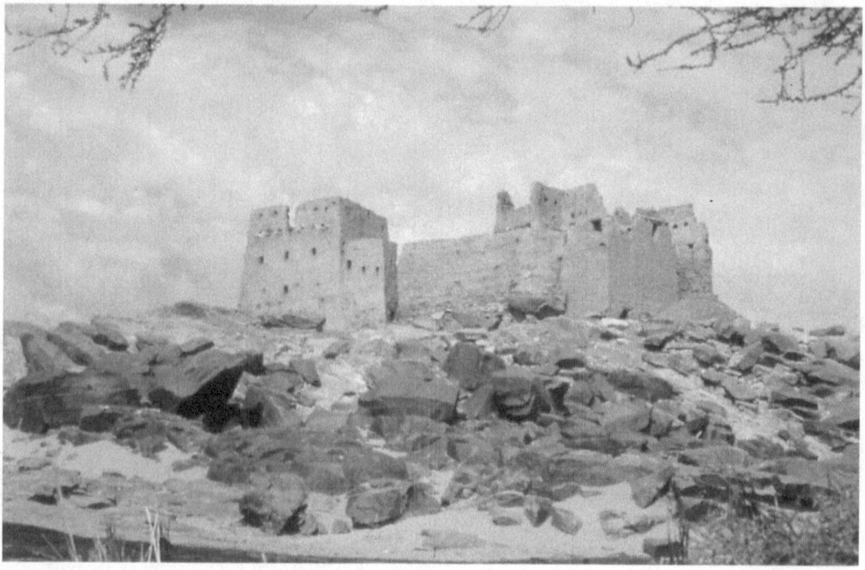
Figure 1.15. Kulubnarti castle.

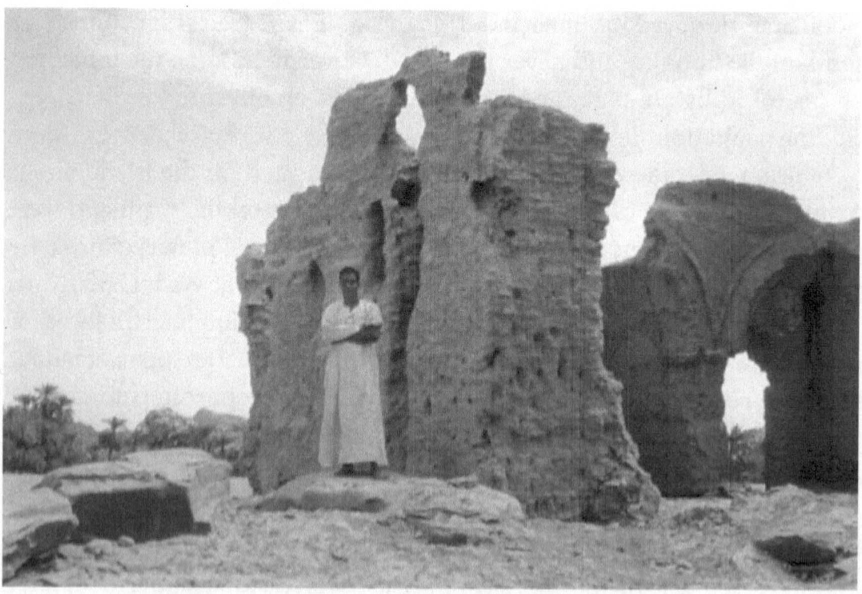
Figure 1.16. Ruins of a Christian church in the mainland cemetery.

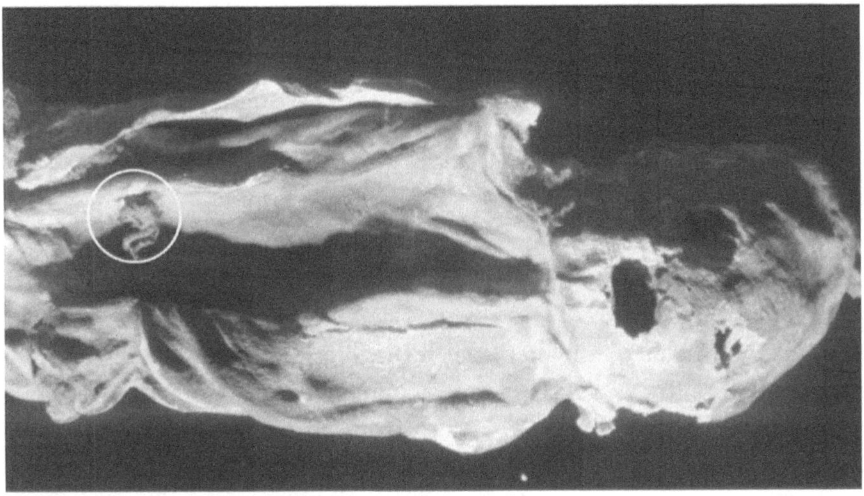

Figure 1.17. Mummified newborn with umbilicus still tied.

I at Colorado obtained funding from the National Science Foundation for excavation of the Kulubnarti cemeteries.

We launched the Colorado-Kentucky Nubia Expedition the day after Christmas that year. Bill joined me for several weeks in Khartoum at the beginning of the expedition while David stayed in Colorado to manage the supply and financial issues that could not be dealt with in Sudan. The paramount reason for my leading the field operation was simple. According to David, he had had his trip to Nubia and it was my turn.

I arrived at Kulubnarti with one graduate assistant from Colorado and one from the University of Kentucky. Bill had visited Kulb a few weeks earlier and arranged for a house complete with living quarters, a kitchen, and laboratory space, as well as a small household staff—most important, a cook—before he joined me in Khartoum. He also hired a local agent to take charge of hiring a crew from several neighboring villages, handle payroll, and arrange for the transport of food and supplies into the village and the skeletons out—north by truck to Wadi Halfa and then south to Khartoum by train. There were no roads in or out of Kulubnarti. Supplies arrived and the human remains were taken out strapped onto 1950s vintage lorries left by the British after independence. The trucks plowed their way along tracks in the sand—breaking down and getting stuck every few miles. The 80-mile trip from Wadi Halfa could take almost two days. The train trip from Khartoum to Wadi Halfa wasn't much more reliable.

I took my first tour around the village and sites the afternoon after we had settled into our house. Houses were semisubterranean with thatched roofs and thick adobe walls. They were excellent at keeping the heat out in the summer, but they also kept the cold in during the winter. January temperatures could drop into the low 40s at night and remain chilly during the day. My room was like an icebox when we arrived in January. Bill had told me that he had never been hotter or colder than he had been at Kulubnarti. He didn't exaggerate.

Looking eastward from the village, I could see the island. Its southern end was dominated by the medieval castle that I had first seen in Bill's living room. Looking westward I could see the mainland cemetery sitting in a wadi some hundred yards downslope from the village. In its center were the ruins of a Christian church. I had our boatman row me to the island at a point near the foot of the castle. The castle was built in late Christian times and may have been used as recently as the Turkish occupation of Sudan in the nineteenth century.

I found the island community cemetery in a narrow wadi about a mile north of the castle. It ran in an east–west direction and ended in an abrupt slope to the channel separating the island from the west bank. The cemetery was poorly constructed. Most of the graves were marked by simple rock cairns, while others had no marker at all. The graves appeared to be randomly strewn across the wadi floor.

The mainland community cemetery was much larger and more complex than the island cemetery. The church was near the center. It was double vaulted, and I could well appreciate why Adams doubted that it could have been designed locally. The surrounding graves were organized into two portions—one Christian and one Muslim. The Christian portion began at the foot of a jebel some hundred yards to the north of the church. It had clearly expanded southward toward the church. As the cemetery continued its expansion toward the river, there was a transition from the Christian to the Muslim graves. The Christian graves are always oriented east–west with the body on its back, head to the west. In pre-Christian times, west was considered to be the land of the dead. Muslim graves had a north–south orientation. The body is flexed on its side facing eastward toward Mecca. The cemetery continues to expand to this day as the villagers of Kulb lay their dead to rest as their ancestors have done since the arrival of Islam, perhaps in the mid-fourteenth century.

Adams estimated that there were likely more than 600 Christian graves in the mainland cemetery. It was financially and logistically impossible

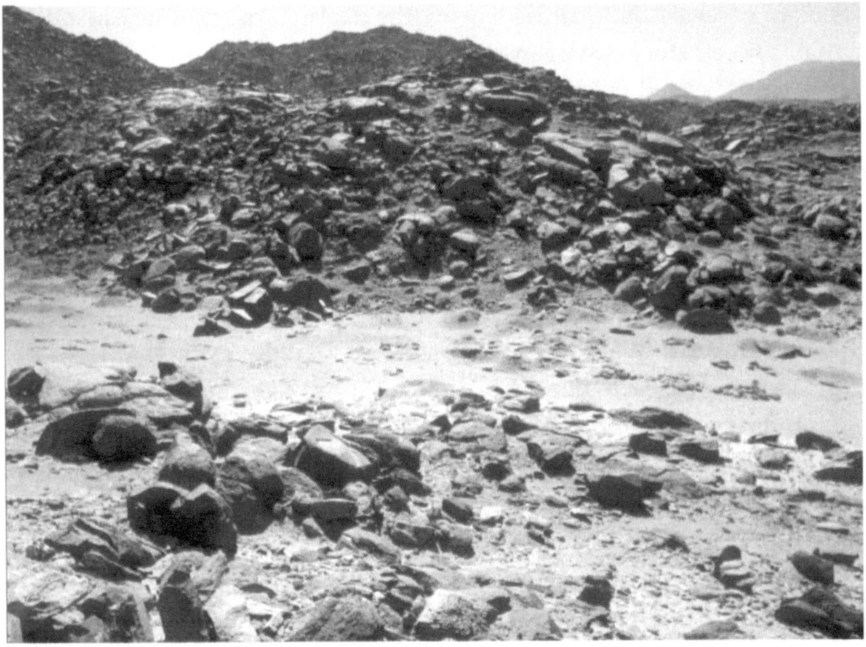

Figure 1.18. The island cemetery 21-S-46.

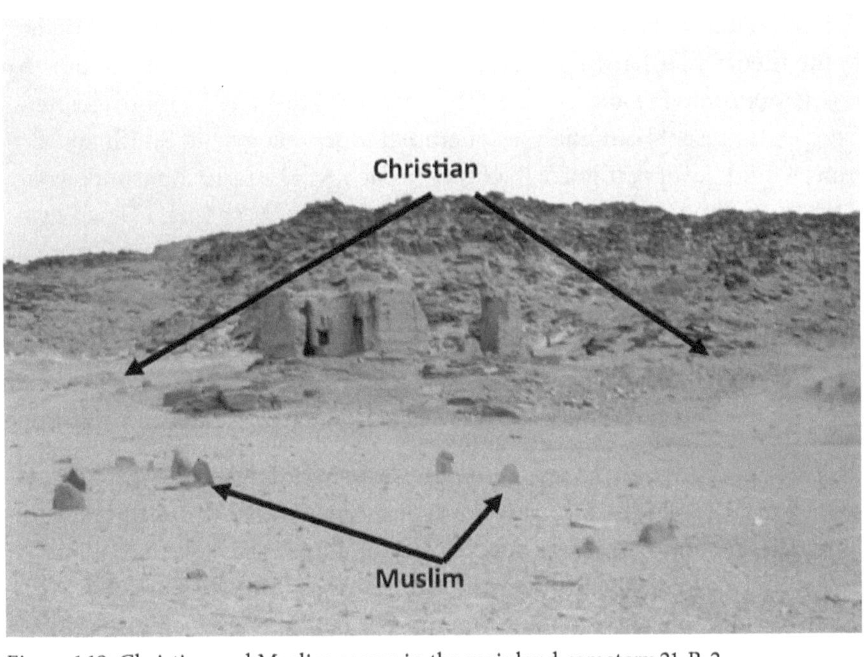

Figure 1.19. Christian and Muslim graves in the mainland cemetery 21-R-2.

for us to excavate them all, so I made the decision to excavate one quadrant of the cemetery east of and flanking the church. Between January and April, we excavated 188 graves from the mainland and 218 from the island cemeteries. As Adams had observed back in 1969, preservation in both cemeteries was excellent. Many individuals were completely or partially mummified. We even discovered fetuses placed in pottery urns prior to burial. It is interesting that where most excavators worry about infant underrepresentation due to factors such as poorer preservation of tiny bones, our modal (most frequent) age at death was birth.

Unlike the earlier Wadi Halfa expedition, we did very little analysis on site. Observations were limited to a preliminary assessment of age and sex and notation of any obvious pathologies. The remains were then inventoried and packaged for shipment to the National Museum of Antiquities in Khartoum, where they were inspected by the Sudanese Antiquities Service. They were then repacked and shipped by plane to the University of Colorado, where they are housed today. Had I not stumbled into George's Introduction to Anthropology class in 1965, followed him to the University of Massachusetts in 1968, gotten my first job at the University of Kentucky in 1971 and my second job at the University of Colorado in 1974, the Kulubnarti remains might still be in the ground.

So now the stage is set. You have the background both to the work and to the theory that has informed it. We can now begin the story of our investigations into life and death on the Nile. The book has six more chapters. Chapter 2 presents our analyses of cranial morphology, but Smith and Batrawi would never recognize it. Our approach will be functional and evolutionary, as opposed to racial. We will be following Washburn's New Physical Anthropology by looking less at descriptive comparisons and more at evolutionary relationships.

Chapter 3 presents our studies of health and disease in the Wadi Halfa and Kulubnarti infants and children. I like to think of them as canaries in the mine shaft. In times gone by, miners often took canaries into the mines. How the canaries sang wasn't important. What was important was when they stopped singing. The canaries stopped singing when dangerous gasses accumulated in the air. Quiet canaries signaled that it was time for the miners to get out. Human culture is one of many ways evolved to enhance reproductive success, and the business end of reproductive success is the survival of infants and children. Infants and children are a culture's canaries. The more they sicken and die, the more trouble the culture is in.

Chapter 4 presents our studies of growth and development as another aspect of subadult well-being. Growth is stunted when infants and children are stressed in a variety of ways, including diseases and dietary deficiencies. The relationship between growth and childhood stress will be of particular importance to us in chapter 4. Chapter 5 extends our investigations of disease (paleopathology) to the adults. Children may be canaries in the mineshaft, but adults produce the canaries. They maintain the cultural system in which the canaries live and die.

Chapter 6 is presented less in the past and more in the present. We present a series of case studies, some of which have never appeared before. These cases are interesting as a kind of detective work, and they also shed light on life and death at its most personal level. Finally, chapter 7 considers what we have accomplished in our quest for a bioethnography of our three Nubian communities.

2

SKULLS, RACES, AND EVOLUTION

An anthropologist will measure a skull at the drop of a hat.

H. L. Shapiro

Skulls

Osteology is one of the most popular courses offered by anthropology departments. The idea of getting to study human bones is fascinating to students. The abundance of television shows, movies, and books featuring forensic anthropologists solving crimes from a few scraps of bone has made interest all the greater. I proposed a new course in forensic anthropology back in the 1990s and the college's course committee expressed concern that the course would be too popular, creating problems at registration.

Osteology courses always begin with the skull. The skull is complex, houses four of the five sensory organs, underlies and gives shape to the face, and is inherently interesting. If you ask someone to name the most fascinating part of a skeleton, the answer, hands-down, will be the skull. Look at a skull, you're looking at a person. Look at a femur and you're looking at a femur.

Learning the skull is often a three-step process. In the first step you learn the bones, features, and landmarks. You learn identification techniques in the second step. These are likely to include age, sex, and possibly race. You are apt to learn, for example, that African populations often have more rectangular-shaped eye orbits. Europeans tend to have a narrow nasal opening. Asians tend to have flat faces with flaring cheek bones. You will then most likely learn to take measurements of the skull.

* * *

Most of the measurements you're apt to learn were invented in the eighteenth and nineteenth centuries, with no concern for how the skull worked. They were invented as a way to describe the skull in numeric terms quite apart from functional consideration. Skulls were measured for practical purposes such as assessing race and diagnosing sex. For those purposes, it didn't matter how a skull worked. What mattered was how it looked. Physical anthropologists had been measuring skulls "at the drop of a hat" in that manner for over a century when Grafton Elliot Smith measured his first Nubian skull.

The Early Days

Petrus Camper had developed a measurement known as the facial angle back in the 1770s (Camper 1791). The angle was produced by the intersection of two lines (figure 2.1). One line was from the base of the nose to the bottom of the ear (the auditory canal in the skull), and the other was from the base of the nose to the glabella. He developed the angle for artistic purposes. According to Camper, the aesthetically ideal angle was 100 degrees. He based this not on any living race, but rather on the ideal represented by Greco-Roman statuary! Art aside, his studies had a far greater impact

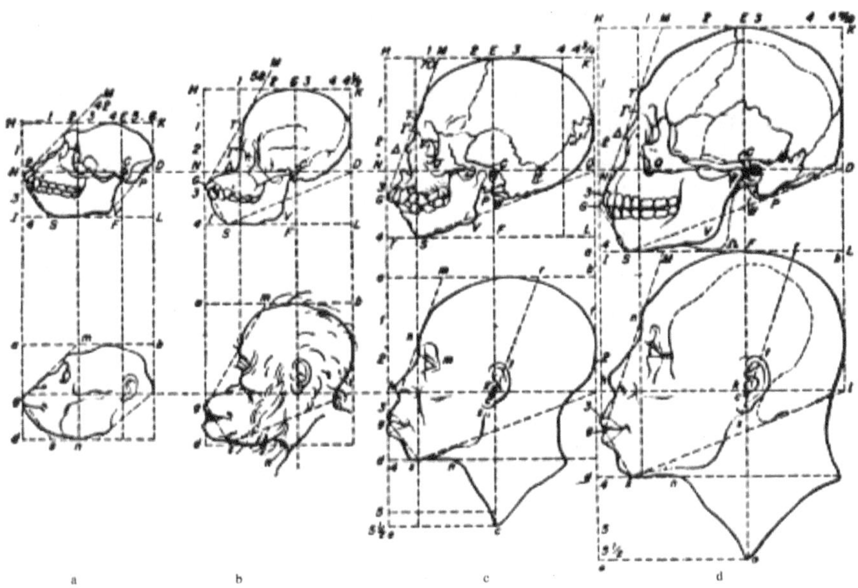

Figure 2.1. Petrus Camper's facial angle (Camper, *Gedagten Van Petrus Camper Over De Misdaad Van Kindermoord; Over De Gemakkelyke Wyze Om Vondelinghuizen In Te Voeren; Over De Oorzaaken Van Kindermoord: En Over Zelfmoord.* Published in 1774 by H. A. de Chalmot).

on the study of race. He found Europeans to have a 90 degree angle, with Orientals at 80 and Africans at 70. Orangutans were included at 58 degrees. According to the facial angle, of all human races, Africans were the furthest removed from classical beauty. Camper's angle would be used by race scientists and eugenicists into the first half of the twentieth century. His comparisons appear in racist literature to this day.

Johann Blumenbach (1795) is best known for a racial scheme based on five colors: white, black, red, yellow, and brown. Color, however, had a serious limitation; it was useless for classifying skeletal remains. He quite naturally turned to craniology as an adjunct to his color scheme. Blumenbach, like Camper, was interested in cranial symmetry and aesthetics, but not with Camper's artistic view. Blumenbach's interest was explicitly racial. He saw a direct connection between cranial symmetry, skin color, and race. In Blumenbach's view, the white race had the most "beautiful" as well as the most symmetrical skull, while the darker races became increasingly less so. The "Negro" was once again the least beautiful and symmetrical of all.

An American by the name of Samuel Morton spent much of his career measuring cranial capacity from thousands of skulls. His approach made perfect sense at the time. After all, who could doubt a natural connection between brain size and intellect? And who could doubt a natural connection between intellect and cultural capacity? He produced a volume (one of several) titled *Crania Aegyptica* (Morton 1844) in which he summarized his comparison of various races.

But for all of their popularity, craniologists cum racial determinists such as Camper, Blumenbach, and Morton were not without their critics. Rudolf Virchow, credited as the father of modern pathology, was extremely critical of craniology and the entire race concept. He had this to say on the subject of race, color, and craniology in 1896:

> Here we must come to clear understanding as to whether we wish to lay greater weight upon skull form or on pigmentation of eyes and skin with its appurtenance, hair or, expressed otherwise, whether we wish to divide mankind more from the standpoint of the osteologist or from that of the dermatologist, the answer seems to admit of no doubt. . . . Even the corrections which have been undertaken in the course of years have not made it possible for even the most practiced craniologist to tell for certain without knowing anything of the provenience of the skull, to which race, let alone stock, it belonged. (reprinted in Count 1950:191)

Franz Boas was as critical as Virchow. In 1911 he discussed the instability of the cephalic index (length of the skull/width × 100)—a favorite of craniologists—as it was used in racial analyses. He made a comparison between the cephalic index of Jewish and Sicilian immigrants raised in the United States and relatives raised in their homeland.

He discovered that the differences between immigrants and their relatives raised in the old country were comparable to the differences between two so-called races (Boas 1911). Boas's research was what Kuhn (1962) would describe as normal science designed to test the race paradigm. Boas found the paradigm wanting. But his study did not bring down the paradigm. There is still an ongoing debate as to whether environmental responses obliterate biological relationships among populations (Relethford 2004).

Criticisms notwithstanding, craniology and racial typology continued to be a powerful force. There is no better example than Earnest Hooton's 1930 study of crania from the site of Pecos Pueblo in New Mexico (Hooton 1930). In the course of his analysis, Hooton identified a "pseudo-Negroid" type. The skulls appeared to be a diluted form of the "Full African Negro" type. How could this be? Racial typology combined with theories of migration admitted but one explanation. "Negroid" invaders must have worked their way up from Northeast Asia across the Bering Strait down into the American Southwest, producing a minor infusion of Negroid blood that had trickled in from the tropical parts of the Old World (Hooton 1930). We couldn't contrive a better example of how a failed paradigm can bend conflicting evidence to its will.

Bones, Bodies, and Statistics

"Marley was dead. This must be distinctly understood, or nothing wonderful can come of the story I am going to relate." Charles Dickens (1843) wrote these two simple sentences at the beginning of his classic story *A Christmas Carol.* He told us everything we needed to know in language that a clever five-year-old could understand. What a terrific thing to do. We begin the presentation of our research on the Wadi Halfa crania in the spirit of Dickens. Here goes: *You need to know some statistics. Unless this is clearly understood, nothing wonderful can come of the story we are going to relate.* Be assured, however, that we are going to focus only on how statistics can be used to understand measurements of the skull. We are going to keep it as simple as we can within the bounds of accuracy.

There are many kinds of statistics. Some, like the mean (average), are descriptive. We can describe 50 Nubian skulls by their average length. Length is a variable, and the mean is a statistic describing one quality of the variable. The mean is useful, but it can be misleading. Suppose we had two samples of skulls—let's say 50 skulls in each sample. Now suppose that the two samples had identical mean cranial length. Here's a question that the mean can't answer: How typical is the mean? That is to say, how well does the mean represent all of the skulls in the sample? The answer depends on how different (variable) the skulls are from one another. The mean can be very typical if all of the skulls are very much like it, but far less typical if the skulls vary widely from it. The study of variability has become a cornerstone of evolutionary biology and a concept worth spending some time on.

We have been using the term "typology" a lot. Grafton Elliot Smith's comparison of "Negroids" and "Caucasoids" was typological because it ignored variability. The comparison was between two idealized forms representing the Negroid and Caucasoid racial types. In formal typology, one specimen is selected to be the type. It is often the first specimen discovered, whether it is actually "typical" or not. Comparisons are then made using type specimens. In the Nubian case, the entire reconstruction of racial migrations was based on the comparison of racial types. There was no consideration of natural variation within the so-called races. Variation was irrelevant.

Darwinism shifted the focus. From an evolutionary perspective, variation is the raw material on which natural selection acts. To paraphrase Darwin: Any individual, if it *varies however slightly* in a manner profitable to itself, will propagate its kind and thus be naturally selected. Without variation, evolution would run down like a $2 watch.

The study of relationships among populations and the evolutionary transformations they undergo, regardless of whether they're ancient Nubians, house cats, or artichokes, requires a measure of variability as a statistical companion to the mean. The companion is the standard deviation (figure 2.2). The standard deviation is in turn the companion of the normal distribution, or so-called bell curve.

The bell curve is one of the most common patterns of variation in nature. Droppings under a bird's nest are distributed as a bell curve (Kranzler et al. 2006). Most drops hit under the nest, but occasionally they don't—their frequency of "misses" drops off with distance from the nest. If you graph the frequency of droppings using the nest as the bull's-eye, you get a bell curve. Biological variables such as height and weight are commonly distributed as bell curves for the same reason arrows miss the bull's-eye and

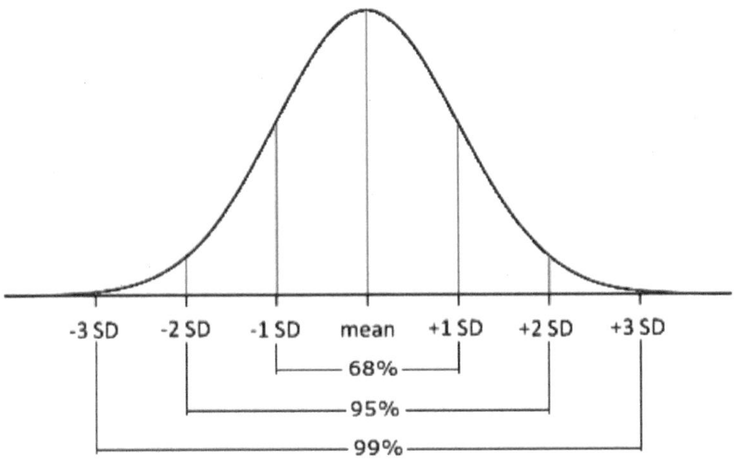

Figure 2.2. Standard deviations in a bell curve or normal distribution function.

bird droppings fall away from the nest. The underlying causes of variation in height and weight are numerous and largely random. Most people are average or near average in height and weight for their population. Individuals become taller or shorter, or heavier or thinner, as the causes become increasingly extreme. Again, if there is no bias in those underlying causes, individuals are no more likely to be extremely short than they are to be extremely tall, or extremely thin. The bell curve is most commonly referred to as a normal distribution.

For statistical purposes, the normal distribution has been divided into areas known as standard deviations. The divisions are standardized for all normal distributions in the following way. By definition, 68 percent of the total area under a normal distribution lies within the bounds of one standard deviation above and below the mean (34 percent on each side of the mean). This means that 68 percent of the population is expected to fall within one standard deviation of the mean if the variable is normal. It also means that the probability of having a height within one standard deviation of the mean is 68 percent. It also means that the probability of being one standard deviation above the mean or one standard deviation below the mean is 34 percent. Two standard deviations encompass 95 percent of the total area (frequency–probability), and 99 percent is encompassed by three. The probability of being more than three standard deviations above the mean is 0.5 percent. The same goes for being more than three standard deviations below the mean, and so on.

The key to the standard deviation is that those percentages never change when a variable is normally distributed. What changes are the actual standard deviations calculated for a given variable in a sample. Let's make an example. Suppose we have two samples—A and B—of 50 skulls each. Both A and B have an average cranial length of 19 centimeters (cm), but sample A has a standard deviation of 2 cm while sample B has a standard deviation of 4 cm. If that were the case, 68 percent of the skulls in A would be expected to lie between 17 cm and 21 cm. In the case of sample B, you would have to go above and below the mean twice as many centimeters (15 and 23 cm) to encompass the same 68 percent. Group B is clearly more variable than group A. The standard deviation gives a numerical expression of variation to go along with the mean.

There are statistical tables that measure areas under the normal distribution in fractions of standard deviation units, and these can be translated into frequencies and probabilities. Virtually every standardized test you have ever taken has placed your score under a normal distribution of scores in standard deviation units. Those units are then converted to percentiles telling you how typical or unusual you are. Unusual can be good or bad, depending on whether you are above or below the mean! The average American male is approximately 70 inches tall with a standard deviation of about 4 inches. That places me 1.5 standard deviations below the mean. Only 7 percent of American men are shorter than I am—a fact that pains me to this day.

Statistics can do more than describe; they can help a researcher make inferences from samples to populations. Samples are subsets of individuals drawn from a larger population of individuals. We see this connection every day. Pollsters sample 1,500 potential voters to estimate how an entire population of voters is apt to vote. Samples, of course, are never identical to the population they come from. They are also never identical to each other if the samples are taken several times from the same population. A pollster will announce that 71 percent of voters intend to vote for candidate X ± 3 percent. That ± is the standard deviation.[1] The standard deviation (calculated as a standard error for samples) tells us that if the poll was taken many times, the estimates would fall somewhere between 74 percent (one standard deviation above the mean) and 68 percent (one standard deviation below the mean) 68 percent of the time. The estimate would fall somewhere between 77 percent and 65 percent 95 percent of the time, and between 80 percent and 62 percent 99 percent of the time. The most reliable polls have the smallest standard deviations.

Now let's return to 50 male and 50 female skulls. These samples are hopefully representative of a larger Nubian population. Exactly what population they represent is determined by the researcher. For example, she may use them as samples of the population of an ancient city, or a geographic region or cultural horizon. It's up to the researcher to define the population. The connection between the population and the samples should be thoroughly explained.

For our purposes, our samples of male and female Nubian skulls were excavated from the mainland cemetery at Kulubnarti. We will be using them as a sample of the people who died in that community in early Christian times. Unlike the carefully constructed samples used by pollsters, our samples often (not always) come to us as fate provides.[2]

Suppose we found that the female skulls averaged 20 cm in length ± 4 cm, while the males averaged 22 cm ± 9 cm. From a statistical standpoint, there are two possible reasons for the difference. First, males and females are actually the same length, but the samples are creating a false impression that they aren't. Alternatively, the samples express a real difference between males and females. In both cases the researcher is using the samples of 50 males and 50 females to make an inference about the larger male and female populations. Whenever samples are used to make inferences concerning populations, the statistics are referred to as inferential. The problem is this: the researcher has to make a choice between the two inferences concerning males and females.

No matter which inference she chooses she is taking a chance. She can conclude that the males and females are actually different, when they in reality aren't; or she can conclude that they are the same, when they are actually different. What she needs is a way to increase the odds that she will make the correct inference. The solution to her dilemma is easier to illustrate if we step away from Nubian skulls for a moment and think about a similar problem where the differences are far more dramatic—house cats and African lions (figure 2.3).

Ask anyone whether house cats are different from lions and they'll say yes. Ask them why and they will state the obvious: they look different. But that doesn't actually answer the question. House cats look different from each other also, as do lions. The answer is that we all *appreciate* that house cats look more like each other than they look like lions, and vice versa. The term "appreciate" was used by a statistician named Carl Pearson to refer to differences we observe without actually measuring them. Every culture has a system of taxonomy for classifying plants and animals based on the

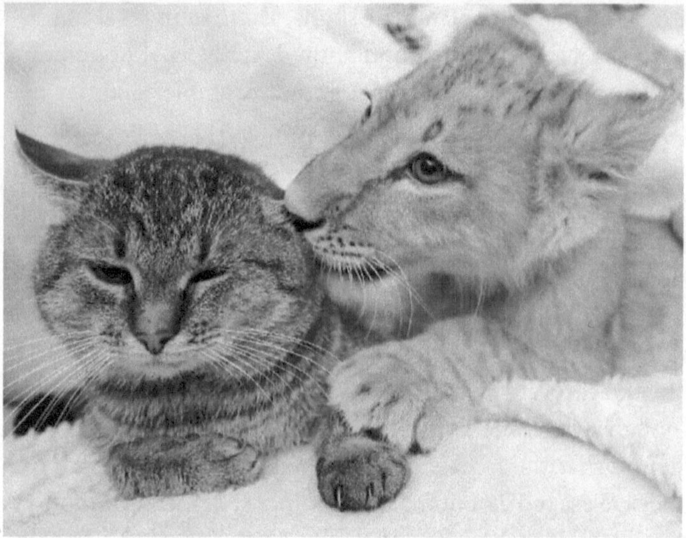

Figure 2.3. Cat and lion.

appreciation of differences within and between groups. The differences are usually of cultural importance.

We don't need a statistic to conclude with confidence that house cats and lions are different, so let's go back to the less apparent difference between our male and female skulls. We had calculated a mean of 22 cm ± 9 cm for the males and 20 cm ± 4 cm for the females. What we want to know is, are males sufficiently alike and different from females, and vice versa, to classify them into separate groups from the standpoint of length? There is a way to answer the question with numbers rather than by appreciation. We can use our means and standard deviations to create a ratio between one mean subtracted from the other (a measure of the difference between groups) in the numerator and within group variation (the standard deviation) in the denominator. The ratio will calculate what we did by appreciation in the case of the lions and house cats. A large ratio means a large difference between males and females relative to how different they are among themselves. The statistical formula calculates a value called Student's t, where $\overline{X}$ represents the means and S represents the standard deviations. As t gets bigger (as the numerator gets larger relative to the denominator), the likelihood that the males and females are different increases. It is traditional to wait until you are 95 percent confident[3] in the decision before concluding the difference is real.

Our statistical comparison of the male and female skulls is referred to as a *univariate* comparison. Univariate refers to the number of variables

$$t = \frac{\bar{X}_1 - \bar{X}_2}{\sqrt{\frac{s_1^2}{N_1} + \frac{s_2^2}{N_2}}}$$

$$3.92 = \frac{22 - 20}{\sqrt{\frac{9}{50} + \frac{4}{50}}}$$

Figure 2.4. Student's *t* test for cranial length.

used for the comparison. If we had wanted to compare males and females for several measurements, such as cranial height, length, facial height, and mandible length, we would have had to calculate a separate Student's *t* test for each measurement.

There's a problem with a univariate approach. Again, let's use an analogy to illustrate the problem. Suppose we compared two desks using three measurements—height, depth, and length. Desk A is higher than desk B. It is also longer and deeper. Are there three kinds of differences between desk A and B? No. Desk A is bigger than desk B, and we have measured size three times.

Human skulls vary a great deal in size, and like desks, big skulls have larger measurements than small skulls. The effect of size can make many measurements redundant to each other. As a result, there are inevitably differences in shape that individual measurements miss (Tabachnick and Fidell 2013). Small skulls may be shaped differently than larger ones. They may have rounder vaults and narrower, less projecting faces. Individual measurements may also interact with one another in complex ways—some contributing more to size and others contributing more to shape. Some measurements may also relate more closely to some areas of the skull than others. Comparing measurements one or two at a time is like pulling all those relationships apart. This does violence to cranial anatomy, which in turn does violence to comparisons based on biologically meaningful differences and similarities.

Multivariate statistics were invented to solve that problem (Tabachnick and Fidell 2013). Many were created in the first decades of the twentieth century but were too complicated to calculate until the advent of computers.

Multivariate statistics that used to require days of computation can be now performed in seconds. George and I routinely gave our osteology students multivariate problems due at the end of class that took me over a week when writing my dissertation. The students use their laptops. I used a computer that filled a room.

So, armed with a computer, let's create a multivariate (multiple variable) statistic to discriminate between our male and female skulls. Let's ask the computer to create a formula using cranial vault height, cranial breadth, cranial height, and mandibular length to make the discrimination. First, we place the skulls in their actual groups. Second, we take our measurements for each skull. The computer uses the data to calculate a formula called a discriminant function. The formula looks like this: Y = measurement 1xλ_1 + measurement 2xλ_2 + measurement 3xλ_3 + measurement 4xλ_4. The formula is designed to transform each skull's measurements into a single value Y with one property. The Y's are as similar within groups and as different between groups as is mathematically possible. The expectation is that the Y's will discriminate male skulls from female skulls better than any of the individual measurements. Here's an example. We have taken our 100 skulls (males and females combined) and computed a formula with the following λ values: .87, .27, -.02, -.70. We have a skull with the following measurements: vault length = 19 cm, cranial breadth = 14 cm, cranial height = 11 cm, and mandibular length = 10 cm. The measurements are converted to the Z scores we discussed earlier.[4] This puts all of measurements on the same scale. The skull's Y value will be $Y = .87 \times 1.7 + .27 \times 1.4 + .02 \times 1.8 + .70 \times 1.7 = 3.28$.

Creating a formula to discriminate skulls whose sex is already known may seem pointless, but it is valuable for two reasons. First, suppose we come across a new skull of unknown sex. We can take the four measurements, run them through the formula, and compute a Y score for the skull. We can then assign the skull to a sex category based on its Y value. We can even calculate the probability that the skull belongs to one or the other of the sex categories and make the assignment on statistical grounds.

Discriminant functions have a second quality that has been far more important to our research than assigning specimens to their proper groups. The λ values are called eigenvectors (or canonical coefficients), and their size and sign indicate how each associated measurement is contributing to the discrimination. This makes it possible to interpret what the discriminant function means.

Table 2.1. Hypothetical eigenvectors

Variable	Eigenvector
Cranial Length	+.87
Cranial Breadth	+.27
Cranial Height	-.02
Mandible Length	-.70

Let's examine the eigenvectors that were just calculated to distinguish our male and female skulls (table 2.1). Their sign and size reflect how much and how each variable contributed to the discrimination of our male and female skulls. According to size, the most important variables were cranial length and mandible length. Cranial height and cranial breadth contributed almost nothing. Second, the signs reveal a shape difference. Males and females are different in the proportion of their cranial length to the length of their mandible. One group has longer vaults (positive sign) and shorter faces (measured as length of the mandible) than the other. We would know which group was which if we calculated each sex's average Y score. The group with the largest average Y score would be the one with greater length (larger positive contribution) and shortest face (larger negative contribution). Reading eigenvector signs and sizes can be more important to understanding why groups differ the way they do than telling skulls apart. That has certainly been the case with our Nubia research.

Discriminant functions have played an important role in anthropological investigations for over a half century. A physicist by the name of Jacob Bronowski (Bronowski and Long 1951, Bronowski 1952) was one of the first to apply discriminant function to an anthropological problem. In the 1950s there was considerable debate regarding the status of *Australopithecus*—Raymond Dart's famous fossil specimen from Taung, South Africa. The question was whether it was a humanlike ape or an apelike human. Bronowski saw an opportunity to apply a discriminant function to the question. He measured a series of human and ape teeth and created a discriminant function to discriminate the two. He then ran the Taung specimen through the function, and found its Y to be closer to the human sample. This provided major support for Dart's interpretation that *Australopithecus* was more human than ape.

Craniofacial Evolution in Ancient Nubia

We are now prepared to present our analyses of Nubian craniofacial evolution from Mesolithic (c. 9000 BCE) through Christian (1450 CE) times. The research we will be sharing developed in two phases beginning with the United Nations Educational, Scientific, and Cultural Organization (UNESCO) work and continuing through our analyses of the Kulubnarti remains. The first phase was directed toward understanding the long-term transformations from Mesolithic through Christian times. The second phase examined the differences between the Wadi Halfa and Kulubnarti Christian populations. The strategy of both took shape from two perspectives. One was cultural-historical and the other theoretical.

The Cultural-Historical Context

The cultural-historical setting for our analysis begins with the Mesolithic (often referred to as the Epipaleolithic). It describes a subsistence economy based on broad-spectrum hunting and gathering. Animals such as wild cattle were hunted, and fishing occurred in riverine environments. The inhabitants of some sites produced harpoons. Wild grasses were gathered and processed with grinding stones. Populations practicing a Mesolithic economy were present in Nubia some 15,000 years ago (Sadig 2013)—some 6,000 years before our Mesolithic sample.

Given their heavy mineralization, direct dating of our Mesolithic material wasn't possible. The associated artifacts were, however, similar to artifacts known as the Qadan Industry (Wendorf et al. 1979; Becker and Wendorf 1993). According to Wendorf and coworkers (Wendorf and Chmielewski 1965), Qadan produced C^{14} dates between 11,959 and 6400 BCE. David Greene and George (Greene and Armelagos 1972) used the Qadan dates to suggest a date for the Wadi Halfa remains of approximately 9000 BCE. Animal and plant remains associated with the burials were indicative of a heavy reliance on large game hunting, with some reliance on fishing and seed gathering. It is likely that the Mesolithic Nubians were also a low-density, dispersed population.

The transition to a food-producing (Neolithic) economy in Nubia occurred during A-Group (3800–2800 BCE) times and was unusual in two regards. First, whereas the Neolithic in most places around the world produced village-living farmers from nomadic hunter-gatherers, the Nubian Neolithic produced nomadic pastoralists from less nomadic Mesolithic hunter-gatherers. Second, unlike the Neolithic elsewhere, the transition in Nubia was gradual (Edwards 2007).

According to Edwards, domestic livestock was present in riverine north and central Sudan by 4000 BCE and barley and wheat by 3000 BCE. The evidence, however, indicates that with the exception of an emphasis on domestic cattle, the economy remained essentially Mesolithic (Gatto 2009). It would appear that populations practicing a hunting and gathering economy continued for centuries in some areas and even millennia in others (Edwards 2007).

Agriculture was intensified during the C-Group period (2500–1500 BCE), but its relationship to pastoralism is a subject of discussion (Hafsaas-Tsakos 2010). One source of evidence for the intensification hypothesis is dental. C-Group populations show increased tooth wear and associated dental diseases relative to their A-Group forebears. It's been argued (Beckett and Lovell 1994) that this most likely resulted from increased use of grinding stones associated with increased grain processing. Not only did stone-on-stone grinding deposit grit into the grain, but additional grit was often added to enhance the grinding process.

Irrigation based on a waterwheel known as the saqia transformed agriculture into a dominant economic activity in Lower Nubia during Meroitic (350 BCE–350 CE) times.[5] Irrigation made it possible to grow multiple crops each year, which in turn brought more produce to the table than ever before. Based on his own work, Adams (1977) argued that saqia-based agriculture had changed little to this day. Agriculture didn't, however, replace pastoral economies. Isotopic analyses indicate that a major source of protein continued to come from herbivorous animals (White and Schwartz 1994).

As we discussed in chapter 1, we have every reason to believe in a genetic continuum linking Nubia's populations from Mesolithic through Christian, and even modern, times. As we mentioned previously, the continuity hypothesis has been supported by Greene's discovery of some 13 dental traits shared among the Nubian populations. All of the traits are known to be under strong genetic control (Greene 1965, 1966, 1967a, 1967b; Greene and Armelagos 1972). Adams's (1967:29) interpretation of the cultural transformations associated with the human remains supports Greene's interpretation and bears repeating:

> We are conscious now of a continuum of cultural evolution within the borders of Nubia, heavily influenced by events and ideas from

> abroad, but involving the same basic population from beginning to end. There is no reason why the Nubians of today should not claim to be the direct descendants, culturally as well as racially, of their Neolithic, and perhaps even their Paleolithic, forebears. (Adams 1966)

The cultural context of the Kulubnarti remains is far simpler than that of Wadi Halfa. Based on recent C^{14} dates, the island and mainland community cemeteries are contemporaneous, with a mean date for the island cemetery of 716 CE and a mean age of 752 CE for the mainland cemetery. The dates place both cemeteries within the first centuries of Nubia's medieval period (Adams 1966). The dates also place Kulubnarti earlier than the Christians at Wadi Halfa.

As discussed in chapter 1, the Kulubnarti folk provide an important cultural-ecological contrast to their northern counterparts. Located as they were to the south of Wadi Halfa in the *Batn el Hajar* (Belly of Rock), the people of Kulubnarti lived on the fringes of both Nubia's northern and southern centers of population. The difficulty of their physical circumstances, combined with their isolation, gave us a treasure trove of opportunities for comparative analyses in all of our studies.

The Theoretical Context

It's useful to think of research as a series of ongoing conversations among scholars. Published articles represent the durable record of those conversations. Conversations wax and wane. Topics come and go. Conflicts and controversies shift focus. As we discussed in the previous chapter, the Nubian First Survey started a conversation about ancient Nubian races and their role in the rise and fall of Nubian civilizations. The Second Survey shifted the conversation away from racial determinism but continued to focus on the importance of constructing and refining racial typologies.

The conversation began to shift again following the UNESCO survey. The shift was driven by a combination of influences. Archaeologists shifted their focus from cemeteries to villages. This new "peasant archaeology" (Adams 2004) provided, for the first time, a more wide-ranging cultural context for a biocultural approach to the human remains. This in turn encouraged a more population-based orientation to the human remains. Genetic information from living populations was incorporated as an adjunct to osteological analyses. And last but not least, multivariate statistics were becoming easier to apply with the advent of new computer technologies.

All of this brought the conversation concerning the ancient Nubians to a crossroads. Some researchers chose to continue a focus on racial relationships aided by multivariate statistics. For example, Michael Crichton (1964)—who would later become a world famous author of medical thrillers—used discriminant function to compare pre-Dynastic and Dynastic Egyptian skulls to a sample of Negroid skulls. He found that the pre-Dynastic Egyptian skulls were more like the Negroids than were the Dynastic Egyptian skulls. He also found that the Dynastic Egyptians were more Caucasoid than were the pre-Dynastics. Putting old wine in new bottles.

Three years after Crichton's study, D. R. Burnor and J. E. Harris (1967) applied multivariate statistics to a similar question of racial affinity. Although they acknowledged that Nubian populations had remained stable over the last several thousand years, they proposed a massive penetration of Negroid Africa by Caucasoids some 14,000 years ago.

Eugene Strouhal (1971) continued to address questions of racial affinity, but with a combination of craniometric and genetic data. He argued for a post-Paleolithic Negroid invasion into Upper Egypt and Lower Nubia. He based his argument first on blood type comparisons among living Egyptians and then on comparisons of ancient Egyptian crania. According to Strouhal, a majority of the skulls examined showed mixed Europoid-Negroid features. One-third showed a dominant presence of Negroid features, and one-third possessed a predominance of Caucasoid traits. The remaining third were either well balanced or possessed characteristics of the neutral range common to both races. Take out the blood group data, and the analysis could have been conducted by Batrawi.

The Colorado Mesolithic material provided an opportunity to take the conversation in a different direction by asking a different question. Could a nonracial, functional approach to the craniofacial variation in our Nubian populations provide the evolutionary insight envisioned by Washburn's "The New Physical Anthropology" and Livingstone's analysis of sickle cell in West Africa? The question gave us the motive; what we needed was the means.

The Visit

The Mesolithic project began with David Carlson's visit to my lab in 1976. David had just finished his doctoral dissertation in which he had analyzed the craniofacial evolution of A-Group through Christian populations excavated by the Joint Scandinavian Expedition to Sudanese Nubia (Vagn Nielsen 1970) during the UNESCO Campaign. David had taken a functional approach based on measurements taken from cephalograms of the

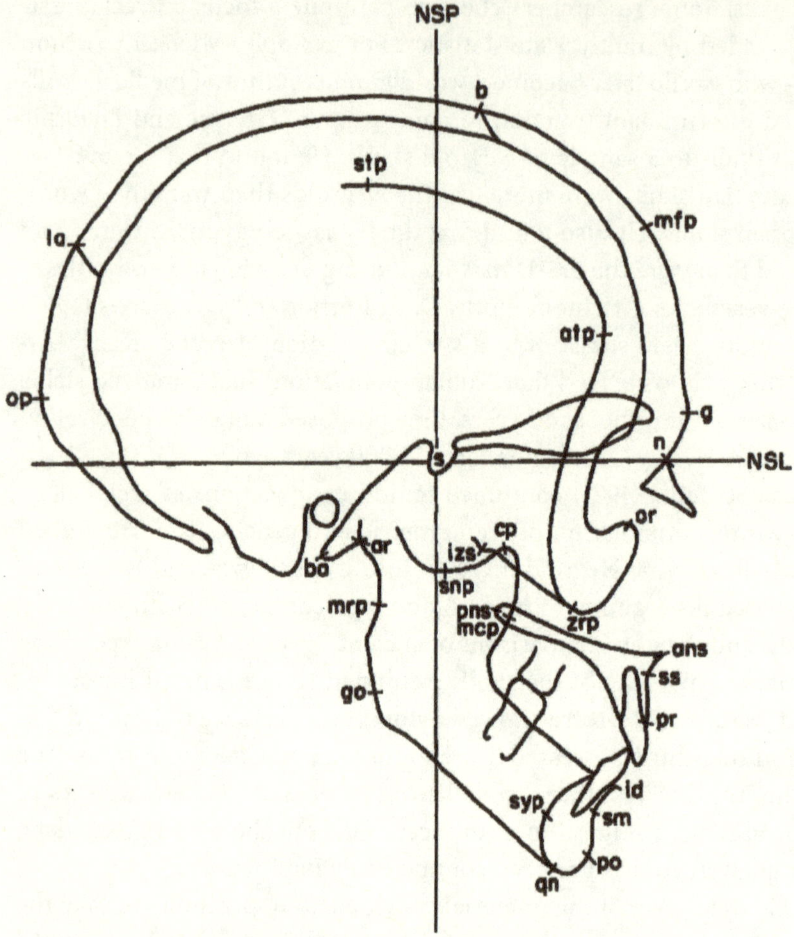

Figure 2.5. Cephalogram with points of measurement.

skulls (figure 2.5). The method was developed as a clinical technique for measuring craniofacial growth in living children. Using the new technique, he had demonstrated a morphological transformation in the Nubia craniofacial complex toward a more rounded skull with a smaller face and reduced muscle attachments—most particularly the chewing muscles. He attributed this change to an evolutionary response to changes in functional demands placed on the chewing apparatus associated with an intensified use of agricultural food resources. The Colorado data combined with the Mesolithic crania provided the means to expand David's study.

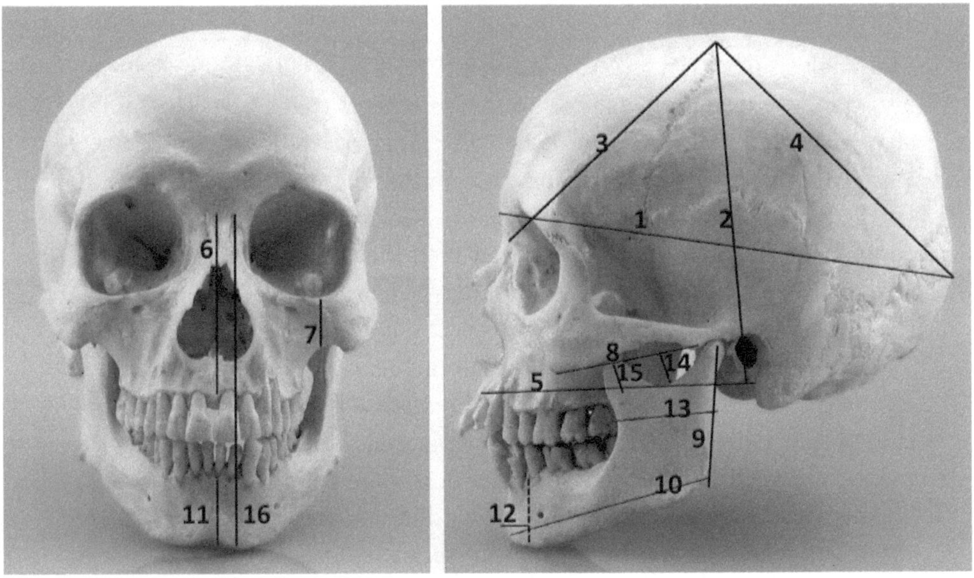

Figure 2.6. Sixteen cranial measurements.

The Analysis

Our plan was to extend David's analysis back in time by incorporating the Mesolithic remains. We would also increase his Meroitic-Christian samples by adding the data collected in the field by the Colorado team. There were, however, two problems. First, the Wadi Halfa data had been collected in the field and consisted of standard cranial measurements. Many (fortunately, not all) of David's data were not comparable to the Wadi Halfa data. Second, many of the Mesolithic skulls were incomplete, thus reducing the number of measurements available. We ended up with 16 measurements (figure 2.6; table 2.2).

Table 2.2. Sixteen cranial measurements

1. Cranial Length	9. Ramus Height
2. Cranial Height	10. Corpus Length
3. Frontal Chord	11. Symphesial Height
4. Parietal Chord	12. Symphesial Thickness
5. Facial Length	13. Ramus Width
6. Upper Facial Height	14. Sygmoid Notch Height
7. Cheek Height	15. Coronoid Process Height
8. Masseter Origin Length	16. Total Facial Height

Phase 1: The Mesolithic Analysis

Our analysis (Carlson and Van Gerven 1977) began with the basic means and standard deviations for our 16 measurements (table 2.3). The sample sizes were as follows: A–C Groups = 52 crania; Meroitic–X-Group = 329 crania; Christian = 154 crania. The means allowed us to measure how much (as a percent) each measurement changed through time. We did this by comparing the percent differences between the Mesolithics and the A–C Groups, then to the combined Meroitic–X-Group and Christian crania (table 2.4).

The principal changes (indicated in boldface) (figures 2.7 and 2.8) fell into two clusters moving in opposite directions. The positive changes included cranial height and the frontal and parietal chords. By these measurements, the skull was becoming higher and more rounded through time. The negative changes all involved the mandible and its articulation with the skull. The mandible was becoming shorter as indicated by a reduction in body (corpus) length. The mandible was also becoming less robust. Bone at the symphysis (chin) buttresses the mandible against twisting forces associated with heavy chewing across the molar teeth. The most notable changes,

Table 2.3. Means and standard deviations for Mesolithic, A-C Group, and Meroitic–X-Group–Christian crania

	Mesolithic		A-C		M-X-Ch	
	Mean	Sd.	Mean	Sd.	Mean	Sd.
Cranial Length	18.58	0.32	18.18	0.64	18.27	0.82
Cranial Height	12.75	0.56	13.91	0.66	13.64	0.64
Frontal Chord	10.57	0.29	11.71	0.45	11.47	0.55
Parietal Chord	11.32	0.35	12.48	0.49	12.35	0.71
Facial Length	10.36	0.35	10.11	0.47	10.28	0.57
Upper Facial Height	6.63	0.33	6.68	0.41	6.66	0.43
Cheek Height	2.57	0.23	2.42	0.26	2.37	0.27
Masseter Origin Length	4.31	0.52	3.38	0.34	3.18	0.32
Ramus Height	4.75	0.62	4.51	0.42	4.55	0.45
Corpus Length	9.25	0.41	7.37	0.57	7.21	0.51
Symphysis Height	3.35	0.22	3.19	0.38	3.28	0.37
Symphysis Thickness	1.69	0.17	1.48	0.14	1.44	0.18
Ramus Width	4.29	0.37	3.71	0.38	3.73	0.31
Sygmoid Notch Height	4.67	0.64	4.41	0.41	4.28	0.37
Coronoid Height	6.13	0.54	5.98	0.53	5.95	0.53
Total Facial Height	10.92	0.61	11.55	0.61	11.46	0.65

Table 2.4. Percent changes from Mesolithic through A-C and Meroitic–X-Group–Christian periods

Measurement	Meso/A-C	Meso/M-X-Ch
Cranial Length	-2.2	-1.7
Cranial Height	**8.4**	**6.4**
Frontal Chord (curve)	**9.7**	**7.9**
Parietal Chord (curve)	**9.3**	**8.4**
Facial Length	-3.5	0.8
Upper Facial Height	0.8	0.5
Cheek Height	-5.9	-7.8
Masseter Origin Length	**-21.6**	**-26.3**
Ramus Height	-3.8	-4.3
Corpus Length	**-20.4**	**-22.8**
Symphysis Height	-4.8	-2.1
Symphysis Thickness	**-12.5**	**-8.4**
Ramus Width	**-13.8**	**-13.1**
Sigmoid Notch Height	-5.8	**-8.4**
Coronoid Process Height	-2.7	-3.1
Total Facial Height	5.5	4.8

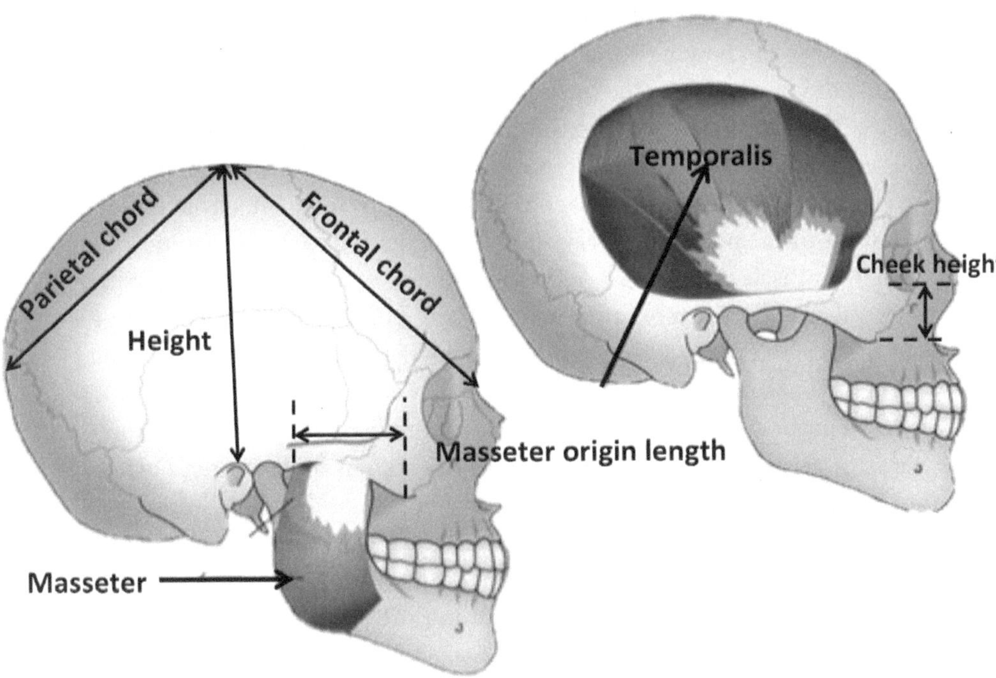

Figure 2.7. Measurements indicating substantial changes.

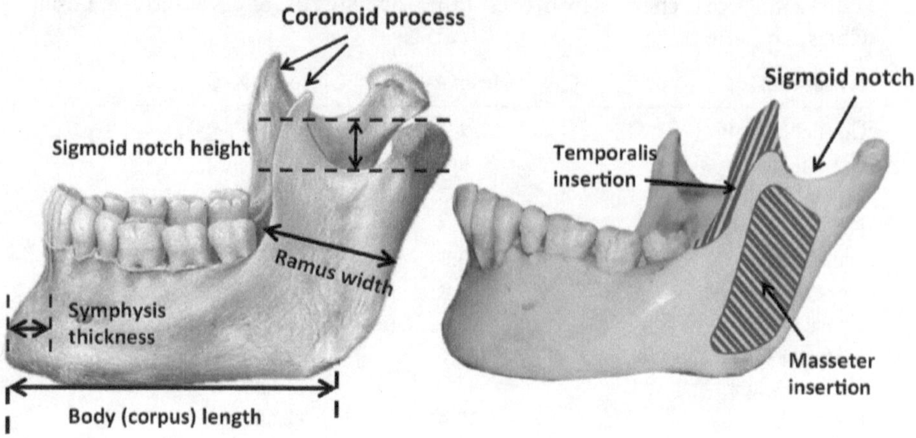

Figure 2.8. Mandible measurements and muscle insertions.

however, are those associated with the chewing musculature. The greatest reduction among all of the measurements taken was masseter origin length. We saw this as extremely important, because the size of a muscle's attachment is an excellent indicator of a muscle's size. The masseter produces powerful chewing force over the molars. You can feel it bulge on the side of your jaw near the back when you clench your teeth. A reduced muscle indicates reduced power in that aspect of chewing.

There appeared to be a pattern of change. The masseter originates on the zygomatic arch (the cheek bone) and descends to an attachment along the ramus of the mandible. The reduction suggested to us the evolution of a smaller muscle. And last, a reduction in cheek height also suggested a smaller masseter. The most anterior (forward) point of the masseter's origin is at the front corner of the zygomatic near where the cheek height measurement is taken.

The temporalis is a second major chewing muscle. It originates as a fan-shaped sheet spreading along the side of the cranial vault. It then narrows into a tendon as it descends behind the zygomatic arch, where it inserts at the top of the ramus onto the coronoid process. The temporalis works with the masseter by producing bite forces over the front teeth. We interpreted the reduced sigmoid notch height as an indication of a smaller coronoid process associated with a smaller temporalis insertion.

Even with all of its limitations, our univariate approach told us a lot about how the skull was evolving. It was getting shorter, higher, and more rounded through time. And most important, the masticatory system was becoming reduced. We could see with our simple univariate approach the same pattern of craniofacial evolution that David had seen in his dissertation analysis. Our next step was to determine if a multivariate approach based on actual measures of association among the variables would produce a comparable result. Before we go on, we need to explain one more aspect of discriminant function.

When there are more than two groups, more than one function may (but not always) be required. There is always one fewer function than groups. Here's a hypothetical example. Suppose we take ten measurements on 24 skulls belonging to three groups and ask the computer to discriminate the groups. Two functions will be calculated, even though only one may be necessary to discriminate the groups. In our illustration (figure 2.9), function I separates group A and function II distinguishes B from C. The circles are two-dimensional standard deviations representing the 95th percentiles for each group.

In the case of our Nubian populations, viewed graphically (figure 2.10), it's clear that the first function produced virtually all of the discrimination. The eigenvectors associated with the first function (table 2.5) indicate that eight variables (boldface) were of primary importance to the discrimination. They formed two groups—one positive and one negative. The positive group included mandible corpus (body) length, symphesial (chin) height, cranial length, masseter origin length, sigmoid notch height, and coronal process height.

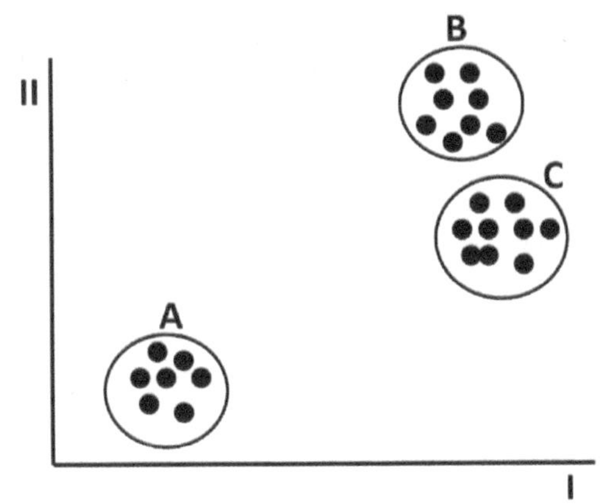

Figure 2.9. A hypothetical discriminant function for three groups.

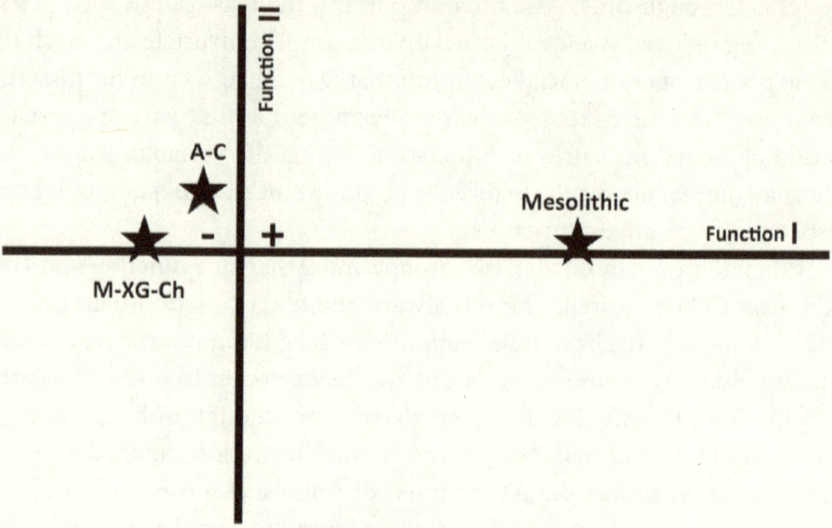

Figure 2.10. Discriminant function distances between the Mesolithic, A-C, and Meroitic-X-Group-Christian crania.

Table 2.5. First function eigenvectors for the Mesolithic through Christian discriminant function

Measurement	Eigenvectors
Cranial Length	**0.40**
Cranial Height	-0.04
Frontal Chord	**-0.42**
Parietal Chord	0.22
Facial Length	**-0.49**
Upper Facial Height	0.2
Cheek Height	0.24
Masseter Origin Length	**0.48**
Ramus Height	0.17
Corpus Length	**1.15**
Symphysis Height	**0.53**
Symphysis Thickness	0.14
Ramus Width	0.05
Sigmoid Notch Height	**0.5**
Coronoid Process Height	**0.5**
Total Facial Height	**-0.98**

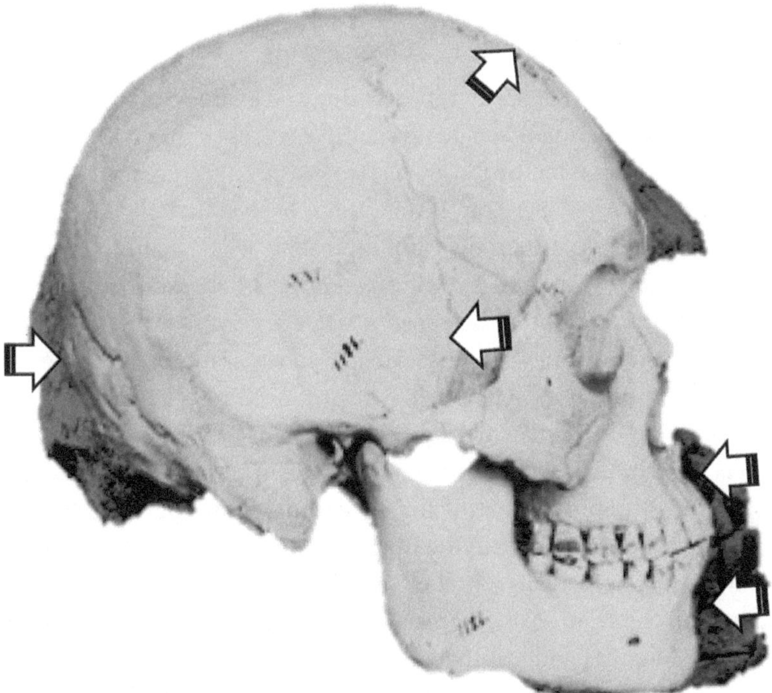

Figure 2.11. Changes in the Nubian skull.

The negative group consisted of frontal chord, facial length, and upper facial height. In other words, individuals with long, low skulls (cranial length +, frontal chord -) had large mandibles with large masseters, and large temporal muscles (sigmoid notch height +, coronal process +). Individuals with shorter, higher skulls had smaller jaws and jaw muscles. Our univariate and multivariate analyses had supported the same interpretation.

Taken together, they had revealed three trends in the evolution of the Nubian skull. First, the vault became shorter, higher, and more rounded (spherical). Second, the position of the face shifted backward farther under the vault. The result was a less projecting[6] facial profile. Third, the robusticity of the face, especially in features associated with mastication, was reduced. In other words, the Nubian skull became increasingly modern (figure 2.11).

Before we move on, there was one additional feature of the discriminant function that we found intriguing. The first function arranged the samples in temporal order. While certainly not a temporal scale, we felt that the arrangement provided additional support for our interpretation.

Biocultural Interactions

The last phase of our analysis was to interpret the biological evidence in its cultural context. We began by representing the evolutionary process as a flow chart of interacting mechanisms and processes (figure 2.12). The chart illustrates what has been proposed as two paths to craniofacial evolution. The first path is represented on the left. It has been called the dental reduction hypothesis. The path on the right represents what has been referred to as the masticatory-function hypothesis. Perhaps because they have been given separate names, there has been a tendency to treat them as though they were in opposition. This bears further consideration.

The dental reduction hypothesis was proposed by David Greene back in 1967 (Greene 1967a). He argued that the dietary shift away from highly abrasive foods, such as the consumption of grasses during Mesolithic times, toward the production of higher carbohydrate foods beginning in A–C Group times and intensifying by the Meroitic period, selected in favor of smaller, morphologically simpler teeth. This dental reduction hypothesis was based on the relationship between tooth size (particularly molars) and the number of cusps and grooves on the chewing surface (figure 2.13).

Large teeth (particularly molars) have more cusps and grooves than do smaller teeth. By providing a larger enamel surface, they are more resistant

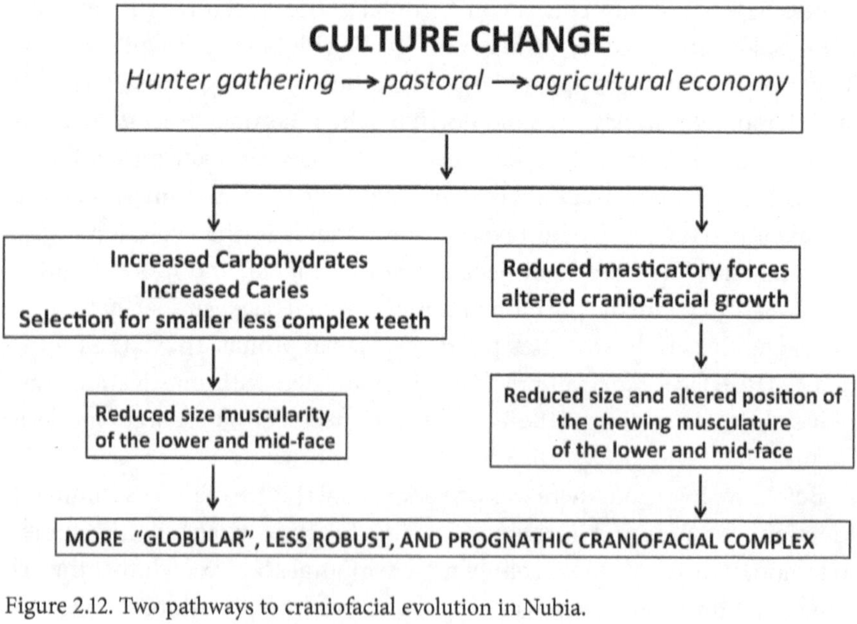

Figure 2.12. Two pathways to craniofacial evolution in Nubia.

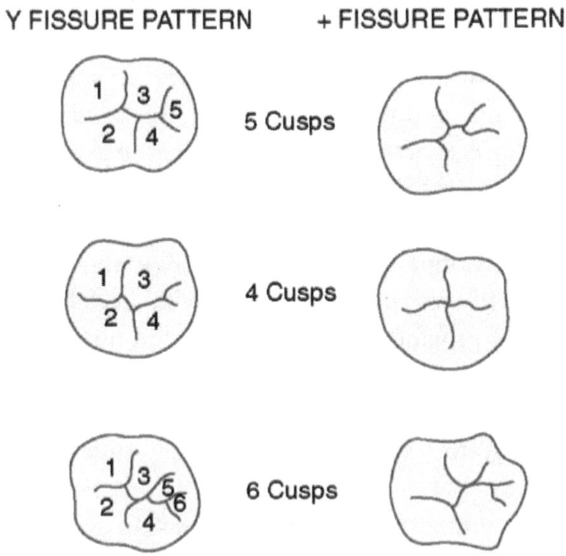

Figure 2.13. Patterns of molar cusps and fissures.

to wear—a major challenge created by the highly abrasive Mesolithic diet. Smaller, simpler teeth are less likely to trap the higher carbohydrate foods typical of an agriculture-based diet. Carbohydrates support the growth of caries-causing bacteria (Greene et al. 1967), which are a far more important cause of tooth loss among the Nubian agriculturalists than wear.

Whereas the dental reduction hypothesis was still widely accepted, David Carlson and I decided that an additional perspective was in order.[7] This became referred to as the masticatory-function hypothesis (Carlson and Van Gerven 1977). The masticatory-function hypothesis was based on two facts concerning the biomechanics of chewing in relation to the dentition—particularly tooth size. First, changing mechanical forces can alter facial morphology; and second, a reduction size of the bones supporting the dentition can reduce the size of the teeth. A number of scholars had presented evidence that reduced tooth size during the course of human evolution may have been the *result* of, rather than the *cause* of, a reduction in size of the face (Sofaer et al. 1971; Sofaer 1973; Anderson et al. 1975; Wolpoff 1976).

Using that information, we interpreted our evidence for facial reduction in the same cultural context as did the advocates of the dental reduction hypothesis. The difference was our emphasis on the contribution of domesticated foods to a decrease in mechanical demands on the masticatory complex. The associated reduction in mechanical demands (reduced muscle activity) resulted in less stimulation of the periosteal membrane, which in turn reduced mandibular and maxillary growth. This resulted in a compensatory reduction in the size of the teeth. These were the two principal hypotheses at the time we reported our research. The question is, are they in opposition? We believed the answer was no.

The dentition and masticatory apparatus obviously share a number of joint functional requirements. The teeth have to fit the musculo-skeletal apparatus, and the apparatus must provide adequate support and functional (occlusal) space for the teeth. The consequence is simple. Craniofacial evolution demands give and take from both the dentition and the skeleton. Both the dentition and the masticatory system were most likely undergoing simultaneous changes.

The advent of irrigation agriculture led to an intensified use of domestic food resources with a higher carbohydrate content. The new foods were also more highly processed, resulting in a lower amount of stress on the masticatory system. Under these conditions, there is no reason to presume that dental and facial reduction operated independently or that either necessarily had priority. It is interesting to note that the pattern evidenced in the evolution of the Nubian skull from Mesolithic through Christian times parallels a global pattern of craniofacial evolution since the Pleistocene. We believe that Nubia provides a microcosm of the pattern with its own historical and biocultural features.

Phase 2: Wadi Halfa and Kulubnarti

The second phase of our research focused on the post-Mesolithic populations (Van Gerven 1982). My goal was to determine whether the long-term changes that David and I had documented appeared in a similar way in the shorter Meroitic through Christian time frame. If that were the case, it would strengthen our argument for in situ evolution. By including data from Kulubnarti, I was also able to add a geographical dimension unavailable to our earlier analysis.

Figure 2.14 and table 2.6 present the results. As you can see, virtually all of the discrimination is produced by the first discriminant function, and once again mandibular length dominated group differences. It is interesting that the function once again separated the Wadi Halfa populations in a temporal sequence. The Meroitics had the longest mandibles and the Christians the shortest. It was also satisfying to see the Kulubnarti samples

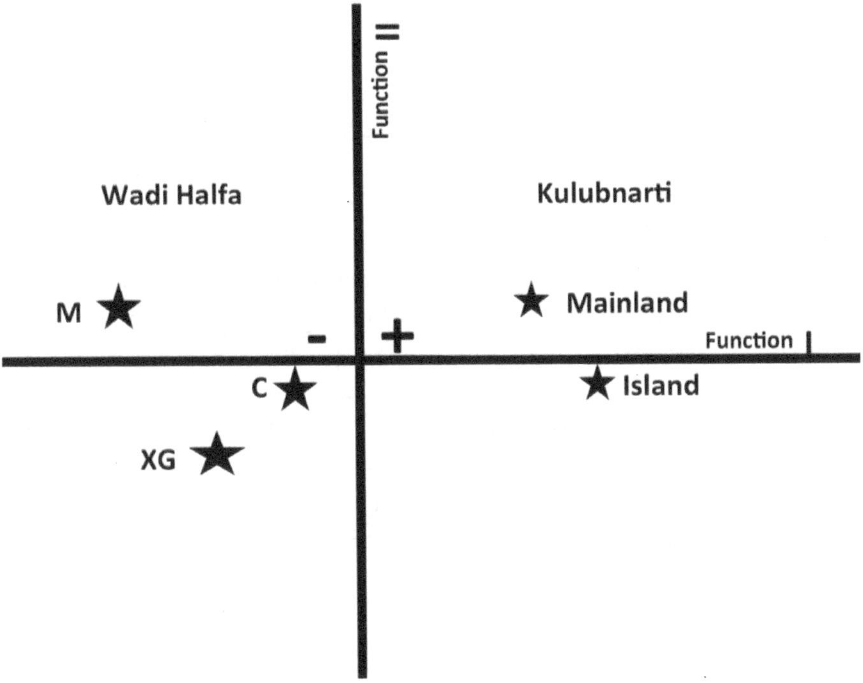

Figure 2.14. Distances between the Kulubnarti and Wadi Halfa populations.

Table 2.6. Eigenvectors for the Kulubnarti and Wadi Halfa crania

Measurement	Eigenvectors
Max. Cranial Length	0.15
Max. Cranial Breadth	-0.17
Basion-bregma Height	0.04
Auricular Height	0.16
Facial Length	0.18
Bizygomatic Diameter	0.41
Nasal Height	0.14
Palatal Length	0.31
Palatal Width	0.36
Mandible Corpus Length	**-1.31**
Mandibular Body Thickness	-0.09
Bigonial Width	0.01

produced their own cluster consistent with their geographic isolation. This raised an interesting question for future research: How would Kulubnarti compare to populations to the south? Perhaps remains excavated by the Merowe Dam Archaeological Salvage Project will provide answers.

The Merowe Dam project, like the salvage archaeology at Wadi Halfa, has been associated with the construction of a dam. In this case the dam is north of Khartoum at the 4th cataract. The first surveys began in 1999, followed by an international program of excavation. The skeletal remains recovered promise to provide new understanding of the biological relationship between Nubia's northern and southern populations.

Although there is much more to be learned, we believe we accomplished what we set out to do almost 40 years ago. We produced analyses that we believe demonstrated the value of a nonracial approach to craniofacial evolution. Our results added one more confirmation of V. Gordon Child's notion that humankind is as much a product of culture as culture is a product of humankind.

A Postscript

Issues concerning the relationships among Nubia's various populations have not gone away. A biological anthropologist by the name of Joel Irish has questioned our interpretation of genetic continuity in Lower Nubia (Irish 2005). His argument is based on an analysis of a number of discrete dental traits, many of which were analyzed by David Greene. Irish has argued that changes in the frequency of several of these traits indicate a replacement of a Nubian population somewhere around 5,600 years ago. He sees a great deal of genetic continuity after that. His conclusion is that populations such as our Mesolithics from Wadi Halfa aren't the ancestors of our later Nubians.

Let's assume for the sake of argument that Irish is correct. Is that a problem for our analysis of craniofacial evolution? Our reasoning is based on a classic paper written by an anthropologist named Leslie White back in 1945 (White 1945). The article was titled "History, Evolutionism, and Functionalism: Three Types of Interpretation of Culture." White argued that phenomena can be analyzed from three perspectives each capable of answering different questions. We can illustrate his argument using our analyses of the crania.

Let's start with a historical approach. According to White, a historical approach is based on giving specific concrete events coordinates in time and space. Virtually all of the early questions concerning Nubian populations were couched in historical terms. The focus was on where and when specific events occurred. For example, questions such as "where did the X-Group people come from" and "when did they arrive in Lower Nubia" were inherently historical. Cranial data was used to help answer those questions.

A functional approach incorporates no coordinates in time or space. Here's an example from physics: $E = MC^2$. The functional relationships between the speed of light, energy, and mass are not true just here and there and now and then. The relationships are true independent of time and space. The function of the masseter muscle is to close the jaw and produce direct compression forces between the lower and upper molars. Here again, the function of the masseter is true independent of time and space.

An evolutionary approach, according to White, brings function and history together. Our analysis of craniofacial evolution in Nubia is an example. We were interested in understanding how the skull was transformed morphologically in response to changing functional demands, which were in turn produced by changes in the cultural environment. Our evolutionary approach gave functional anatomy coordinates in time and space.

Irish's approach is historical. Having established to his satisfaction a genetic break between Nubia's earlier and later populations around 5,600 years ago, his questions are these: Where did the resident populations go, and where did the new people come from? Irish's questions are historical, ours are evolutionary. One is not better, more important, or more interesting than the other. Are the two approaches in conflict? No. They are asking different questions.

Suppose there was a genetic break between our Mesolithic and post-Mesolithic populations. Would that perturb the evolutionary changes we have documented? Only if the mixing or displacement of one population by another involved anatomies as divergent as to defy the evolutionary changes we have proposed. The question boils down to this: What did the arriving population look like? The most likely answer is that they looked pretty similar and were most likely experiencing similar environmental demands and evolutionary responses. The people may have moved from here to there, but the process of craniofacial evolution would have continued.

3

HEALTH AND DISEASE

The Children

There can be no keener revelation of a society's soul than the way in which it treats its children.

Nelson Mandela

In times gone by, miners took canaries with them into the mines. It wasn't because they enjoyed the birds' song. They knew that when the canaries stopped singing the air had gone bad and it was time to get out. Children are society's canaries in the mine. When infants and children die in great numbers, the cultural system designed to sustain them is going bad. Culture, after all, is one of many kinds of social organization designed by evolution to promote reproductive success—the survival of infants and children. Childhood disease and mortality represent defects in the biological response and cultural adjustments people and populations must make in their struggle to maintain reproductive success. For example, biological anthropologists have discovered that populations making the transition to agriculture were less healthy than their hunting and gathering forebears (Cohen and Armelagos 1984; Steckel and Rose 2002). How do we know? We see an increase in the frequency of infectious and nutritional diseases, most particularly among infants and children.

This chapter begins our discussions of disease in ancient Nubia (Armelagos 1969). Diseases are the rock stars of osteology. They are what the public wants to see. They are what people want to hear about. People don't come to our talks hoping to learn about cranial morphology and multivariate statistics. They come hoping to see broken legs and fractured skulls. They want to see horrible infections and terrifying cancers. Diseases are dramatic, mysterious, and frightening. The study of disease in ancient people is frightening but safe, like a roller coaster.

Fortunately, diseases are as important to skeletal biologists as they are fascinating to the public. In terms of natural selection and the evolution of human populations, diseases are the point of the spear. Diseases have shaped the course of human history. Bubonic plague helped end the Middle Ages and set the stage for the Renaissance (Gottfried 1983; Herlihy 1997). Contagion brought down the Roman Empire as surely as barbarian invaders. Smallpox, measles, influenza, and cholera brought to the Americas (Crossby 2004) by European invaders killed more indigenous people than the weapons and armies that came with them. Syphilis (Baker and Armelagos 1988; Harper et al. 2011), transported to Europe by those same invaders, returned the favor. But these are diseases on a grand scale. It's the small-scale diseases—the relentless, daily whittling away of infants and children by microbes and parasites of all shapes and sizes—that drive the course of biocultural evolution.

Our Nubians lived in the world of small-scale diseases. Theirs were the diseases of village life—intestinal parasites, bacterial infections, and nutritional deficiencies. The evidence these conditions have left behind on bones and teeth is often subtle, but there to find if you know what to look for. Learning what to look for has a long history.

The Early Days of Paleopathology

One of the earliest studies in paleopathology goes back to the late eighteenth century. It reported a cancer (sarcoma) in a cave bear. One thing turned out to be true, and one false. The bear was truly dead, but it didn't have cancer. What looked like cancer was a callus caused by an old fracture. The bear gave paleopathology its first lesson: diagnosing a disease from ancient bones is a complicated business.

The nineteenth century was the age of the dilettante physician paleopathologist. After all, who would make a better paleopathologist than a doctor? Doctors diagnosed and treated diseases for a living. They may not be able to cure ancient diseases, but they could certainly diagnose them. Debates concerning the best diagnosis dominated the literature. They were often heated, but they were far from fruitless. Developing good diagnostic techniques was essential. Without diagnosis, paleopathology is a dead-end street. Diagnosis, of course, required material, and skeletons were hard to come by. Paleopathologists needed specimens. Colonialism lent a hand. It's interesting when you think about it. Colonialism wasn't only followed by cultural collapse and political chaos; it was followed by paleopathology!

The French invasion of Egypt (1798–1801) created a fascination with pyramids, temples, tombs, and mummies that swept across Europe. There was a particular interest in the techniques and religious significance of mummification—an interest we have to this day. Mummy movies are still big box office. On the scientific side, A. B. Granville's "An Essay on Egyptian Mummies" (Granville 1825) and Thomas Pettigrew's "A History of Egyptian Mummies" (Pettigrew 1934) still remain authoritative.

Mummies fueled an ever-growing interest in ancient diseases. They were mysterious corpses. How did these ancients live, and how did they die? Physicians became increasingly attracted to the study. The colonial connection didn't stop with the French. Egypt became a British Protectorate in 1915, and Britain founded the English-language School of Medicine in Cairo soon thereafter. The faculty included Grafton Elliot Smith (Armelagos 1997) in the Department of Anatomy, Marc Ruffer (Sandison 1967) in the Department of Bacteriology, and Alfred Lucas (Gilberg 1997) in the Department of Chemistry. They all became fascinated with mummies, and each devoted a great portion of his career to their study. We know Smith from the First Archaeological Survey of Nubia. Ruffer became a pioneer in paleopathology, and Lucas became known as the Sherlock Holmes of Egyptology. By the 1930s, paleopathology became a recognized, legitimate science due largely to their influence.

Defining achievements of the period include the first diagnoses of infectious diseases such as syphilis (Lortet 1907), tuberculosis (Smith and Jones 1908), and leprosy (Smith and Derry 1910). New technologies were also being brought to bear. Wilhelm Roentgen discovered the X-ray in 1895. Soon thereafter, A. Dedekind in Britain and W. Koenig in Germany were using X-rays to examine mummified remains (Chhem 2008). Flinders Petrie used radiography on an Old Kingdom mummy excavated at the site of Deshasheh in 1898. It was taken by taxi to the X-ray facility. His X-ray analysis led to the discovery of lines of interrupted long bone growth (near the growth plates) known today as Harris lines (Sandison 1972).[1] Ruffer (1909) brought histology to paleopathology. He and his coworkers discovered histological evidence for a host of conditions. These included dwarfism, tuberculosis, arteriosclerosis, pneumonia, smallpox, and bilharzias (a parasitic disease of the liver). The diagnosis of each was a monumental achievement for paleopathology. Ruffer was not alone in his study of histology. G. S. Shattock reported arterial disease (Shattock 1909) in the mummy of an ancient king (King Merneptah), and A. R. Long (1931) reported a case of cardiovascular and kidney disease in a 3,000-year-old Egyptian. J. K. Mitchell (1900) found what may be a case of poliomyelitis.

It wasn't all histology. Rare gross pathologies were also discovered.

Gallstones and gout (Smith and Dawson 1924), scrotal hernia, rectal and vaginal prolapse (Jones 1908), achondroplastic dwarfism (Keith 1913), hydrocephaly (Derry 1913), and carcinoma were all discovered in little more than the first fifteen years of the nineteenth century. For the young science of paleopathology, the nineteenth century was the age of discovery.

In his book *The Common Sense of Science*, Jacob Bronowski (1967) describes how sciences develop from their earliest days to their maturity. The first stage is discovery. The discovery stage can be brought about by the invention of a new instrument, such as the telescope or the electron microscope. It can also be brought about by the discovery of new phenomena. In anthropology, it can be the discovery of a new fossil, a new culture, or a new prehistoric period. In paleopathology, it was often the discovery of new diseases or the discovery of new diagnostic methods. During the discovery stage, the dominant focus of investigation is description, with very little interest in further analysis. A point is reached, however, when description alone ceases to be worthy of interest. Beyond that point, there has to be further analysis typically leading to new theoretical perspectives. By the second half of the twentieth century, paleopathology's age of discovery and description was coming to an end. The modern era of problem-oriented analysis was starting to emerge. Bronowski would say that paleopathology was becoming a mature science.

Paleopathology Today

The modern age of paleopathology is often defined by E. A. Hooton's (1930) *The Indians of Pecos Pueblo*. Hooton's *Pecos* took the traditional case-by-case diagnostic approach to a new level. He created disease categories and provided frequencies of occurrence. His use of simple frequency statistics made it possible to see beyond cases to patterns of disease in the Pecos community. It made it possible to ask new kinds of questions. For example, reporting 40 cases of fractured femurs was far less useful than reporting 40 fractured femurs out of 300 femurs. Knowing the frequency of fractured femurs can lead to any number of interesting questions. What if 60 percent of the fractures occurred among young adults, or 60 percent of those occurred among women? What might that mean? Answering that kind of question led inevitably to an interest in the biological and cultural contexts within which the conditions occurred. The union of the cultural and the biological aspects of disease in ancient populations gave birth to what has come to be known as a biocultural approach. No one has expressed the spirit of that approach more eloquently than Calvin Wells did back in 1964. Wells said that

> the pattern of disease or injuries that affect any group of people is never a matter of chance. It is invariably the expression of stresses and strains to which they were exposed, a response to everything in their environment and behavior. It reflects their genetic inheritance (which is their internal environment), the climate in which they lived, the soil that gave them sustenance and the animals or plants that shared their homeland. It is influenced by their daily occupation, their habits of diet, their choice of dwelling and clothes, their social structure, even their folklore and mythology. (Wells 1964:17)

Wells's reference to "*the pattern of disease or injuries that affect any group*" captured the essence of the new age of biocultural analysis in paleopathology.

Disease patterns in living populations are in the purview of the epidemiologist (Harper and Armelagos 2010). Paleopathologists would have to adopt a paleo-epidemiological approach. If the approach was to work, information beyond the specimen would have to be gathered and brought to bear. Statistical techniques would have to be developed to analyze the interactions among multiple variables. Excavations would have to operate more like crime scenes, and laboratories more like forensic facilities.

Some years ago, George and I wrote an article titled "Paleopathologist as Detective" (Armelagos and Van Gerven 1993). It was fun to write. We argued that ferreting out an ancient disease is a lot like solving a crime with no witnesses. Crimes without witnesses are not unusual. Think about it. Criminals seldom commit their crimes when someone is looking. A detective has to rely on the clues left behind at the crime scene—fingerprints, blood spatter, fragments of clothing, possibly DNA. Like modern crimes, there are no witnesses to ancient diseases. The paleopathologist has to rely on the clues left behind—the bones and teeth, the residue of a tissue, and the occasional artifact. Both the detective and the paleopathologist use their evidence to build circumstantial cases. They have to assemble the clues into lines of evidence. They have to demonstrate that all of the evidence leads to a single inescapable conclusion. John Doe committed the murder. Tuberculosis killed 15 percent of the children between the ages of 5 and 15 years.

Detectives spend years learning their craft. They have to know what evidence to look for and how to interpret it when they find it. They have to learn the art of deduction. But deduction and circumstantial evidence can never stand alone. Sherlock Holmes made the point back in 1891. In "The Boscombe Valley Mystery," Watson commented, "I could hardly imagine a more damning case. . . . If ever circumstantial evidence pointed to a criminal it does so here." Holmes responds: "Circumstantial evidence is a very tricky thing. . . . It may seem to point very straight to one thing, but if you shift your own point of view a little, you may find it pointing . . . to something entirely different" (Doyle 1891). Holmes was telling Watson that the art of induction is equally important. For example, Holmes studied thousands of cigarette ashes (induction) in order to deduce the source of one ash he found at the scene of a crime. That's the art of deduction based on the science of induction.

Let's elaborate using health and the transition to agriculture mentioned at the beginning of this chapter. Up until the mid-twentieth century, most anthropologists envisioned the transition to agriculture as a good idea various cultures had about 10,000 years ago. Anthropologists assumed that agriculture made life better, and that the benefits were immediate. After all, the food supply became more abundant and predictable. Populations settled down and built permanent villages. Population sizes grew.

But starting in the 1960s, paleopathologists began examining patterns of disease in populations at the transition to agriculture (Cohen and Armelagos 1984). They found again and again that people got sicker, more children died, and life expectancy declined. The inductive evidence became so abundant that the deductions had to change. It became clear that agriculture did not appear because hunter-gatherers had a good idea that had somehow eluded them for a million years. Hunter-gatherers turned to agriculture because they were forced to by a whole series of environmental changes, some of their own creation. The transition to food production cost them dearly. We now use that general understanding to infer a lot of human behavior in ancient times.

In 1964 a scientist by the name of J. R. Platt used the term "strong inference" to describe what he envisioned as the scientific (both inductive and deductive) approach in its purest form. In his view, strong inference was based on four stages (Platt 1964:347):

1. Devise alternative hypotheses.
2. Devise experiments to exclude one or more of the hypotheses.
3. Carry out experiments to get "clean results."
4. Recycle the procedure.

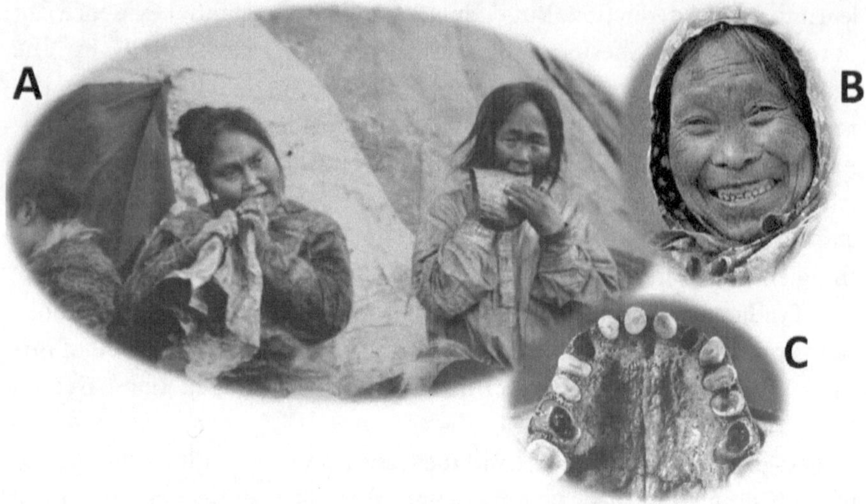

Figure 3.1. Inuit women softening leather clothing in the ethnographic present (A and B), and an archaeological example of teeth showing similar wear (C) (images adapted from www.Gala-re.com).

The question for the paleopathologist is this: how far can we apply Platt's model to a non-experimental science such as ours? The answer is, further than many might think. Paleopathology may not be an experimental science, but it's most certainly a comparative one. Our comparative method takes advantage of *natural* experiments. We can't design experiments to assess the impact of poor nutrition on childhood growth by putting skeletons in experimental groups and varying the quality of their nutrition. But we can measure bone growth among skeletons found in differing nutritional environments. The environments provide what experimentalists call the treatment variable. Growth data provide what is called the response variable. Don't underestimate the power of comparison. Let's look at a couple of natural experiments.

Among the Navajo, weaving is primarily a female task. Hours spent at the loom result in characteristic patterns of joint damage and arthritis in the hands. Female skeletons found in association with the remains of weaving technology show the same pattern of arthritic change (Bridges 1991, 1994). The males do not. While we can't do a laboratory experiment to prove it, we believe a strong inference can be made in support of weaving as a gendered activity in ancient times.

Here's a second example. Hide clothing traditionally worn by Inuit (sometimes referred to as Eskimo) people becomes hard and stiff after it gets wet and then dries. Traditionally, Inuit women had the task of softening the clothing by chewing and pulling the leather with their front teeth. This constant pulling and chewing resulted in a highly specific pattern of wear on the front teeth. This pattern has been observed in ancient skeletal populations, providing a strong inference in support of a gendered activity (Molnar 2011).

Our Navajo and Inuit examples give us an opportunity to make an important point concerning sex and gender. The word "sex" makes a lot of people edgy, including skeletal biologists. Many authors of osteology textbooks have dropped the word "sex" entirely. References are made to the gender of the human skeleton. Skeletons don't have gender. They have sex. A skeleton can't tell us how the owner identified himself or herself, or how he or she performed his or her masculinity or femininity during life. We judge skeletons to be male or female. That doesn't mean that there are only two sexes,[2] and it doesn't mean that we can't study gendered behaviors. We just gave you two examples of how we can. Sex, nevertheless, is a vital point of comparison for both the paleopathologist and the paleodemographer.

Age at death is a second variable vital to both paleopathology and paleodemography. Infant mortality and mean life expectancy say a lot about social well-being. For example, mean life expectancy at birth in the United States is over 70 years; it's about half of that in Sudan today. Infant mortality (death in the first year) is 53 per 1,000 in Sudan. It's 6 per 1,000 in the United States, and that's higher than any other country in the developed world. Those numbers speak volumes. They do in ancient societies as well. As you will see, comparisons by age and sex were important points of departure for both the Wadi Halfa and Kulubnarti research, so it's important to take some time and consider how the two are determined.

The Estimation of Sex and Age

It isn't our intention to teach you how to estimate the sex and age of skeletons. There are any number of excellent manuals and textbooks that can provide that information (e.g., White and Folkens 2005). Our intention is to provide a basic conceptual overview sufficient for your understanding of the various analyses to be presented.

Sex

One aspect of male-female difference is sexual dimorphism—two morphologies. For example, Olive baboons are highly dimorphic in body size.

Females are approximately 30 percent of male size. Humans aren't nearly as dimorphic (Van Gerven and Armelagos 1980). Human males are approximately 15 percent larger than females. Nevertheless, there are dimorphisms in the human skeleton. Males tend to be more heavily muscled than females and consequently have larger, rougher muscle markings on their bones. That said, females from a very robust population may be, on average, more robust than males in a more gracile (lightly built) population.

Pelvic features related to the requirements of childbirth (Sibley et al. 1992) are far and away the most sexually dimorphic, and hence reliable for sex determination. The inlet of the birth canal is larger and rounder in females. The outlet is also larger. Dimorphic features do, however, present a problem. They develop at puberty, making the assignment of sex for infants and children virtually impossible. We can nevertheless study sex differences in childhood health and mortality. Certain kinds of stresses, including nutritional privations and infections, leave lifelong marks on bones and teeth (Goodman and Armelagos 1988). These provide a "memory" of childhood illnesses accessible from the adults that can be sexed.

Age

Estimations of age at death are aided by a wide variety of features. The techniques employed follow the development of several organ systems and are based on patterns of growth and development observed in the living. One of the earliest developing organs useful for estimating age is the dentition. We all know from experience that babies begin to get their teeth at more or less the same time. Their first teeth begin erupting at around five months. Anyone who has been around a teething baby knows what that's like.

By about 18 months the first baby molar is erupted, and so on. Children begin losing their baby teeth around age seven. Most of us get our last adult tooth—the third molar, or wisdom tooth—in our later teens. Because the pattern is highly consistent, we can estimate age at death for ancient children and adolescents up to the point that the third molars have erupted.

Bones grow from their outer surfaces and ends. In the case of limb bones, the growing bone has a cap (known as an epiphysis) at each end, separated from the shaft of the bone by a plate of cartilage. The bone grows as the cartilage expands and is turned to new bone. When the bone is scheduled to stop growing, the cartilage is lost and the cap fuses to the shaft—a process known as epiphyseal union. Union begins at about age nine with the distal end of the humerus and ends in the twenties with the sternal end of the clavicle (White and Folkens 2005:373; White et al. 2011:391). Again, this

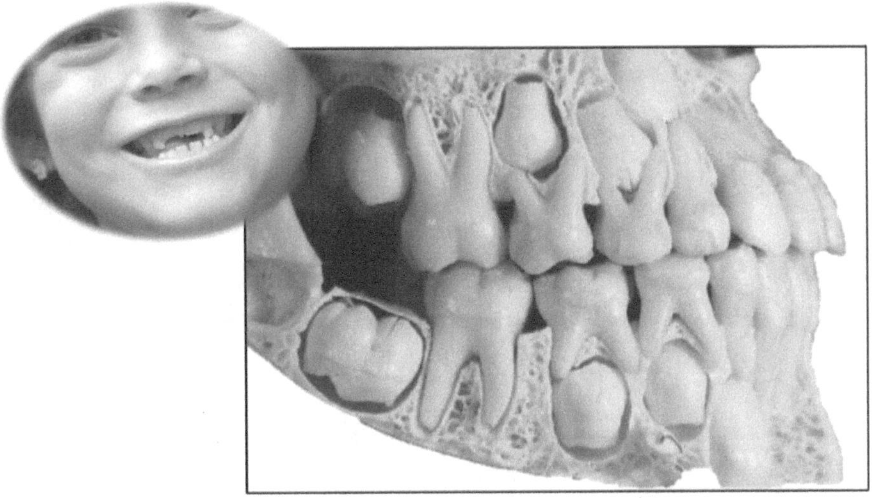

Figure 3.2. Dental eruption.

Bone	Estimated age of fusion	
	Proximal/Medial end	Distal/Lateral end
Humerus (upper arm)	10 – 15 years	9 – 15 years
Radius (lower arm)	14 – 19 years	16 – 22 years
Femur (upper leg)	15.5 – 19.5 years	14.5 – 22 years
Tibia (lower leg)	15.5 – 22 years	14.5 – 19.5 years
Clavicle (collarbone)	19 – 30 years	19 – 20 years

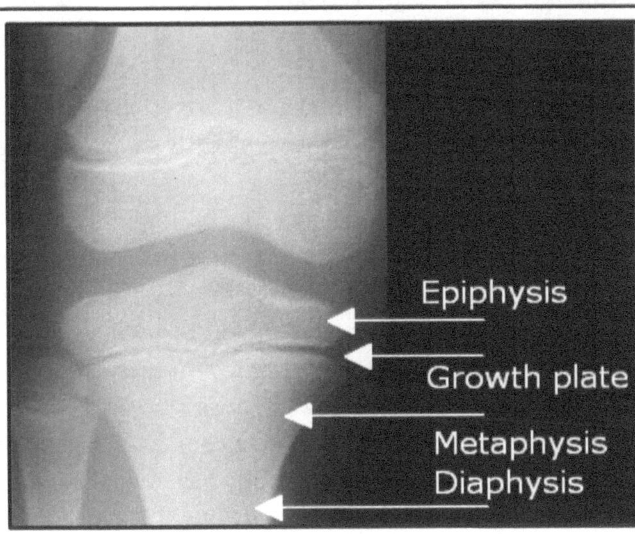

Figure 3.3. Ages of epiphyseal union (adapted from "Forensics 101: Ephiphyseal Union" by Jen J. Danna, 2001, http://jenjdanna.com/blog/2011/12/13/forensics-101-epiphyseal-fusion.html).

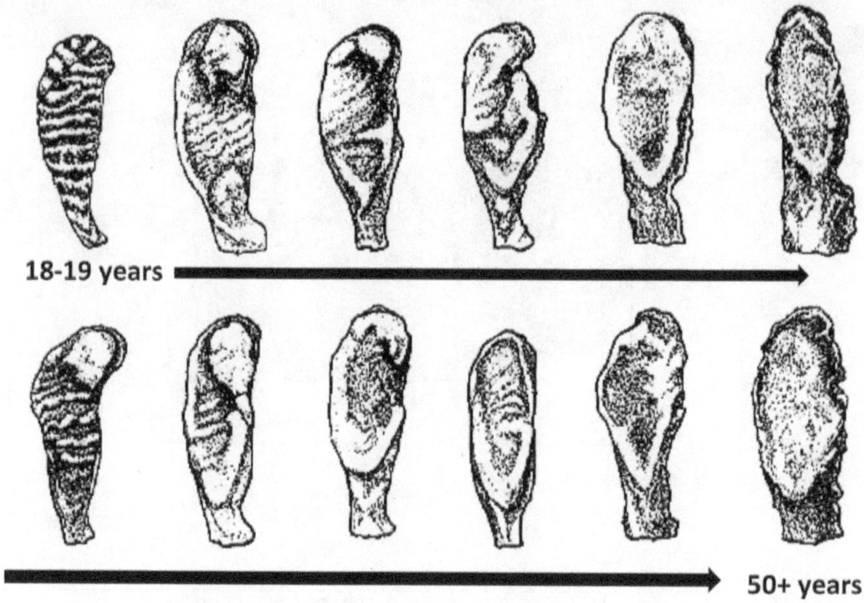

Figure 3.4. Age changes in the os pubis.

process is quite regular, and age at death can be estimated between the time when the first epiphyses begin to fuse and the last fusion is completed.

Estimating age becomes more challenging after all of the teeth are erupted and all of the bones are fused. The most common technique is based on regular changes on the surface, or "face," of the pubic bone, where the two halves come together (White et al. 2011:397). The feature is called the pubic symphysis. The surface of the symphysis changes topographically in a highly regular way with advancing age. A system for estimating age at death based on these regular changes was developed first in 1920 (Todd 1920) and has been revised and refined a number of times (Stewart 1957; Brooks and Suchey 1990). Its usefulness declines with age and becomes difficult to apply beyond the sixth decade of life.

The degree to which the various aging techniques accurately estimate age at death has been a subject of debate. Those who have questioned their accuracy have gone on to question the legitimacy of paleodemographic reconstructions. Critics of paleodemography have argued that reconstructions of demographic variables such as fertility, life expectancy, and survivorship are meaningless due to the unreliability of the age estimates on which they are based. Much of the argument comes down to definitions, interpretations, and expectations of the age estimates. When demographers say that a person died at age 30, they mean 30 years. Paleodemographers use developmental years. When they talk about a seven-year-old child, they are talking about a skeleton that is developmentally comparable to a living seven-year-old child. Nevertheless, the paleodemographer's goal is to make developmental years correspond as closely as possible to calendar years.

Most demographers agree that developmental and calendar years approximate each other quite closely for subadults when multiple features are available. Everyone agrees that estimates become less precise with advancing age. As a consequence, older skeletons are typically placed in age categories such as 25–35 years,[3] whereas the age categories for infants and children may range from months to one or two years. Even with the use of categories spanning multiple years, some demographers use the age issue to reject paleodemography out of hand (Wood et al. 1992). Indeed, some have viewed age estimates as little more than the "random fluctuations and errors of method" (Bocquet-Appel and Masset 1982). While it is not our intent to recount the various debates (Van Gerven and Armelagos 1983), you need to have some confidence in the age estimates we will be using. So let's test the "random fluctuations" assertion.

Inasmuch as most of the criticism is directed toward our ability to estimate adult ages, let's look at how our age estimates performed in one of our studies of an age-related condition known as osteoporosis. As you probably know from the popular media, osteoporosis is a progressive loss of bone tissue with advancing age. Men tend to lose very little bone as they get older, but women may lose as much as 40 percent of their bone volume by the time they reach their seventies.

We conducted several studies of osteoporosis going back over 30 years (Armelagos and Martin 1990; Armelagos et al. 1976; Mulhern 2000). We discuss them in detail in chapter 5. They are relevant here because age estimates are a vital part of the analyses. We can, in fact, test a hypothesis using our bone loss and age data. If our age estimates are nothing more than "random fluctuations and errors of method," we should see absolutely no pattern of age-related bone loss.

Figures 3.5 and 3.6 illustrate bone loss at the femoral midshaft of 120 females from Wadi Halfa. Their ages and sex were estimated using the criteria we have discussed. It's clear that the marrow cavity is expanding and the surrounding bone (known as the cortex) is thinning. This is precisely what is seen in living women of known age. We're not seeing random fluctuations in our bone loss data. What we do see is a coherent pattern of loss consistent with osteoporosis. There is one difference between Wadi Halfa

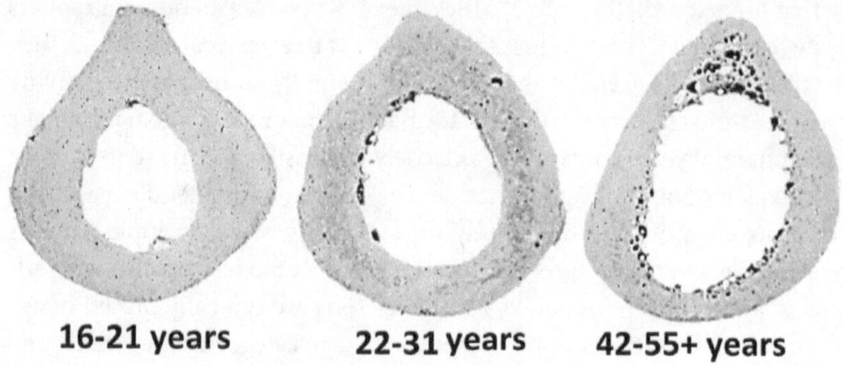

Figure 3.5. Cross sections of femoral midshafts showing bone loss in three age categories.

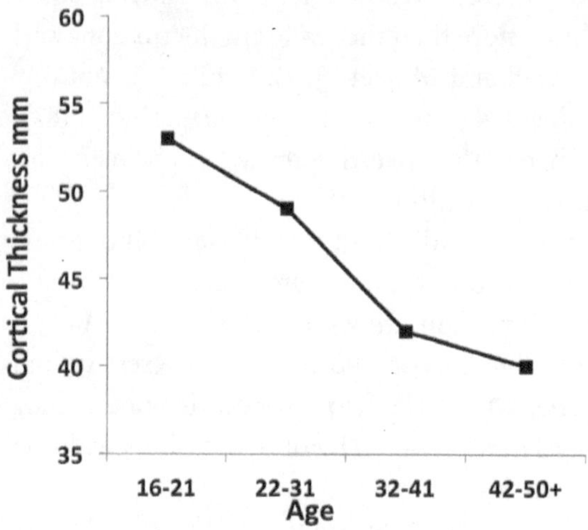

Figure 3.6. Female bone loss with age in the combined Meroitic-Christian samples from Wadi Halfa.

and modern women. The Wadi Halfa women begin losing bone in young adulthood. Modern women lose very little until after menopause. We discuss that difference in chapter 5.

From Skeletons to Communities

No matter how reliable the age estimates and sex assignments may be, a serious issue remains. Calling an assemblage of skeletons—even skeletons excavated from a cemetery—a community, or a population, or even a sample, doesn't make it so. The question is how do paleodemographers take the step from skeletons to communities?

Cemetery remains such as those at Wadi Halfa and Kulubnarti are inevitably samples of samples. The first sample is the cemetery. Unless a cemetery is completely excavated, the skeletons are a sample of all of the dead buried in the cemetery. The island community cemetery at Kulubnarti was in a wadi bounded on three sides by rocky jebel. We excavated every grave we identified from side to side and end to end; however, not every grave had a marking. It appeared that the stones used to mark earlier graves were occasionally moved to mark more recent ones. A few unmarked graves could have been missed. It is likely that there were as many as 600 Christian graves in the mainland cemetery. We excavated 188 graves from one cemetery quadrant.

The second sample is one of the village or community. Not everyone who lived in a community ends up in the community cemetery. People come and go, and people die here and there. Not everyone in the cemetery was born or even raised in the community. There are other factors. Some societies bury infants only after they have attained a certain age. This is often defined as the age of naming. An infant may not be considered a person prior to naming, and may be disposed of outside of the cemetery. That can be a serious problem for a paleodemographer because infant underrepresentation creates the appearance of low infant mortality. Then there is the issue of sample size. Small samples can leave age categories with few or even no individuals. Even reducing the number of categories may not solve the problem. Fortunately, the Wadi Halfa and Kulubnarti samples were quite large.

We have great confidence that the Kulubnarti (Van Gerven 1981) and Wadi Halfa (Armelagos et al. 1968; Armelagos et al. 1965) cemeteries are worthy of demographic analysis for several reasons:

- The cemeteries had clear boundaries and were in close proximity to their villages. Clear boundaries mean less scatter, which in turn enhances recovery. Close proximity enhances the connection between the cemetery and its community.
- Infant underrepresentation was likely to be minimal. Preservation at Kulubnarti and Wadi Halfa was excellent (figure 3.7). Even fetuses are represented at Kulubnarti, and the modal (most common) age at death was birth in both cemeteries.
- While the likelihood of overlooking other fragile remains (pathologies and the elderly) can never be discounted, it is noteworthy that

many individuals at Wadi Halfa and Kulubnarti were completely or partially mummified, and virtually every skeleton was complete.

There is a final point to be made. Critics criticize paleodemographic reconstructions as though they are stand-alone endpoints of analysis. In reality, they are but one line of evidence among many. Like all lines of evidence, they bring strengths and weaknesses to the investigation. Their merit lies in the contribution they make to the totality of an investigation. They are an aid to understanding; they are never an answer or solution in and of themselves. An excellent example of how paleodemography can contribute to a biocultural perspective is George's analysis of social status and survival at Meinarti (Green and Armelagos 1974).

When I asked George what was his dissertation's most important contribution to paleopathology, he said "the mean." I hate to contradict my friend and mentor, but he was wrong. His most important contribution was his analysis of status and mortality at Meinarti (Armelagos 1968). It marked the beginning of his biocultural approach that would define the rest of his career. It was also one of the first biocultural analyses in the literature.

Graves at Meinarti were constructed in two forms. Some were simple with no elaborate covering; others had superstructures (figures 3.8 and 3.9). Most superstructures consisted of a brick "*mastaba*" (Arabic for table)

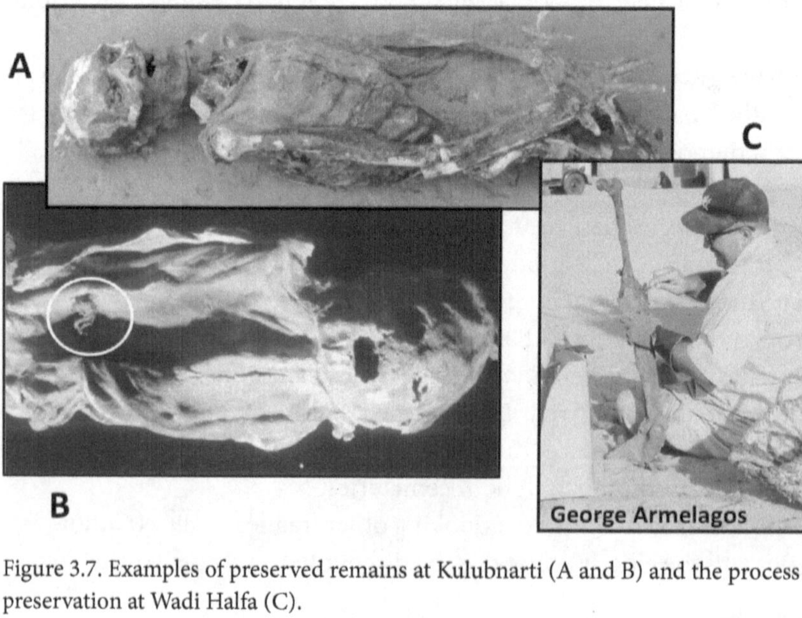

Figure 3.7. Examples of preserved remains at Kulubnarti (A and B) and the process of preservation at Wadi Halfa (C).

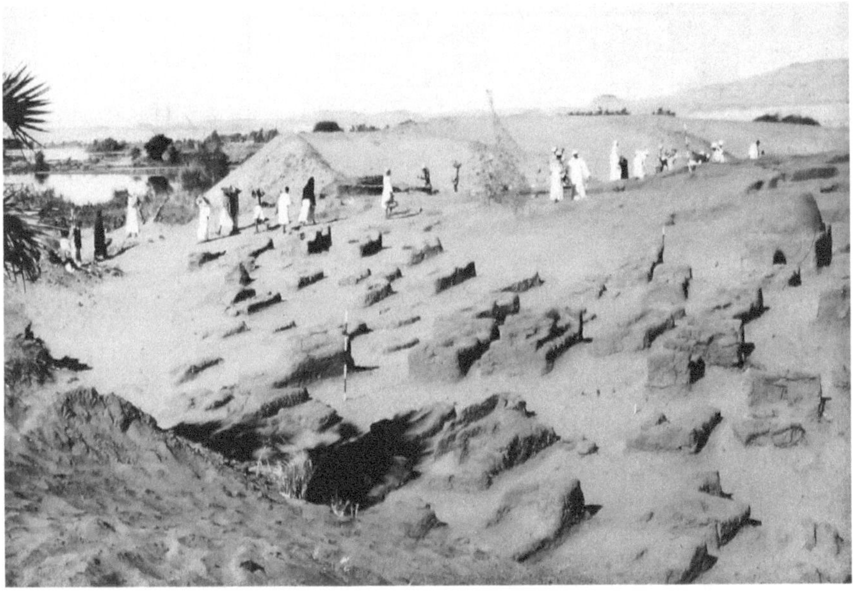

Figure 3.8. Mastaba tombs at Meinarti.

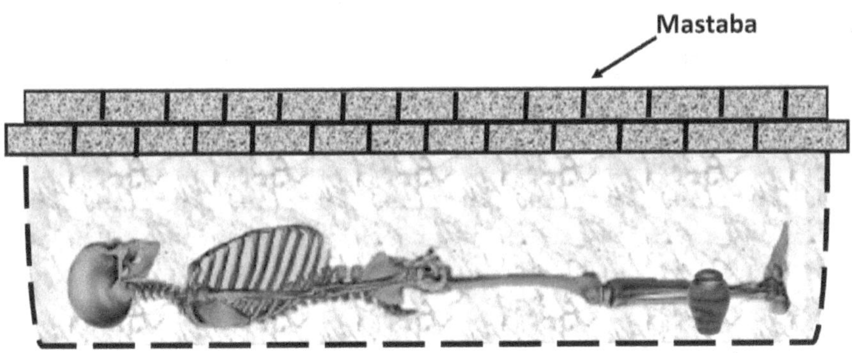

Figure 3.9. A tomb interior from Meinarti.

covering the grave. *Mastabas* were typically 2 meters in length, 1 meter in breadth, and about 60 centimeters in height. They were occasionally constructed to produce a small domed structure that might contain a space for a votive lamp.

George hypothesized that superstructures denoted the status of the interred. They were no doubt costly and took time to build. The fact that not all graves had them supported the hypothesis. He hypothesized further that status would have had a positive influence on health and survival. He then looked to the cultural and biological information to test his hypotheses. Status is commonly obtained in one of two ways. It can be inherited, or

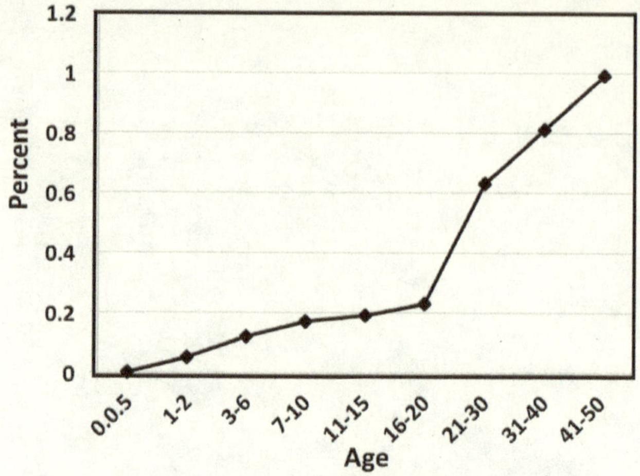

Figure 3.10. Frequency of tomb burial with age at Meinarti.

it can be achieved. His analysis of superstructure frequency with age at death (figure 3.10) suggested the latter. It was clear that the frequency of superstructures was low until adulthood and then increased sharply with advancing years (Green and Armelagos 1974). Status apparently accrued with age.

It is at this point that George took the step to a biocultural analysis. He incorporated mortality data to test his hypothesis concerning the relationship between high status and increased survival. When he graphed survivorship[4] (figure 3.11) for those with and without superstructures, the pattern was clear. Individuals buried with superstructures out-survived those who were not.

George's evidence supported three strong inferences. First, superstructures reflected social status. Second, status appeared to be achieved rather than inherited. And third, higher status contributed to increased life expectancy. According to George, this may have been due to greater social support and access to resources.

It is important to reiterate that George's inferences are not supported by any single source of evidence, but by the body of evidence taken together. It's exciting to note that George's Meinarti analysis continues to spawn research. Emerging dietary analyses based on stable isotopes (Turner et al. 2007; Sandberg et al. 2014) have revealed dietary differences that could bear directly on George's inference regarding social class and access to resources.

We are now going to shift our focus from Meinarti to Kulubnarti. Following the remains arrival at the University of Colorado back in 1979, two graduate students (Mary Kay Sandford and James Hummert) and I began our first demographic analysis (Van Gerven et al. 1981). We found that life expectancy at birth was dramatically different between the mainland and island communities (figure 3.12). The average island newborn lived 10.6 years compared to 18.8 years in the mainland community. The difference in life expectancy continued throughout childhood until the 13–15 year age category.

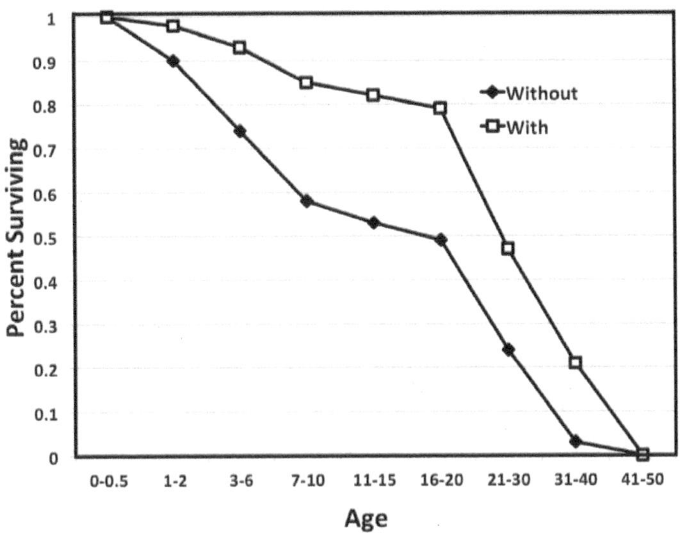

Figure 3.11. Survivorship with and without tombs at Meinarti.

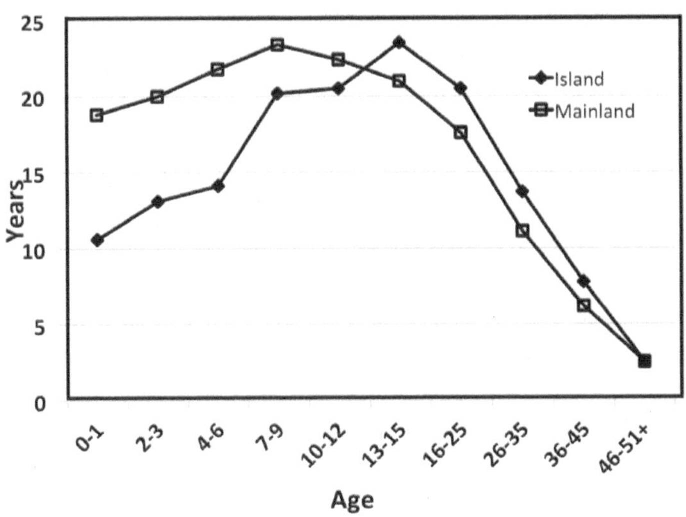

Figure 3.12. Mean life expectancy at Kulubnarti.

There are two possible explanations for the difference in life expectancy. First, the island community may have had a higher birthrate. Our infant frequencies were numerators without denominators. For example, 50 is more than 20; however, 50 out of 300 is smaller than 20 out of 45. On the other hand, there may have been more infants and children in the island cemetery because infants and children were sicker and dying at a higher rate than their mainland counterparts. We hypothesized that the difference in infant mortality was a consequence of the latter alternative (Van Gerven et al. 1990; Van Gerven et al. 1995). Testing that hypothesis set us on a program of research that continues to this day.

We're now going to shift our attention to Kulubnarti and the question of infant mortality in the mainland and island communities. If, as George and I believed, there was a lower life expectancy of infants and children on the island, we should be able to observe poorer health among the island children. You'll notice that we're talking about health, not any particular disease. For paleopathologists, the companion to health is stress.

Skeletal pathologies can be categorized into two basic groups. Some pathologies are related to specific (or at least a small number of) diseases. Diseases such as syphilis and tuberculosis leave their unique and identifiable signatures on bone and are subject to differential diagnoses. Other skeletal indicators are less specific. They have been described as indicators of generalized stress. For example, signs in bones and teeth of interrupted growth do not indicate a specific pathological condition, but rather some assault or assaults on the body capable of interrupting growth. The assault may have been an infection, nutritional deficiency, or some other stressor. Indicators of generalized stress have tremendous value to the paleopathologist because they measure overall health as opposed to specific disease events. We are going to examine three stress indicators at Kulubnarti. They are cribra orbitalia, enamel hypoplasias, and enamel microdefects. If our hypothesis that lower life expectancy among the island infants and children was due to poorer health is correct, we should see higher levels of stress during the childhood years.

Cribra orbitalia appears as one or several lesions on the roof of the eye orbit (Mittler and Van Gerven 1994). The lesions range from a concentration of small pinhole-like perforations (figure 3.13a) in one or both orbits to an outgrowth of fine coral-like bone (figure 3.13b). The lesion has been associated with expansion of red blood producing bone marrow sandwiched between the inner and outer surfaces of the orbital roof (Mensforth et al. 1978).

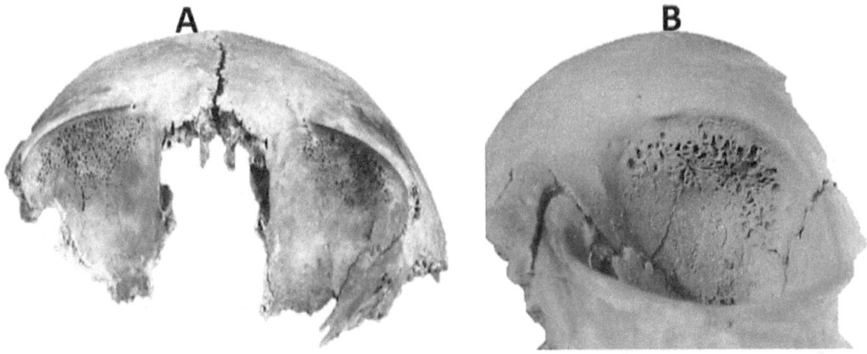

Figure 3.13. Cribra orbitalia.

The condition has been studied in diverse populations, including the American Southwest (Zaino 1967; El-Najjar et al. 1975; Walker 1985), Australia and Papua New Guinea (Webb 1982), Mariana Islands (Stodder 1997), Great Britain (Stuart-Macadam 1991), Italy (Facchini et al. 2004), Egypt (Fairgrieve and Molto 2000), and Nubia (Carlson et al. 1974; Mittler and Van Gerven 1994). It has been most commonly interpreted as a skeletal response to iron deficiency anemia. The connection between cribra orbitalia and iron deficiency goes back to the 1960s (Moseley 1965); it continued to gain traction through the 1970s. Today the lesion and iron deficiency are virtually synonymous. Popularity notwithstanding, the iron deficiency hypothesis must be tested with biological and cultural evidence if a strong inference is to be supported. Let's review the evidence, starting with the biological baseline.

Anemia is defined as too few red blood cells and/or too little hemoglobin. Hemoglobin gives red cells their color. It is the protein responsible for transporting oxygen into, and carbon dioxide from, our tissues. The primary symptoms of anemia are fatigue and loss of energy with a concomitant loss of work capacity. Other symptoms include shortness of breath, dizziness, and headache. Here are some astounding numbers: Each red blood cell contains about 250 million molecules of hemoglobin. The average person has between 20 and 30 trillion red cells circulating through his or her body at any point in time. The average red cell lives for about 120 days, and so each of us has to produce about 46 billion new red cells per day. Each molecule of hemoglobin has to have one atom of iron. Acquiring sufficient iron to support red cell production is a losing battle for the majority of the world's population.

Nubian agriculturalists have been subsisting on an iron-deficient diet for centuries. Their dietary staples are cereals, including millet, wheat, and barley. Such cereals contain reasonable amounts of iron. The problem is that the plants' tissues also contain phytate (Brune et al. 1992). Phytate is used by many plants, including cereals, to store phosphorus. Unfortunately for humans, iron binds to phytate, making the iron indigestible. From a dietary perspective, the vast majority of iron in the Nubian diet might as well be on the moon. It should not come as a surprise then that iron deficiency anemia is the number one nutritional problem from Cairo to Khartoum (May and Jarcho 1961).

The challenges aren't only dietary. High incidences of parasitic (Hibbs et al. 2011) and bacterial infections capable of causing anemia are well documented in modern Egypt and Nubia (May and Jarcho 1961). Hookworm infection and schistosomiasis (Hibbs et al. 2011) in particular are common in both Egypt and Nubia. It has been demonstrated (Eng 1958) that hookworm infection alone can cause iron deficiency anemia, even when dietary intake of iron is normal.

Nubians face their greatest peril during infancy and early childhood. One of the greatest stressors for infants is weaning, and with it, a syndrome known as "weanling diarrhea." As the name implies, "weanling diarrhea" primarily affects infants who are just beginning to utilize solid food (McDade and Worthman 1998). In its most severe form, it causes extreme dehydration and malnutrition, often leading to death. An infant with diarrhea can die of dehydration in as little as three days. In order to survive bout after bout of diarrhea and all of its attendant consequences, the infant must be able to recover quickly after each illness.

Insufficient iron, and its attendant anemia, compromises children of the Nile Valley today, and the same challenges no doubt compromised their counterparts in the past. Today 56 percent of modern Egyptian (and Nubian) women are living on a diet insufficient in iron (May and Jarcho 1961), resulting in iron-poor milk. Nursing is prolonged, perhaps into the second year. Studies on modern children have found that prolonged nursing by mothers with iron-poor milk compromises infant iron levels (Kramer and Kakuma 2004). In addition, weaning infants are exposed to parasitic infections not encountered at the breast. A study of African children (Stoltzfus et al. 1996) found significant association between hookworm infection alone and iron deficiency in children.

If we put these factors together, from the infant's perspective, the consequence is dire. The infant's first meal at the breast begins a life of iron

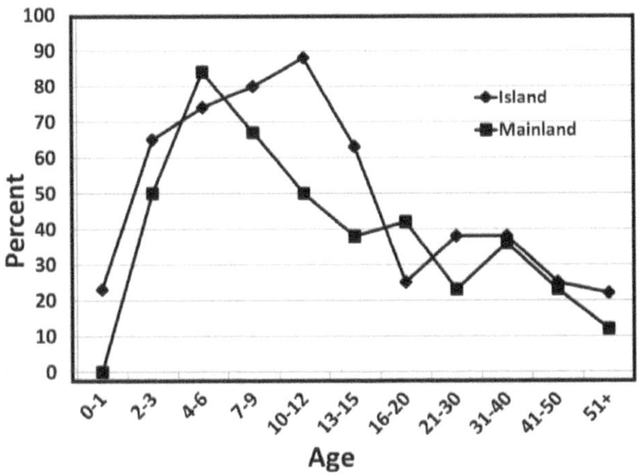

Figure 3.14. Age and frequency of cribra orbitalia at Kulubnarti.

insufficiency, and the situation only gets worse. Mother's milk loses much of its nutritional quality over time, and may be providing very little nutrition by weaning. As a result, the infant is more iron deficient at weaning than it was at birth, and other bodily resources necessary for proper growth and development are compromised as well. The infant is ill prepared for the conditions it's about to face as a freestanding individual.

Cribra orbitalia at Kulubnarti has been the subject of two investigations. The first was conducted as part of our initial demographic analysis. Two of my graduate students (James Hummert and Mary Kay Sandford) and I found that lesion frequencies were concentrated among infants and children (figure 3.14), just as the iron deficiency hypothesis predicted (Van Gerven et al. 1981). Twenty-three percent of island infants in the 0–1 year age group had a lesion compared to none in the mainland community. Also, lesion frequencies peaked at 4–6 years among the mainland children while they continued to rise until 10–12 years on the island. Island children also developed the lesion earlier, and frequencies continued to increase longer. The cribra orbitalia data gave us our first support of our hypothesis that the island children died in higher numbers because they were sicker.

But the data was not as clear as we had hoped. Frequencies peaked among the island children beyond the age of weaning and remained substantial in both communities well into middle age. While we had faith in our interpretation, those aspects of the outcome continued to bother us. Of course, that is precisely the way that old research generates new research. Were there no lingering questions, there would be nothing more to do.

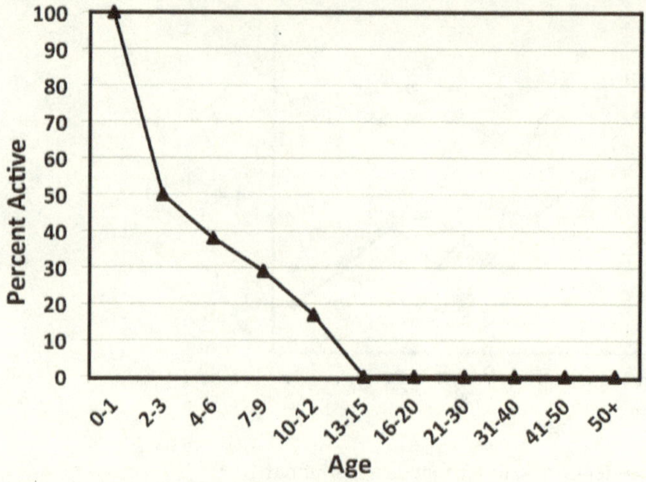

Figure 3.15. Frequency of active lesions for the combined Kulubnarti communities.

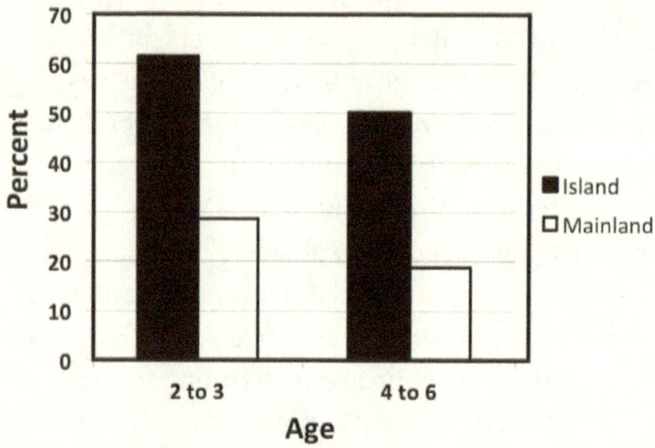

Figure 3.16. Frequency of active cribra orbitalia by cemetery at Kulubnarti.

The issue remained unresolved until 1988. Diane Mittler was a new graduate student looking for a research project for a master's thesis. We discussed the cribra orbitalia research, and I suggested that she do a reanalysis incorporating a distinction between active and healing lesions. Criteria for making the distinction had been established using Native American remains from the site of Libben in Ohio (Lallo et al. 1977). Active lesions had clearly defined porosities with sharp edges, while healing lesions showed round edges and signs of new bone growth within the porosities.

Her analysis produced (figure 3.15) much clearer support for the weanling diarrhea hypothesis. One hundred percent of the lesions present in

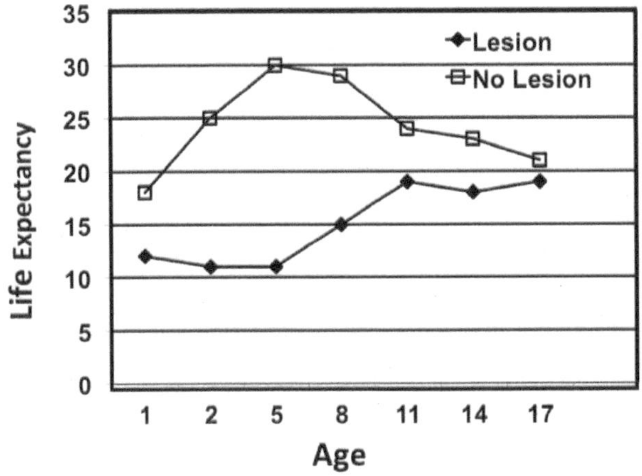

Figure 3.17. Cribra orbitalia and life expectancy at Kulubnarti.

the 0–1 age group were active. The percentage drops to 17 percent among 10- to 12-year-olds. There were no active lesions beyond that point (Mittler and Van Gerven 1994). The samples were too small for her to pursue a cemetery comparison beyond ages 4–6, but the pattern she found (figure 3.16) supported our hypothesis of health differences between the island and mainland communities.

Diane asked one final question. Was there a relationship between the presence of cribra orbitalia and survival? That is to say, did the conditions underlying the lesion have an impact on life expectancy? The answer was clear (figure 3.17). Mean life expectancy was dramatically lower for those with an active lesion at the time of their death. Most important, the disparity began to close in later childhood. The pattern provided even stronger support for our stress hypothesis. Given the higher lesion frequencies in the island community and the linkage between the lesion and life expectancy, one would predict higher levels of infant mortality on the island.

Diane's study revealed a striking continuity between the Nubian past and present. For our Kulubnarti folk, as with their modern counterparts, weaning was second only to birth as a cause of infant mortality (Katzenberg et al. 1996; Armelagos et al. 2009). Babies were no doubt iron deprived in the womb by mothers as deficient in iron as they are today. They were then nursed at the breast by mothers producing milk inadequate in iron. They were taken from the breast abruptly and thrust into the iron-poor diet of adults and assaulted repeatedly by diarrheas compounded by other contributors to iron deficiency. These no doubt included a host of microbes and parasites teeming in the food they ate, the water they drank, and the fields in which they played, just like today.

In the past, our case for iron deficiency would have concluded at this point. There has, however, been a recent challenge to the iron deficiency hypothesis that warrants consideration. Philip Walker and coworkers (Walker et al. 2009) have stipulated that the facts concerning the lesion are not in dispute. What they've disputed is the biological processes necessary to produce the lesion. Their position is simple. Iron deficiency anemia is incapable of causing cribra orbitalia because iron deficiency anemia cannot lead to the increase in red blood cells (RBCs) necessary to induce marrow hypertrophy (expansion). According to them:

> The simple fact that iron-deficiency anemia effectively decreases mature RBC production means that it cannot possibly be responsible for the osseous expression of hemopoietic marrow expansion that paleopathologists recognize as porotic hyperostosis and cribra orbitalia. (Walker et al. 2009:112)

There is, they argue, a nutritional anemia that can produce sufficient marrow hypertrophy to cause cribra orbitalia. According to them, an inadequate amount of vitamin B_{12} results in the production of defective red cells with shortened life spans. The body then attempts to compensate by producing more (but defective) red blood cells. The result is a positive feedback loop; defective cells cause anemia leading to the production of more defective cells. The result is marrow hypertrophy resulting in cribra orbitalia. They go on to argue that the biocultural conditions likely to produce iron deficiency anemia are also likely to produce B_{12} deficiency. Thus, the age and geographic distribution of the lesion are better explained by the B_{12} hypothesis.

The B_{12} hypothesis has been rebutted by Mark Oxenham and Ivor Cavill (2010). They argue that iron deficiency is still a reasonable explanation for cribra orbitalia because an iron shortage does not reduce or eliminate the likelihood of marrow hypertrophy. According to them:

> Because the rate of iron supply to the stimulated red marrow is limited in iron deficiency, there are too many erythroblasts chasing too little iron. The result of this is that an increasing proportion [of red cells] will fail to make sufficient haemoglobin in the time available to become functioning erythrocytes; these are destroyed within the marrow. (Oxenham and Cavill 2010:200)

The result is marrow hypertrophy.

George and I have argued that decoupling cribra orbitalia from iron deficiency is unwarranted; however, that doesn't necessarily mean that the linkage between vitamin B_{12} and hypertrophy is incorrect. Remember, cribra orbitalia is a generalized bony response to anemia. In some cases, the anemia may be caused by B_{12} deficiency, and in other cases, iron deficiency. As for our interpretation, we continued to believe that the Nubian data supports the strong inference of iron deficiency.

While cribra orbitalia has played a central role in the study of dietary stress, it is not the only indicator that has been extensively studied. There are two additional indicators of childhood stress. They are both defects in dental enamel. One is a visible defect known as enamel hypoplasia, and the other is a microscopic defect known as accentuated striae of Retzius (Rose 1977; Rose et al. 1978). Both respond to an even wider range of stressors than does cribra orbitalia. These include starvation, malnutrition, dehydration, and a host of metabolic and infectious diseases. In order to appreciate the nature of the evidence they provide, we once again need a biological baseline.

Enamel is produced by cells called ameloblasts. Ameloblasts appear first on the surface of dentin—a bonelike tissue lying beneath enamel in a mature tooth. Enamel is created as each ameloblast moves in a perpendicular direction away from the dentin. Each creates a rod of enamel as it goes. The rods continue to form until the ameloblasts reach the crown surface. Each completed rod is approximately 0.001 millimeter in diameter and follows the path of the ameloblast that produced it. A completed crown is a dead, rock hard, virtually inorganic material made of between 5 and 12 million rods. Because it is inorganic, enamel can never restore or repair itself once it is made.

Rods would be of no interest to paleopathology were it not for one facet of their production. The ameloblasts making them do not work continuously. They pause or rest on two cycles. The first is circadian (every 24 hours), and the second is weekly (plus or minus a day or two). The circadian (24-hour) pause, sometimes called a rest period, may be linked to other physiological cycles. It is unclear what causes the second cycle. It may reflect some physiological rhythm within the cells. The weekly pauses result in striae of Retzius (figure 3.18).

Occasionally striae of Retzius become accentuated. Accentuated striae (figure 3.19a) are wider and darker—often a dark brown. They have played a key role in our study of childhood stress for two important reasons. First,

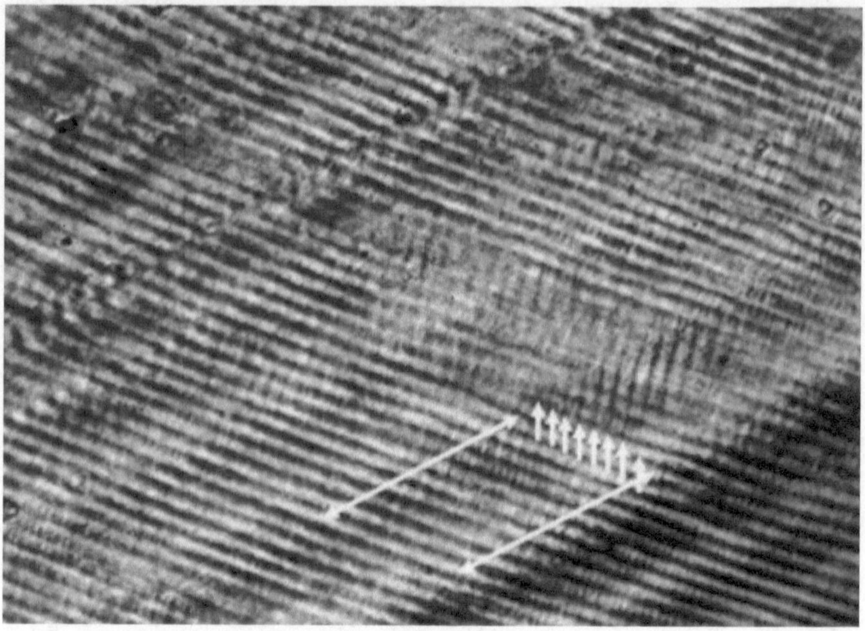

Figure 3.18. Circadian pauses (*short arrows*) and striae of Retzius (*long arrows*) (image by Timothy G. Bromage for *Natural History Magazine*).

they form during periods of physiological stress sufficient to cause growth interruptions lasting one to five days (Condon and Rose 1992); and second, because enamel is incapable of repair, they leave a permanent record of infant childhood stress events. Such stresses include starvation, dietary deficiencies, and a host of nutritional and microbial diseases. We all have at least one accentuated stria. It records the trauma of birth, and is referred to as the neonatal line (figure 3.19b).

Hypoplasias appear as bands (linear hypoplasias) or pits of abnormally thin enamel running across the tooth crown (figure 3.20). While their relationship to accentuated striae isn't entirely understood, a connection between the two seems likely. Some accentuated striae are not associated with hypoplasias; however, hypoplasias are always associated with at least one accentuated stria. This would support a severity hypothesis with a threshold effect (Goodman et al. 1980). The hypothesis states that if a stress becomes severe enough or lasts long enough, the enamel goes from a micro to a macro response. It has also been hypothesized that accentuated striae and hypoplasias may represent responses to different disease etiologies (behaviors). One thing is certain: the Kulubnarti research has been enlightened by both.

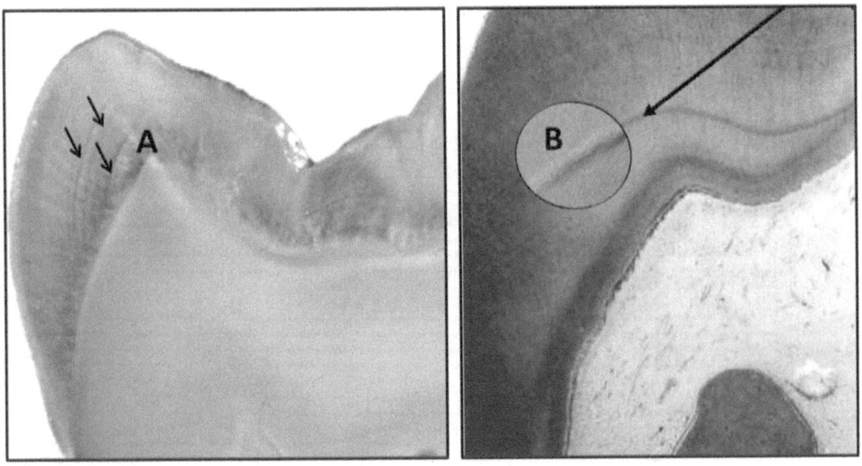

Figure 3.19. Accentuated striae of Retzius (A) and the neonatal line (B).

At the time I began my analysis of hypoplasias, Alan Goodman, a colleague at Hampshire College in Amherst, Massachusetts, had worked out a method for determining the age at which they were produced (Goodman et al. 1984). He did this by measuring each defect's distance from the point at which the enamel meets the root, known as the dental-enamel junction. Using the canine tooth as an example, the enamel begins forming at birth

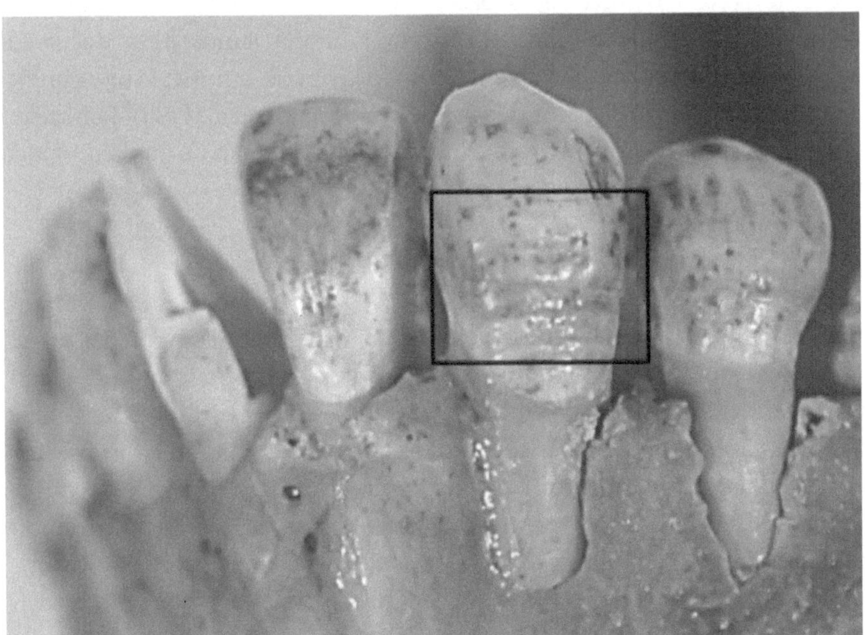

Figure 3.20. Enamel hypoplasias from Kulubnarti.

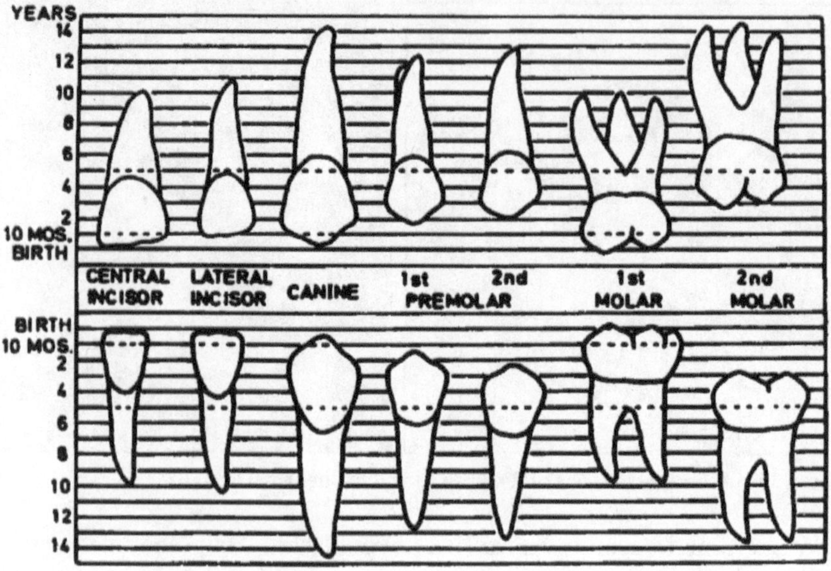

Figure 3.21. Timing of enamel formation (Goodman et al. 1980).

starting at the tip of the cusp. The enamel then advances toward the root until it reaches the dental-enamel junction by age six.[5] The rate of enamel formation (cusp to junction) is reasonably constant. It follows then that if a defect appeared midway between cusp and junction, it most likely occurred at age three. Careful measurement (figure 3.21) made it possible to estimate age of occurrence in six-month intervals (Goodman et al. 1980). I chose to measure the canine for our study, but the technique can be applied to any tooth type as long as its developmental schedule and rate of enamel formation are known.

I had one major problem that had to be dealt with as I began taking my measurements—tooth wear. I experienced this personally while living in the village. If you have ever encountered a small amount of grit in a salad, imagine virtually every mouthful of food you eat containing grit. Sand was everywhere. It filtered down from the palm branch roofs and blew in through windows. It was impossible to prepare sand-free food. I lost enamel down to dentin on my molars in five months. Once the pulp cavity is exposed, the tooth becomes infected and abscessed. The most common request I had for medicine from my workers and even strangers was for toothache. A young boy came to work at the site one morning with his left eye swollen shut from an abscessed tooth. Most Nubians today are virtually toothless by middle age. The same was true in the past.

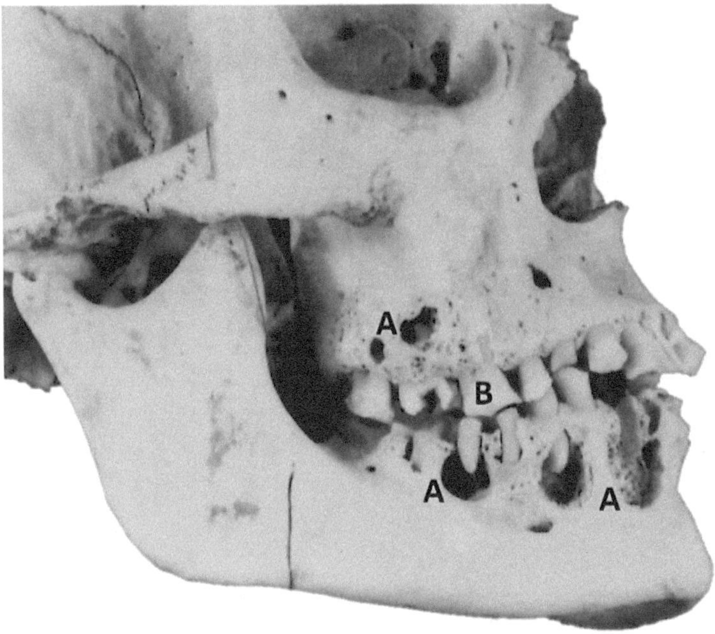

Figure 3.22. Apical abscesses (A) and crown wear (B) at Wadi Halfa.

Tooth wear in the Kulubnarti remains was so rapid that I seldom saw caries on the chewing surface. Wear overtook their formation. Virtually all tooth loss was the result of tooth wear leading to abscess (figure 3.22). The problem for my hypoplasia research was that wear obliterated hypoplasias. As a result, I could only compare individuals with comparable amounts of wear. The consequence was smaller sample sizes than I had hoped for.

My results revealed an interesting pattern of similarities and differences. The cemeteries were virtually identical in hypoplasia frequencies for the first four years, and then diverged sharply (figure 3.23). Frequencies dropped by 42 percent by age five on the mainland, while they remained high on the island for the next two years. The island children also experienced shorter recovery periods between hypoplasias than their mainland neighbors. Eighty percent of the hypoplasias (figure 3.24) in the island children occurred in successive six-month intervals. Only 30 percent occurred successively among the mainland children. On the mainland, the majority (70 percent) were spaced by a least a year.

The higher frequency and consecutive occurrence of hypoplasias among the island children suggested little recovery time between stress events. This corresponded well to their higher frequency of cribra orbitalia and

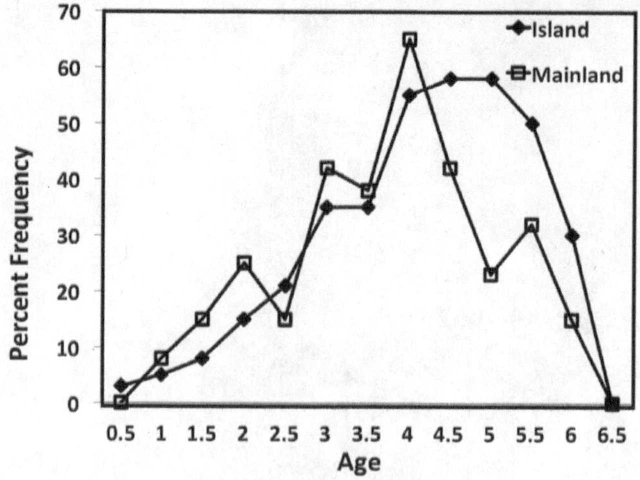

Figure 3.23. Hypoplasia frequencies at Kulubnarti.

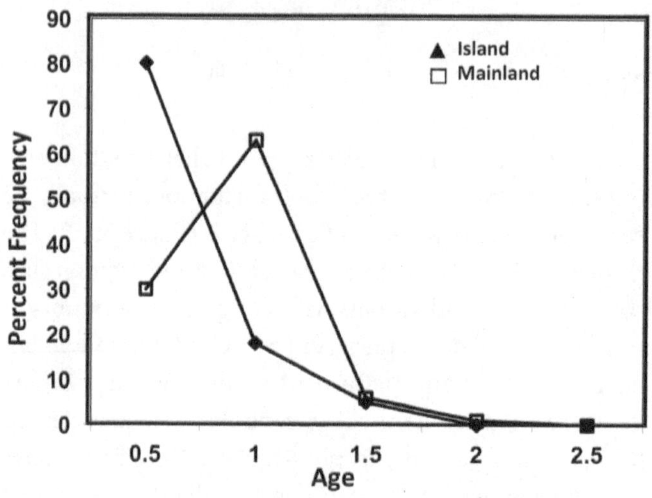

Figure 3.24. Intervals between hypoplasias at Kulubnarti.

again supported our differential health hypothesis. The data also supports a difference between males and females that suggested greater female resilience to stress (figure 3.25). Four percent of the males developed their first hypoplasias at age one, while the first hypoplasias didn't appear among females for another year. It appeared that males were particularly vulnerable relative to females between 1.5 and 2.5 years. This would likely have

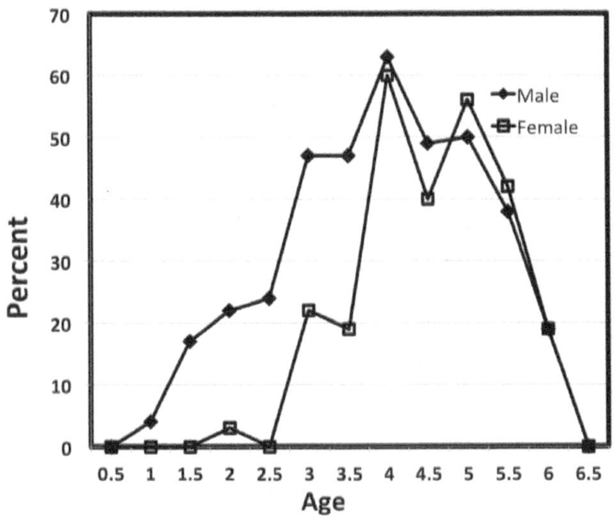

Figure 3.25. Hypoplasia frequencies by age.

bracketed the weaning period. We explore sex differences in stress response in greater detail in the next chapter.

Although both Diane's study of cribra orbitalia and my study of hypoplasia indicated episodes of childhood stress, it was important to assess the extent to which they occurred together as part of an overall childhood stress syndrome. It was also important to determine the extent to which they had an impact on subadult mortality (Mittler and Van Gerven 1994). We chose to use a statistic known as the correlation coefficient to assess the relationship between the hypoplasias and cribra orbitalia. The correlation coefficient is a measure of the degree of association between variables. It can be positive or negative and ranges from -1 to 1. A coefficient of 1 indicates a perfect positive relationship. Diane and I found that the cribra orbitalia/hypoplasia correlation was 0.97 (figure 3.26).

We then measured the association between cribra orbitalia, hypoplasia, and probability of dying (figure 3.27). All three increased, peaked, and declined together.

Putting the data together, it appeared clear to us that the bodies of infants and children were more frequent in the island cemetery because they were sicker than their mainland counterparts. Our results certainly supported that strong inference. There was, however, one more line of evidence that supported our hypothesis.

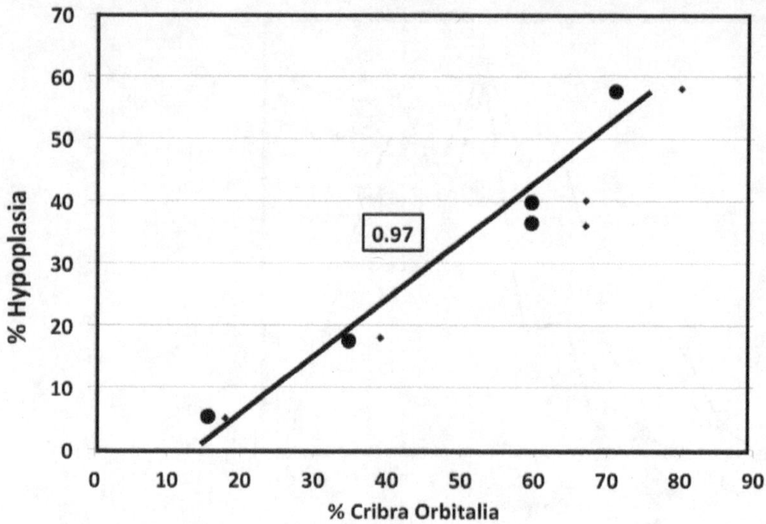

Figure 3.26. The correlation between frequencies of hypoplasia and cribra orbitalia.

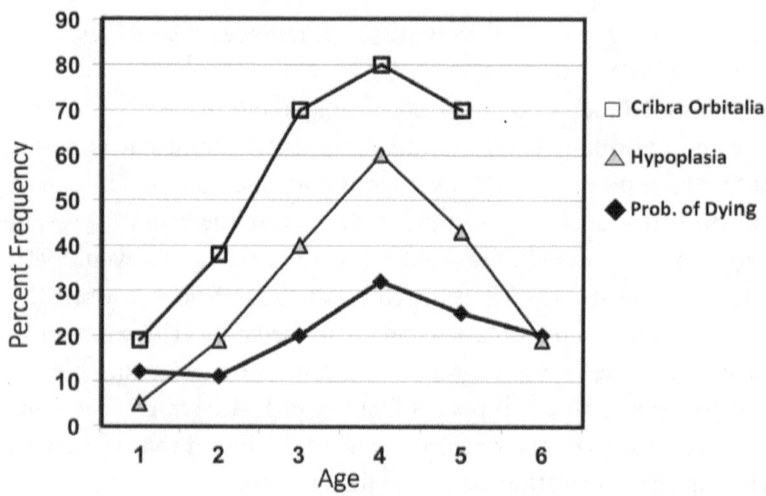

Figure 3.27. Cribra orbitalia, hypoplasia, and probability of dying.

Sandy Karhu decided to analyze accentuated striae of Retzius in the canine teeth for her Ph.D. dissertation in 1991 (Karhu 1991). Given the problem of wear, it was impossible to compare defect frequencies between worn and unworn teeth for exactly the reason that it was impossible in the hypoplasia study. However, rather than limit her study to unworn teeth, she

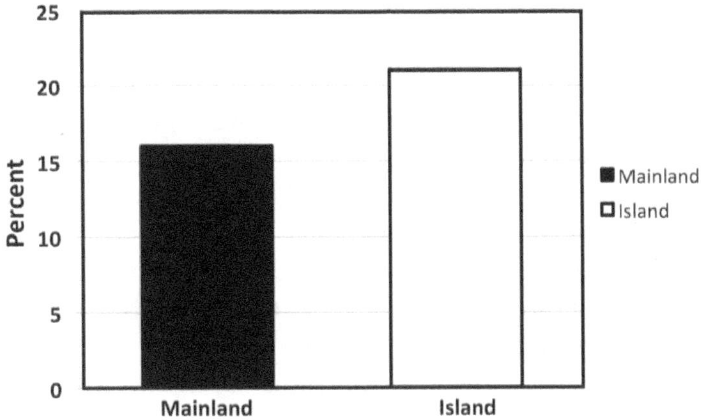

Figure 3.28. Percent of six-month intervals with at least one accentuated stria.

developed a different strategy. She first counted the number of six-month intervals preserved on the crown and then computed the percentage of those intervals with at least one accentuated stria (figure 3.28). Measured in this way, the island children had a higher percentage of defects than their mainland counterparts.

Our studies of cribra orbitalia, hypoplasia, and striae of Retzius, produced by independent researchers using different tissues and techniques, provided powerful evidence in support of our mortality hypothesis. The island children were sicker and died more often than their mainland counterparts. And it may not have been the severity of any one illness event that made the difference. Continuous illness with little time for recovery can draw a child down to death more quickly than a child who has a chance to recover between bouts of illness.

Our research focused on struggles common to all of the children. There can be no doubt that weaning was a challenge to them all. That said, the health and well-being of the island children suffered even more from the impoverished culture that supported them. Greene and coworkers (Greene et al. 1986) estimated that fertility rates on the island would have had to have reached the maximum observed among living populations just to maintain their numbers. The descendants of the mainland community are still living in the village of Kulb. The island community has been long abandoned. While we can never know what became of them, the children—the canaries in the mine—were telling them to leave or die.

The Coffins Are Small

George never loved research more than when he could relate it to modern issues. He was tireless in his opposition to the race concept, not only as an issue in prehistory but in modern times as well. The images of famine today struck us both in relation to our studies of the Nubian children. Search Google images for famine and count the number depicting infants and children. It's the vast majority, and not only because they dramatize the tragedy. There are more of them. Again and again, the coffins going to the graveyard are small. From the standpoint of health and disease, our Nubian children, particularly those living on the island, lived in the same world as the impoverished children of today.

We felt that every aspect of infant and childhood health available for analysis supported the strong inference that the island children died in greater numbers because they were sicker (more stressed) than their mainland counterparts. The obvious next question is why? Why were the canaries in the mine sounding the alarm on the island? The answer to that question requires the cultural context, and that is a focus of the next chapter. But first there is one additional line of evidence to present—growth and development.

4

GROWTH AND DEVELOPMENT

Just think of it as another growth opportunity.

Two years before George finished his dissertation, he was already sharing his data to support student research. In 1966, while he was working as a senior instructor at the University of Utah, one of the graduate students approached him wondering if he might use some of George's data for his master's thesis. His name was Paul Mahler, and he wasn't considered to be among the top students in the program. But George couldn't have cared less about departmental opinions regarding students. He saw something in Paul. Paul worked hard without big rewards, and, most important, he was willing and sincere. He and George got the idea to do a growth study using femur length. Only one study of the kind had been done at that time. Frank Johnston had done an analysis using remains from the site of Indian Knoll in Kentucky (Johnston 1962).

Virtually no studies had been done because adequate samples of infants and children were hard to come by, and almost no one believed that growth could be studied using dead children.[1] Even Johnston was cautious. He made it clear that some degree of error was introduced because the remains did not represent normal healthy infants and children. He went on to suggest that an adequate investigation would require an extremely large sample in order to represent all age groups. The big concern, however, was the nature of the sample. How could the study of dead children tell us anything about growth in their living counterparts? After all, students of childhood growth (Maresh 1955) measured normal living children to establish growth standards for the comparison of populations living under various conditions of health and nutrition (Gorstein et al. 1994). Standards were also used to evaluate the growth of individual children (Eveleth and Tanner 1976). George acknowledged that while the studies of "paleogrowth" had limitations, they still had a potential worth pursuing. Paul's thesis explored that position, and, in so doing, laid the foundation for our Kulubnarti growth studies that followed.

The Wadi Halfa Growth Study

Paul's first step was to compare the Wadi Halfa children to modern growth standards. He made the comparison by first measuring incremental increases in femur length as a proxy for stature (Armelagos et al. 1972) for a combined sample of 57 infants and children ages six months to 16 years (figure 4.1).[2] His results revealed a rate of increase in femur length similar to stature increase in living children. His data even revealed an adolescent growth spurt common in living adolescents (arrows).[3] A signal of normal growth appeared to have been retained. He then moved to a comparison of growth velocity. Velocity is measured as the percent change from one age category to the next. Changes in velocity undergo a characteristic pattern of deceleration and acceleration in living children (Maresh 1955). Deceleration typically occurs during infancy and early childhood. This is followed by a moderate increase leading up to the adolescent growth spurt in the early teen years. With the exception of the 9–10 year age categories, the Wadi Halfa children followed the same pattern (figure 4.2). In the Wadi Halfa children, growth deceleration stopped at ages 7–8, and the growth spurt began at ages 11–13. Paul interpreted the abrupt increase in the age 9–10 value as an anomaly most likely due to small sample size. Whatever

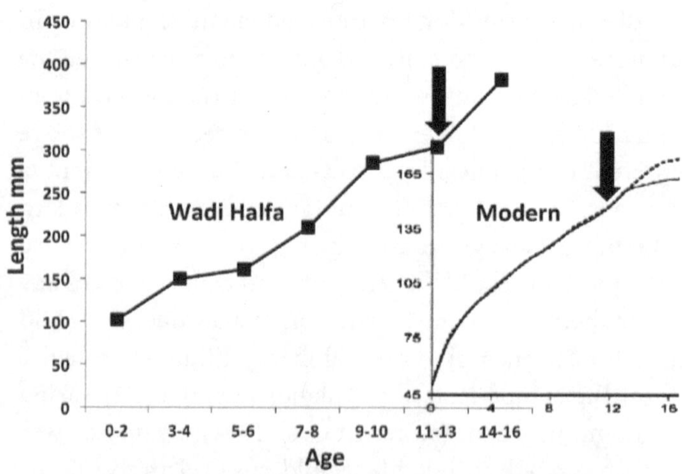

Figure 4.1. Wadi Halfa incremental growth in femur length and modern stature. The arrow indicates adolescent growth spurt.

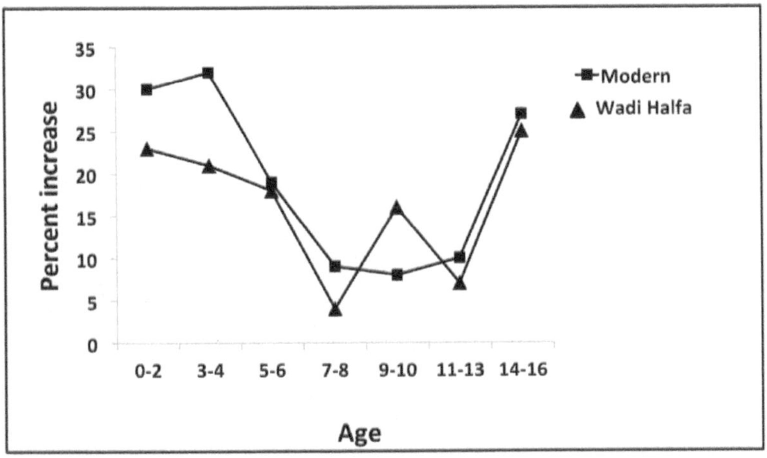

Figure 4.2. Wadi Halfa growth velocity compared to modern stature velocity.

the case, the point he made for incremental growth also applied to growth velocity. Meaningful information regarding typical growth velocity appeared to have been retained. Paul concluded that whatever conditions were causing subadult mortality, they weren't sufficient to entirely obliterate growth patterns observed in living children. The signal that Paul discovered anticipated what has become a fruitful area of study (Jantz and Owsley 1984; Pinhashi et al. 2006; Schillaci et al. 2011; Pinhashi et al. 2013).

The Kulubnarti Study

As with the Wadi Halfa analysis, the Kulubnarti study was part of a thesis. James Hummert had recently joined our graduate program with an unusual background. He left a career as an actor. He had played in a long-running soap opera titled *The Doctors* and was in the cast of a Tony Award–winning Broadway play titled *The Changing Room*. Not surprisingly, he became a terrific lecturer.

Given the growth signal that Paul discovered at Wadi Halfa, we were hopeful that a study of the Kulubnarti children would yield some informative results. The project was provided a larger sample of infants and children than was available at Wadi Halfa. The modal (most frequent) age at death in both cemeteries was birth. Ironically, the biggest problem Jim faced was preservation, but not in the way you would expect. There wasn't too little preservation; there was too much (figure 4.3). Infants and children were mummified more often than adults. I suspect the difference was a matter

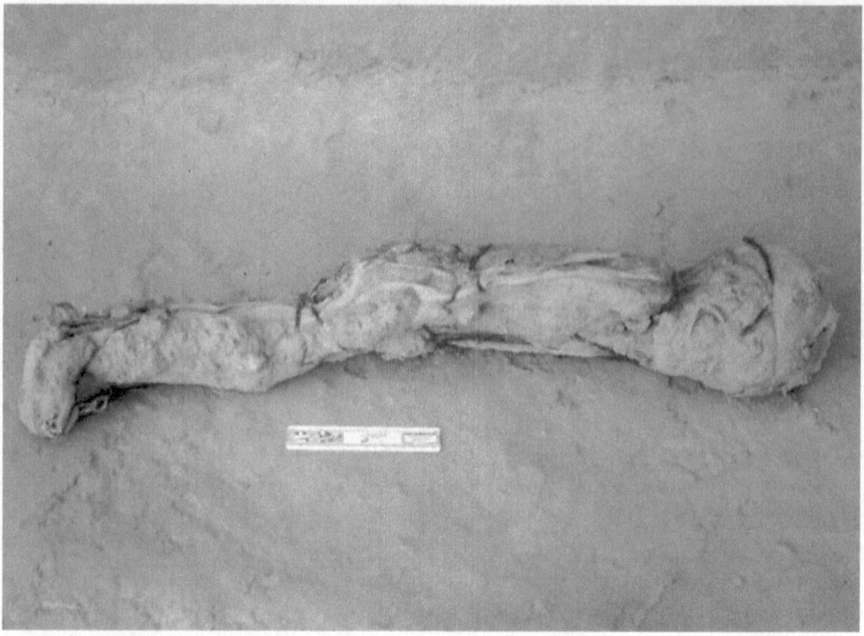

Figure 4.3. Mummified child with shroud, from the mainland cemetery.

of surface area–to–volume ratio. Infants and children have a much larger surface area relative to their volume than do adults. Their larger surface allows moisture to escape more rapidly. This is one of the reasons why hands and feet mummify more often than torsos in all cases of natural mummification. It is also a likely reason why Egyptian embalmers removed the wet internal organs from the body cavity as part of the embalming process.

A major goal of Jim's analysis was to provide a comparative framework for both the Wadi Halfa and the two Kulubnarti populations. He therefore began with the same measures of incremental growth and growth velocity that Paul had used (Hummert and Van Gerven 1983). The island community provided 124 subadult skeletons, and the mainland 56. Ages ranged across the growth period from birth through 16 years.

Jim discovered the same similarity between the Kulubnarti and modern children that Paul had observed at Wadi Halfa (figure 4.4). It was particularly reassuring that a growth spurt appeared at the same age. Growth velocity also followed the modern pattern (figure 4.5). In fact, it fit the modern pattern more closely than did Wadi Halfa. Of course, Jim was well aware of dangers in comparing dead Nubian children to the living. But he was convinced that a comparison of the Nubian communities to each other would be worthwhile. He began with a comparison between Wadi Halfa

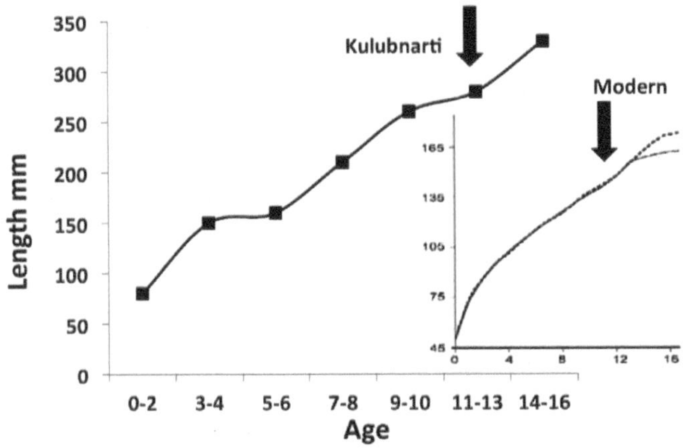

Figure 4.4. Kulubnarti incremental growth in femur length and modern stature. The arrow indicates the adolescent growth spurt.

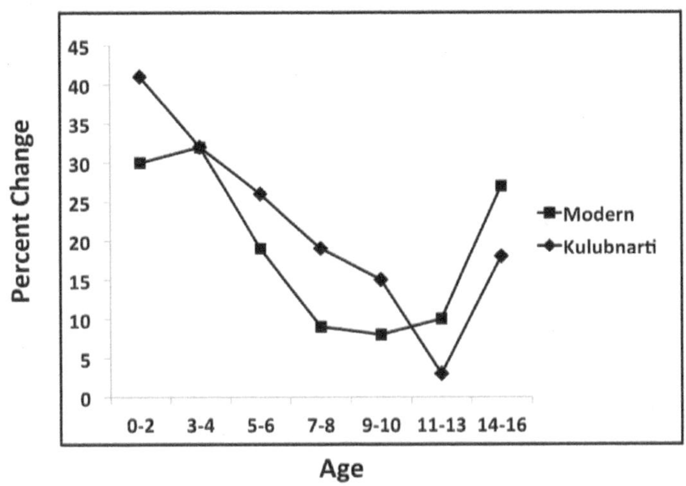

Figure 4.5. Kulubnarti femoral growth velocity compared to modern.

and the combined Kulubnarti sample (figure 4.6) and then compared the Kulubnarti communities to each other (figure 4.7).

The incremental growth data turned out to be particularly revealing. Femur lengths and incremental growth remained virtually identical in both comparisons until the 7–8 year age category. At that point, Wadi Halfa diverged from Kulubnarti just as the Kulubnarti communities diverged from each other. In a sense, Wadi Halfa was to Kulubnarti as the Kulubnarti communities were to each other. Jim's results fit extremely well with our studies of childhood stress at Kulubnarti. To the extent that growth was affected

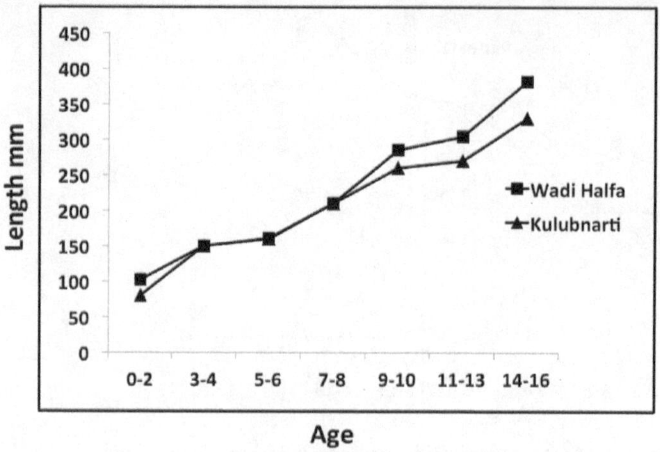

Figure 4.6. Incremental growth at Kulubnarti and Wadi Halfa.

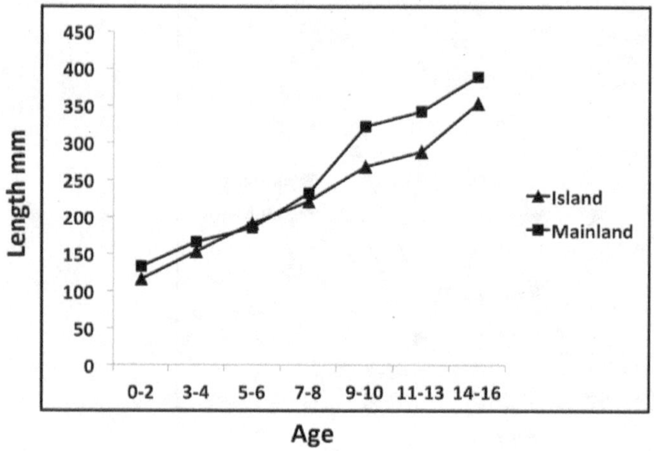

Figure 4.7. Incremental growth in the mainland and island Kulubnarti communities.

by stress, the impoverished children in both Kulubnarti communities experienced higher levels of stress than their Wadi Halfa counterparts, and the island children at Kulubnarti were more stressed than their mainland neighbors.

One of the most innovative growth studies on the Kulubnarti children was conducted by Midori Albert, one of David Greene's doctoral students. She looked at bilateral (left–right) asymmetry in the timing of epiphyseal union in the subadults. While we are all bilaterally symmetrical, we aren't perfectly so. We are all asymmetrical to some, usually unnoticeable degree.

Asymmetry increases when children are stressed during growth. Midori measured asymmetry in the Kulubnarti adolescents by determining the timing of epiphyseal union in left-right pairs of long bones. Once again the island children were more asymmetrical than their mainland counterparts (Albert and Greene 1999).

There was one aspect of the relationship between growth and stress that Jim's data couldn't address—differences between the sexes. This was a logical next question, given that greater female resistance to stressful conditions had been demonstrated across a wide variety of taxa, including humans (Washburn et al. 1965; Stini 1979). The problem was finding a way to measure male-female differences. As we have discussed, diagnosing sex from subadult skeletons is virtually impossible. Solving that problem became a research project for Katherine Moore (a doctoral student) and Susan Thorp (an undergraduate). They were lab partners in my osteology class back in 1985.

Together they developed a research design from the following information: previous research had demonstrated that skeletal growth and development were more sensitive to environmental stress than was the dentition (Owsley and Janz 1985). More specifically, skeletal growth showed considerable interruption relative to the dentition in populations undergoing nutritional privation. This was likely due to differences in genetic program and phenotypic expression between the two systems. Skeletal (body size) response to environmental stress would certainly be more advantageous than a dental response. No one would contest that a reduction in body size had a greater impact on caloric need during a period of food shortage than a reduction in tooth size.

Also, the functional demands on the dentition were unlikely to change with perturbations in the dietary environment. Katherine and Susan then reasoned that as both dental development and skeletal growth proceed with age, the two should approximate each other under normal environmental conditions. During periods of interrupted growth, on the other hand, dental development would likely advance ahead of skeletal development. They hypothesized further that this lack of correspondence should be measurable by comparing estimates of age based on skeletal and then on dental development (Moore et al. 1986).

Their problem was how to diagnose sex using a subadult sample. The Kulubnarti remains provided a way around that problem. Some of the mummified children retained their sex organs.[4] While the samples weren't large, 10 males and 13 females were sufficiently well preserved. Katherine

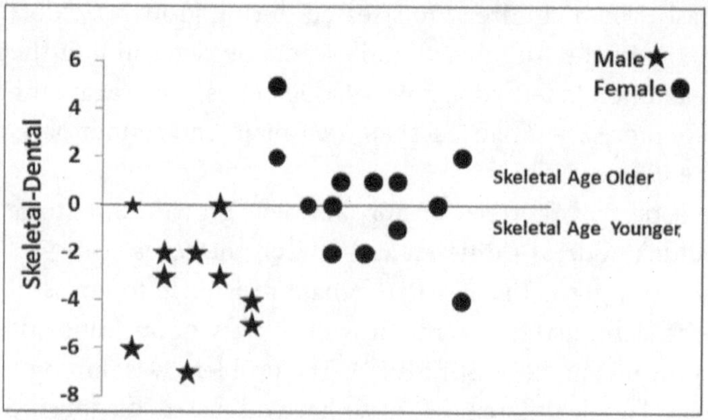

Figure 4.8. Skeletal age compared to dental age at Kulubnarti.

and Susan's methods of analysis were straightforward. Estimates of dental and skeletal age were made independently using published criteria. The categories were refined using population-specific patterns of dental wear. They then calculated the difference between the two age estimates. Only 3 of 13 females had a skeletal age that was less than their dental age (figure 4.8). Three were equal, and six had a skeletal age greater than their dental age. In sharp contrast, no male had a skeletal age greater than his dental age. Two out of ten were equal. The results suggest that the Kulubnarti females were more stress-resistant.

Their linkage between skeletal growth and dental development has recently gained support by a study of living Portuguese children. Hugo Cardoso compared skeletal growth to dental development in two groups—one from low economic status families and one from high. He found greater growth retardation relative to dental development in the low-status group (Cardoso 2007). He argued, as we did, that the difference is due to greater buffering of dental development against environmental stressors.

Childhood Stress in Our Wadi Halfa and Kulubnarti Communities

Our studies of childhood stress in Wadi Halfa and Kulubnarti revealed a consistent pattern of difference. The Wadi Halfa infants and children were better off than the infants and children at Kulubnarti. The children living in the mainland community at Kulubnarti were likewise better off than their island neighbors. This is a good time to move away from biology and consider the cultural environments in which these differences played out.

Wadi Halfa

The people of Wadi Halfa experienced their share of political and social changes. The town of Meinarti was transformed from an administrative center of some importance during Meroitic times into an agrarian village during the subsequent X-Group period. Through it all, however, the Meinarti community enjoyed greater material well-being in a more hospitable setting than did their Kulubnarti neighbors. The Kulubnarti folk were eking out a living in the *Batn el Hajar*, a region that Adams had described as the most barren, inhospitable region of the Nile Valley. His description presented in chapter 1 bears repeating:

> The tortured landscape of bare granite ridges and gullies which characterizes this part of Nubia begins at the bank of the river itself; alluvium exists not as a continuous floodplain, but only in protected pockets and coves. Fields and tiny hamlets hug the banks wherever such soil is available, but for long stretches neither natural nor cultivated vegetation is to be seen. The narrow channel and steep riverbanks make agriculture difficult even where alluvium is present, because of the extreme differential between high and low Nile levels. At the slack season the surface of the stream may be fifty feet or more below the neighboring fields; in these circumstances irrigation is a practical impossibility without the aid of modern pumps. (Adams 1977:26)

There can be no doubt that, compared to the population of Wadi Halfa, the people of Kulubnarti lived impoverished lives in an impoverished environment. It would be unreasonable to suppose that the circumstances of their lives wouldn't have had an effect on the health of their children. Taken together, the entirety of our research into stress, including mortality and responses to disease and nutritional deprivation and growth, supports that conclusion.

Kulubnarti Island and the Mainland

Our research at Kulubnarti was directed by our initial measures of life expectancy in the two communities. There were two possible explanations for the substantially lower life expectancy on the island. The island folk may have a higher birth rate. Alternatively, they may have experienced a higher rate of infant mortality due to the circumstances of their lives. We hypothesized the latter. We proposed that if differences in health were driving the difference in life expectancy, we should see higher levels of stress among the island children. We have met that expectation using multiple measures of stress involving different organ systems. Our hypothesis is also supported by the economic circumstances of the two communities revealed by the archaeological evidence. According to Adams:

> The Nubians of today are mostly a population of small, freehold farmers, living in scattered villages up and down the Nile. Both archaeology and history suggest that this has been true at least since Meroitic times. Here and there among them, however, one finds groups of landless semi-nomadic persons who act as sharecroppers or seasonal laborers for the landholding families. . . . They are generally impoverished, poorly housed and dressed and looked down on by members of the landowning class. (Adams and Adams 2006–2007:11)

There is architectural evidence at Kulubnarti supporting Adams's interpretation. Itinerant communities were consistently located on small islands like Kulubnarti. The island houses are literally shanties (figure 4.9) with walls made of little more than stacked rocks. They had doorways less than a meter high. The contrast between the island and mainland communities is best illustrated by two churches—one on the island (figure 4.10) and one

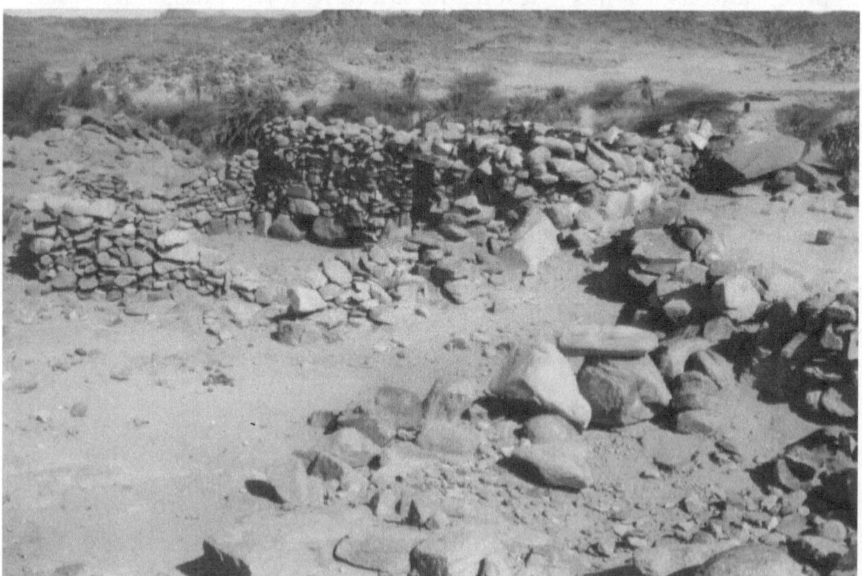

Figure 4.9. An island house at Kulubnarti.

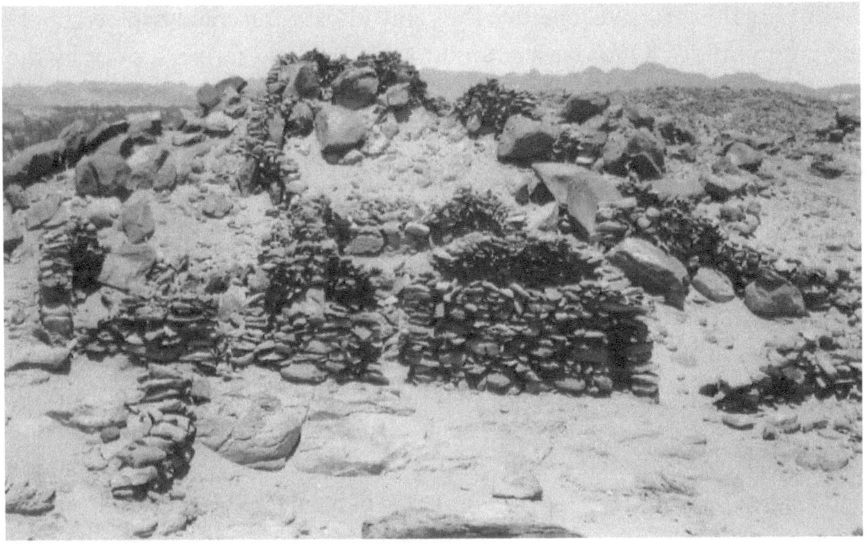

Figure 4.10. An island church at Kulubnarti.

on the mainland (figure 4.11). The island church was literally built among the large boulders dominating the island's terrain. Its floor sloped so much that one end was a full 2 meters lower than the other. The mainland church stands in stark contrast. It is made of brick and mortar, and its double-vaulted interior was decorated with murals. It was almost certainly a product of a professional builder (Adams and Adams 2006–2007).

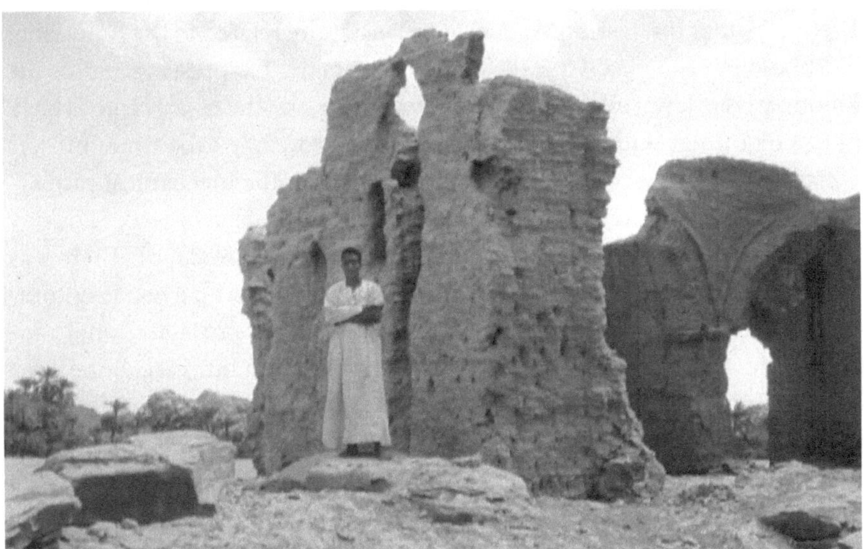

Figure 4.11. The mainland church at Kulubnarti.

Putting the evidence together, the cemeteries represented two neighboring communities. One was a community of freehold farmers, poor by the standards of Wadi Halfa, but well-off in comparison to their island neighbors. The island folk were a landless, itinerant underclass—socially distinct and economically deprived (Adams and Adams 2006–2007). Now, suppose we measured the frequency of dietary deficiencies, enamel defects, and growth retardation in a modern community of migrant farmworkers in California's Simi Valley compared to the children of their employers. What would you predict? Our studies of the infants and children have given us a window on the health of the communities in which they lived. They remind us that the costs of poverty and diminished opportunity transcend time and space. The children of ancient Nubia paid no less a price for the impoverishment of their communities than do the children of the slums and shantytowns today. George and I also believe that our studies provide an example of the synergy between physical anthropology and archaeology in their common goal—an understanding of the human condition across time and space. We also believe that the osteological and archaeological evidence together have shed an ethnographic-like light on the lives of our three Nubian communities.

Growth and Morphology

Not all of our research on the infants and children has focused on stress. There are other interesting aspects of growth more related to the functional morphology of the growing skeleton. The remarkable preservation of the Kulubnarti children allowed us to analyze that also. The research goes back to Jim Hummert and his study of long bone growth. At the time Jim was doing his analysis, there was a growing interest in the mechanical properties of bone in relationship to its external and internal geometry (Lovejoy et al. 1976; Martin and Atkinson 1977; Ruff and Hayes 1983a, b). There was a particular interest in bending strength. The basics aren't particularly complex. For example, bending strength—known as the cross-sectional moment of inertia (CSMI)—increases as the material (in our case, bone) in a cross section moves away from the center. This is obvious if you compare the strength needed to bend a rod as opposed to a pipe—even if they are made from the same amount of material. Shape also affects CSMI. A bone with a round shaft has equal bending strength in any direction, as long as the thickness of the material is equal. An elliptical shape is stronger along its long axis than its short. The tibia becomes increasingly elliptical with its long axis in the anterior-posterior direction.

Jim and I decided that the Kulubnarti children would be ideal subjects for studying the mechanical aspects of bone growth. No one had done an analysis of infants and children in that way at the time, and Jim had already measured lengths, diameters, and percent cortical areas for the tibia as part of his dissertation.[5] The length and diameter measurements were straightforward, but the measurement of percent cortical area requires a little explanation. It consisted of laying a 1 millimeter by 1 millimeter grid over a cross section of the shaft.

Because Jim knew the number of line intersections per area of the grid, he could measure the surface area of a bone by counting the number of grid intersections laying over it. He then calculated percent cortical area as a percentage of bone within the total area.

While bending strength could have been calculated from Jim's measurements, we had access to a far more effective way. David Burr volunteered to measure CSMI using his Norland-Cameron bone mineral analyzer. David was my first doctoral student. His dissertation examined the effects of sexual dimorphism on the biomechanics of bipedal locomotion. At the time David had taken a faculty position in the Department of Anatomy at the West Virginia University. He had purchased a Norland-Cameron bone mineral analyzer for the bone biology laboratory he was in the process of building. The device worked by passing a photon beam across a subject's bone (often the wrist bones), the signal from which reflects a number of properties, including CSMI (Martin and Burr 1984).

The technology was developed for clinical application, but its potential utility for the study of archaeological remains was clear. The same attributes measured for clinical purposes could be used to investigate skeletal architecture as an adaptation to the mechanical forces associated with physical activity. This made it ideal for our purposes. Thus, a Van Gerven and Hummert project became a Van Gerven, Hummert, and Burr project (Van Gerven et al. 1985). Tibias from 172 individuals from the combined Kulubnarti cemeteries were sent to David for analysis. They ranged in age from birth to 14 years. Beyond having been part of Jim's research, the tibia was an ideal choice because the shaft undergoes considerable changes in geometry during growth. The shaft is round in infancy and early childhood, and then becomes increasingly elliptical front-to-back with age. You only need to feel your "shinbone" to verify that.

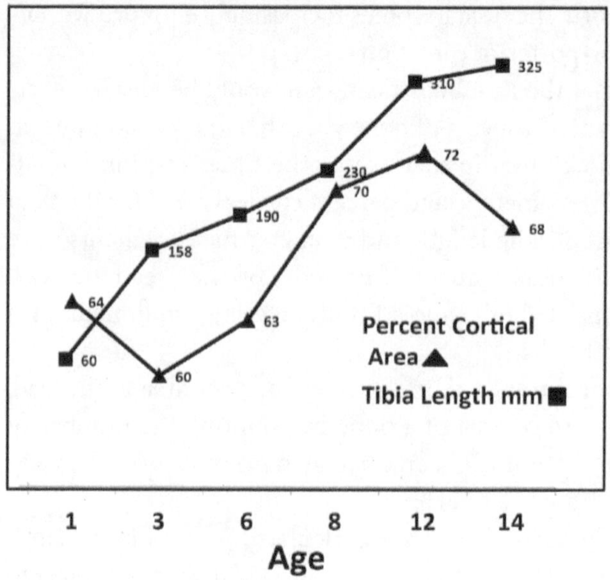

Figure 4.12. Age changes in femur length and percent cortical area.

The tibia showed the same pattern of incremental growth observed for the femur in our earlier research. There was rapid growth in infancy, followed by some decline, followed by a second increase starting at age 8 (figure 4.12). Growth then slowed as the end of the growth period approached. Percent cortical area behaved differently. As incremental length increased at age 8, percent cortical area began to slow and then dropped sharply at age 12, when growth in length increased once again. Indeed, from age 8 onward, length and percent cortical area became mirror images. This led us to two questions: first, what impact did this have on the mechanical properties of the bone; and second, what aspect of growth physiology might it reflect? The mechanical aspect was clarified when we examined changes in midshaft diameters (figure 4.13). There was a consistent increase in both anterior posterior (AP) and medial lateral (ML) diameters until age 8, when the AP diameter growth increased rapidly ahead. At that point, the shaft changed shape from round to elliptical. The CSMI data revealed the consequences (figure 4.14). The strength of the tibia (bending strength) at midshaft increased equally until the AP diameter increased ahead of the ML diameter. As expected, the tibia shaft became increasingly stronger along the AP axis. We interpreted this as a likely adaptation to AP bending forces associated with leg extension during bipedal locomotion.

An adaptation of this sort made sense. Children don't just get bigger; they mature. They do new and different things, and the skeleton must have ways to respond. What we saw in the tibia—and, by extension, the skeleton—was a superb economy of energy. Redirecting bone growth to areas of increased stress is certainly more economical than simply growing more bone. We had no way to know if this growth pattern is normal for all

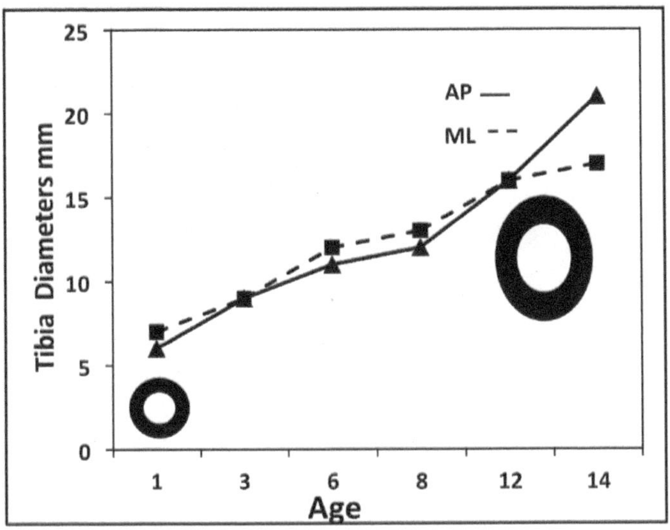

Figure 4.13. Age changes in midshaft diameter of the tibia.

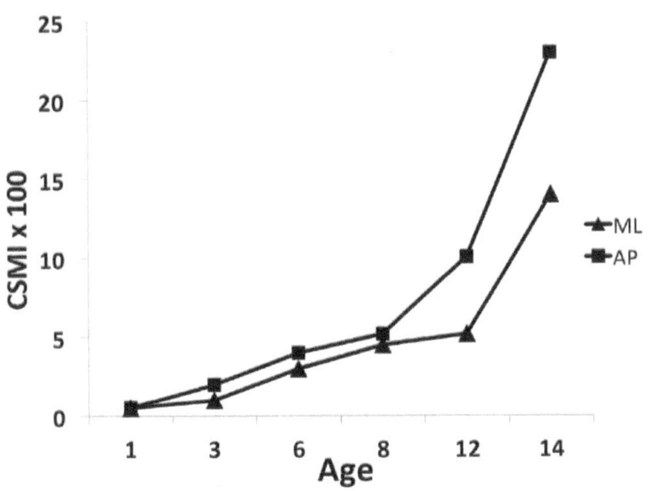

Figure 4.14. Anterior posterior (AP) and medial lateral (ML) bending strength with age.

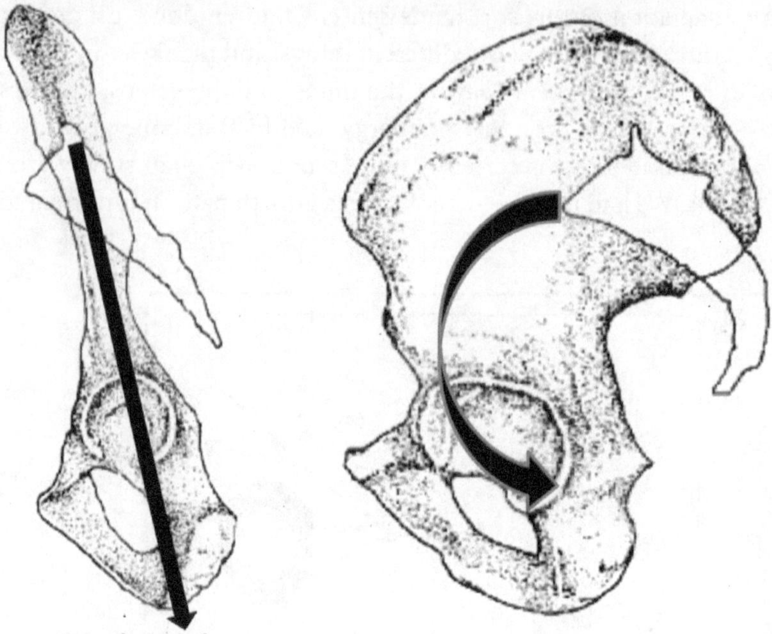

Figure 4.15. The quadrupedal and bipedal pelvis.

children. However, it seemed to us that for a poorly nourished child, the economy could be important to survival.

What we have seen in the growing tibia is an example of an important principle in biology—a principle that is central to all of comparative anatomy and most of paleontology: form follows function (Thompson 1942). Without that linkage, we could learn nothing about an extinct animal from its bones. Comparing the anatomy of a chimpanzee to a monkey or a human would be pointless. But the form follows function principle does not mean that the two are always in perfect harmony. The tension between form and function stems from a simple fact. Evolution builds what *is* from what *was*. The sleek bodies of whales and seals evolved from terrestrial ancestors. Snakes have quadrupedal ancestors, the ancestors of horses had toes, and our roots go back to a quadrupedal monkey-like ancestor.

Many years ago, a wonderful article was written by an anthropologist named Wilton Krogman titled "The Scars of Human Evolution" (Krogman 1951). The article looked at the many imperfect compromises that went into building our biped form from a quadrupedal ancestry. Krogman pointed out that we suffer from high blood pressure and strokes because our blood has to be pumped uphill to our brain. Our knees are prone to injury, and we are wracked by problems of the lower back. The list goes on. Evolution builds what it can from what's at hand. The process has been referred to as creative scavenging (Dorit 1997).

Perhaps the best example in biological anthropology of Dorit's scavenging metaphor is the human pelvis (Lovejoy 1981; Tague and Lovejoy 1986). No one can escape an introductory course in osteology without learning about the transformation of the quadrupedal pelvis into a bipedal one. It's the story of a quadruped with a well-designed pelvis becoming a biped with a pelvis that does the best it can. For our purposes, the quadruped's pelvis is built for two things—supporting its hind limbs in locomotion and giving birth to babies. The locomotor features work harmoniously with the obstetric features. The pelvis is long and tubular, providing relatively straight passage for birthing (figure 4.15).

The evolution of bipedal gait required a new pelvic design. As an accommodation for the muscles of locomotion, the pelvis became flexed back upon itself. The pelvic canal ceased to be a canal, but rather became two chambers—an upper (the inlet) and a lower (the outlet)—with a turn between the two. This required the baby to make a turn as it traveled from the inlet through the outlet. The consequence was a compromised and often dangerous delivery. The challenge was made worse with the rapid expansion of the human brain following the evolution of bipedal gait. God's curse (Genesis 3:16) on Eve was "I will greatly multiply your pain in childbirth, in pain you will bring forth children." And there is the connection to our studies of the Nubian infants. Our focus to this point has been on the growth process. This is a good point to introduce a study of a growth outcome—an outcome of vital importance to the youngest Nubians of all.

The Obstetric Pelvis Project

Studies of pelvic morphology are divisible into three basic categories. The first is clinical, having to do with obstetrics and gynecology. The second is paleontological, having to do with the evolution of bipedal gait (Tague and Lovejoy 1986; Rosenberg and Trevathan 1995, 2002; Rosenberg 1992; Trevathan 1988). The third is forensic, having to do with the diagnosis of sex from skeletal remains (Krogman 1962; Bruzek 2002). The diagnosis of sex has been a dominant theme in the analysis of archaeological remains, with most of the literature involving technique. What has been notably absent was an analysis of pelvic morphology within a single archaeological population using all three areas of inquiry.

One of the most exciting things about a new generation of students is the life experiences they bring. Jim Hummert brought his background in the theater and became an outstanding classroom teacher. Lynn Sibley came to us as a practicing nurse midwife. Her training drew her almost immediately to the Kulubnarti pelvic remains. Here were dozens of individuals with all of their pelvic bones preserved. She became convinced that if she reconstructed the pelves, she could measure and evaluate them just as was done for living women. She was particularly interested in using the measurements to understand the connections between growth, nutrition, gestation, and childbirth at Kulubnarti. We were all convinced that such an analysis would make an important contribution to the literature.

She set about the project in 1989. The sample she selected to study consisted of 36 adult females from the combined island and mainland cemeteries. The measures (figures 4.16 and 4.17) represented those taken in the course of a standard prenatal examination. As a result, Lynn was able to reach across time and make a clinical evaluation of these 36 women as

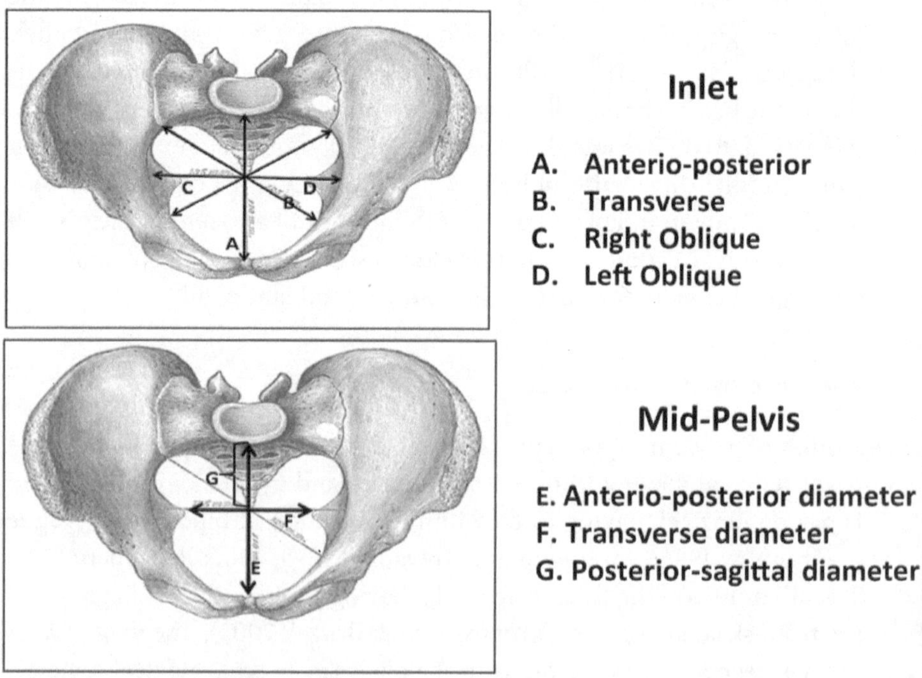

Figure 4.16. Inlet midpelvic dimensions.

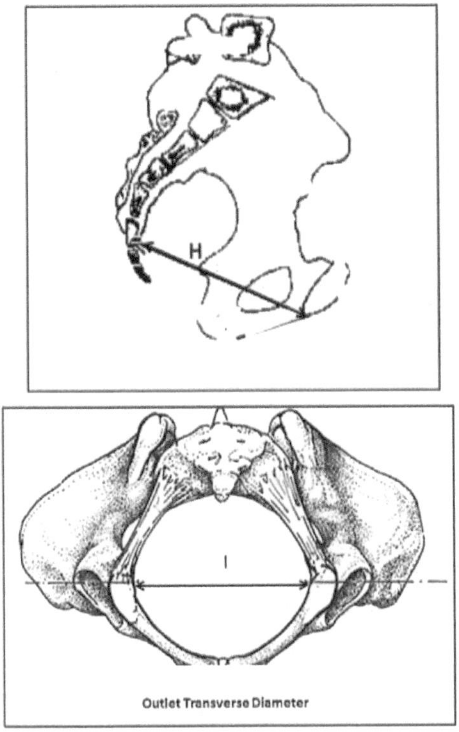

Figure 4.17. Outlet dimensions.

though they were her patients. She was also able to estimate the likely impact of pelvic morphology on newborns as would be expected in a clinical setting (Sibley et al. 1992). The results weren't surprising, but were more pronounced than Lynn expected.

Compared to normal U.S. females, the Kulubnarti females were smaller in every dimension (figure 4.18). A great portion of this difference was no doubt due to a body size effect. But that couldn't explain all of the differences. For example, the difference in midplane posterior sagittal diameter was far too great to explain by a body size difference only. That was also true for inlet transverse diameter and midplane transverse diameter. The Kulubnarti women differed in the same way when compared to other archaeological populations (figure 4.19). With the exception of AP inlet and midplane postsagittal diameter (Kulubnarti is larger than Pecos), the Kulubnarti females are small. But here again, simple body size cannot be the only contributing factor. The results raised an important question: could some aspect of the reduced dimensions at Kulubnarti have had obstetric consequences important to both the babies and their mothers?

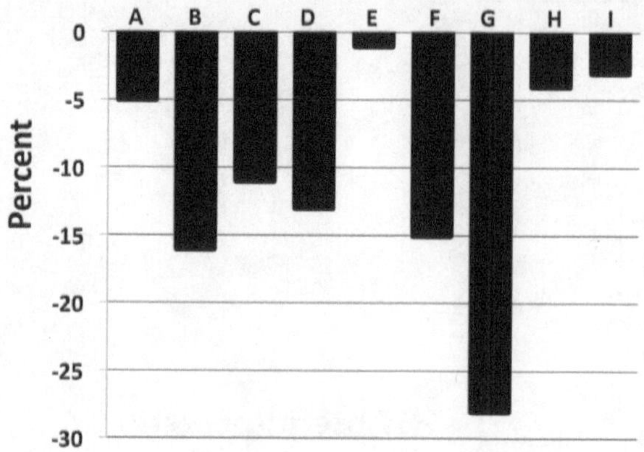

Figure 4.18. Size differences between Kulubnarti and U.S. normal (A = anterior-posterior inlet; B = transverse inlet; C = right oblique inlet; D = left oblique inlet; E = anterior-posterior diameter; F = transverse diameter; G = posterior-sagittal diameter; H = anterior-posterior outlet; I = transverse inlet).

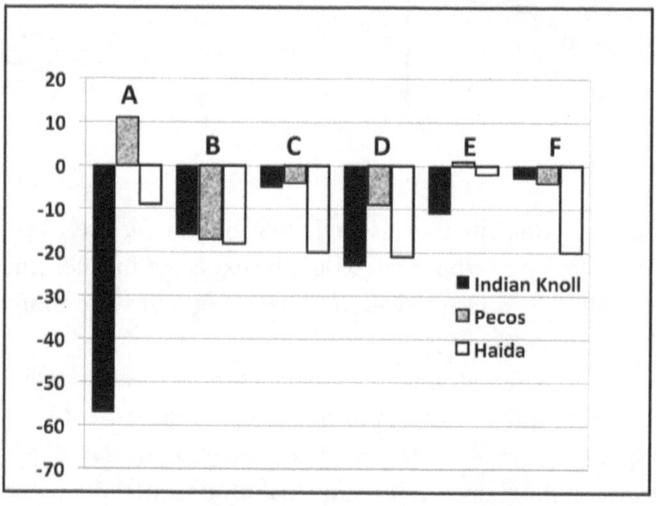

Figure 4.19. Size differences between Kulubnarti and three archaeological populations (A = anterior-posterior inlet; B = transverse inlet; C = anterior-posterior midplane; D = transverse midplane; E = posterior midplane; F = anterior-posterior outlet).

One way to approach the question was to compare the Kulubnarti pelves to modern American clinical standards. Clinically, if an obstetric measurement drops below a certain value, the pelvis is considered contracted in that dimension. The prevalence of contracted dimensions at Kulubnarti is striking (figure 4.20). But beyond the number, the dimensions involved are

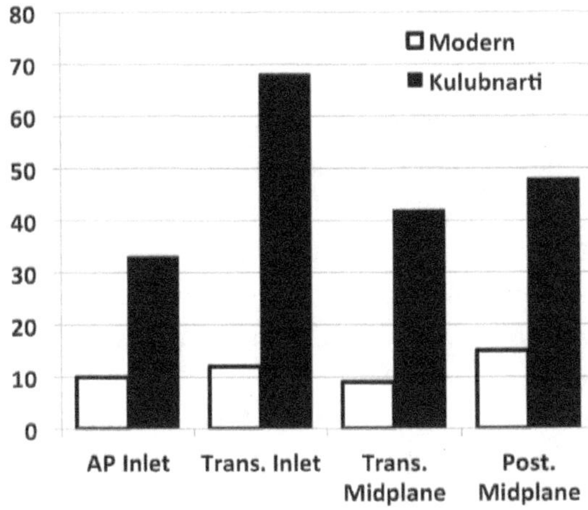

Figure 4.20. Frequency of contracted pelves at Kulubnarti compared to modern American women.

noteworthy. The inlet sagittal and transverse dimensions bound the space through which the fetal head must pass as it engages the birth canal. Engagement, in which the baby drops into the pelvic inlet, is the first critical step in delivery. The posterior sagittal and midplane transverse dimensions define the narrowest points through which the fetus must pass as it negotiates the pelvic curve. Indeed, the midplane transverse is the narrowest point along the birth canal and is a reference point in the assessment of delivery. Lynn concluded that the Kulubnarti women were contracted at those points where contraction was apt to present the greatest challenges. The question was if such challenges had important consequences on the life and health of the Kulubnarti children.

Lynn placed the question in the context of previous research. The Kulubnarti pelves were small relative to both modern and other archaeological populations. There was abundant evidence for nutritional stress provided by our earlier studies of cribra orbitalia (Van Gerven et al. 1981) and enamel hypoplasia (Van Gerven et al. 1990). This was particularly significant given the strong relationship between nutrition and birth. There was also the evidence for high infant mortality. Recall that the modal age at death was birth. In Lynn's view, that was the most important context of all.

Lynn observed that "for moderately contracted [pelves] the prognosis for a successful delivery of a term size fetus is borderline, and for the severely contracted the prognosis is considered hopeless." There is a last, poignant piece of evidence—a possible breech delivery. This obstetric tragedy has its own implications. A young adult, though poorly preserved, was found supine on what appeared to be a fiber mat. A fetus was lying on her pelvic floor extended across the pelvic inlet in a breech position. It is likely that this young woman labored to death. Upon observing this burial, Sibley noted: "The possible breech delivery at Kulubnarti bears silent witness to this grim fact [of obstetric tragedy]. It is possible that individuals S-224, R-85, and R-99, or others like them with markedly reduced pelvic dimensions, suffered untold reproductive morbidity and, perhaps, mortality" (Sibley et al. 1992:428).

It wasn't unreasonable to make the strong inference that the Kulubnarti women were delivering small babies and that this contributed to the high rates of infant mortality. And this told us something important about life and death in this tiny medieval village. Survival for these simple folk was always a complex negotiation between the relentless challenges of the environment and the capacity of frail human beings to respond.

Birth demanded a balancing act between the risks of obstetric tragedy on one hand and the challenges of poor nutrition on the other. This was a balancing act that no doubt reverberated throughout the childhood years and beyond. Just as adverse conditions prior to birth lead to poorer health during infancy and childhood, poor childhood health increases the risk of poor health across the adult years. Indeed there are a number of studies showing that growth during infancy and early childhood can also affect adult health. We turn to our studies of adult health in the next chapter.

5

HEALTH AND DISEASE

The Adults

Getting old isn't for sissies.

In chapters 3 and 4 we concentrated on childhood stress and disease and their impact on growth and development in infants and children. As we said before, the youngest members of a community are the most vulnerable, and, like canaries in the mine, they are the first to sound the alarm when their society begins to fail. They thus provide a measure of cultural success apart from the trappings of material achievement. That has had important implications for our understanding of the Wadi Halfa and Kulubnarti communities. As we have seen, the X-Group period has often been considered a time of cultural decline. In material terms, that may be true. However, our investigations have challenged that view when applied to the well-being of the populations. Measured in terms of reproductive success, X-Group populations may have been better adapted than their Meroitic counterparts. But this doesn't mean that adults are irrelevant. They build and maintain cultural systems. They devise technologies, social organizations, and systems of belief designed to ensure the survival of future generations. It's important to know how the adults, as well as the infants and children, were doing.

Compared to the infants and children, the Wadi Halfa and Kulubnarti adults provided us fewer opportunities to inquire into health. Grown tissues are less responsive to environmental perturbations, and many conditions, such as the neoplasms (benign tumors and cancers) discussed in the next chapter, operate at the individual level (Wallace 1992). The conditions seen among adults most commonly involve degenerative changes, three of which we present in this chapter. They are dental pathologies (Brothwell 1963; Hillson 2007), age-related bone loss (Dewey et al. 1969; Armelagos et al. 1976), and fractures (Kilgore et al. 1997). Dental pathologies are important because they involve both infection and wear and tear (Hillson 1979, 2007). Age-related bone loss (osteoporosis) is interesting because it provides an important measure of the stresses associated with female reproduction (Martin and Armelagos 1979), and fractures reflect the challenges of daily activities (Buzon and Richman 2007; Judd 2000). Let's begin with dental pathology.

Dental Pathology: The Biological Baseline

In order to discuss dental pathology, we need to know some basics about teeth and the conditions that afflict them. Teeth are principally composed of enamel, dentin, and cementum. Enamel is not a living tissue. It is virtually inorganic and harder than jade. And as any hockey player will tell you, once damaged, enamel is incapable of repairing itself. Dentin makes up the bulk of the tooth. It is a living tissue beneath the enamel layer. It is softer than enamel, but harder than bone, and deforms enough under compression to make the enamel less brittle. Dentin contains small tubules connecting it to the pulp cavity. The pulp cavity houses the tooth's neuro-vascular bundle (vein, artery, and nerve). There is also a layer of tissue known as cementum lining the space between the bony wall of the tooth socket and the root. Cementum helps anchor teeth in their sockets. We will be examining three important sources of dental pathology.[1] They are caries, wear, and abscess (figure 5.1).

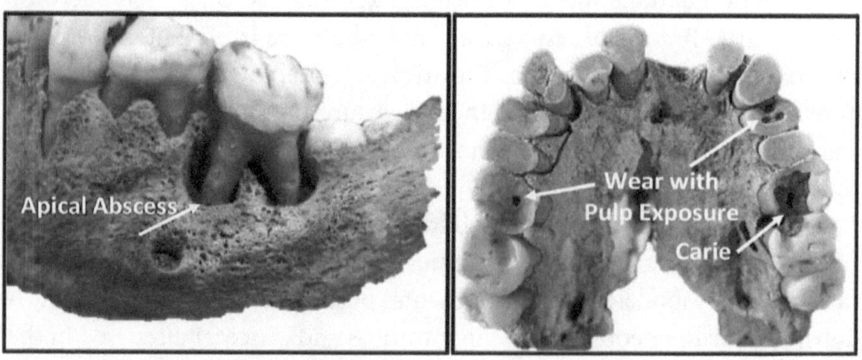

Figure 5.1. Dental pathologies.

Caries

Dental caries, commonly known as cavities, are an infectious disease caused by several species of *streptococcus* bacteria. The most common is *Streptococcus mutans* (Loesche 1986; Marsh 2004). Millions of the bacteria cover dental surfaces in a thin film known as plaque (Marsh 2004). The bacteria consume carbohydrates left on tooth surfaces after eating. Consumption produces acid by-products capable of demineralizing and then destroying enamel, leading to dental caries. We learn that a sure way to prevent caries is to remove plaque either by brushing or by applying an antibacterial mouthwash containing fluoride. Fluoride is a naturally occurring substance that reduces caries by inhibiting enamel demineralization (Featherstone 1999). Programs for introducing low levels of fluoride into drinking water were started in the United States in the 1950s and 1960s and are now present in some 30 countries (Iheozor-Ejiofor et al. 2013). Most toothpaste products are also fluoridated.

The addition of fluoride to drinking water and toothpastes had an unexpected consequence for dentists and dental schools around the country. An 80 percent reduction in caries produced a dramatic drop in visits to the dentist. Dentists quit doing business, and some dental schools actually closed for lack of students. The "clinical gap" has now been filled by a growing emphasis on orthodontics, periodontics (the treatment of gum diseases), and aesthetics, such as tooth whitening. Retainers and braces have made many a house payment for orthodontists. As a side note, there is anecdotal data suggesting a resurgence of dental caries due to the use of unfluoridated bottled water. This is another example of diseases never being a matter of chance.

Wear

A second source of dental disease, particularly in prehistoric times, is tooth wear. While enamel is rock-hard, it is still subject to wear and tear over the course of a lifetime of chewing. The rate of wear increases rapidly once the enamel is worn through and the dentin is exposed. Once wear reaches the pulp cavity, the tooth becomes infected, leading to abscessing and eventually death of the tooth. Not surprisingly, natural selection favors dental designs capable of resisting wear over an organism's normal life span. This is well illustrated in the case of dentures for cows. Argentine dentist Osvaldo Errobidart (Errobidart 2013) discovered that a typical 1,000-pound cow's teeth are good for about eight years. After that, its

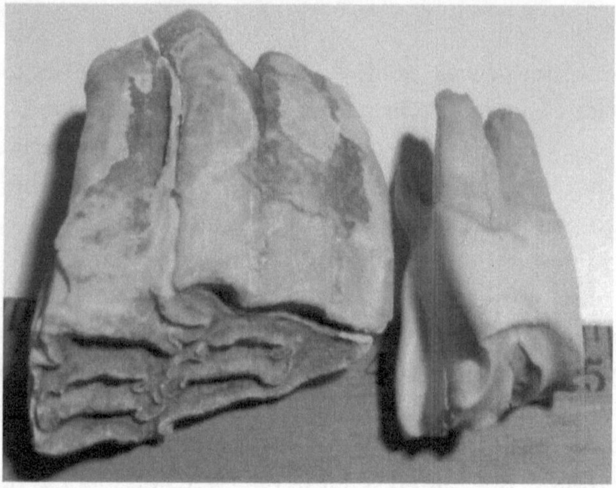

Figure 5.2. Horse molar tooth.

teeth are so badly worn that the cow can't chew well enough to maintain a level of nutrition adequate for milk production. The cow is then typically slaughtered. Errobidart found a solution: fit "geriatric" cows with stainless steel dentures. Fitted with new teeth, the cow's years of milk production are significantly extended.

In the natural world of denture-free animals, evolution has selected for a wide variety of dental designs based on life span and diet. Animals with long life spans typically have more wear-resistant teeth than do those with short lives. Abrasives in the diet also play an important role, and, of course, life span and diet interact. Features enhancing wear-resistance include enamel thickness, complexity, and surface area. Morphologically complex teeth with many cusps and fissures have more surface area than do less complex teeth of the same size. In terms of complexity and surface area, consider the horse's tooth in figure 5.2.

These principles apply just as well to us and our ancestors. Figure 5.3 shows a comparison of molar sizes between a modern chimpanzee, a four-million-year-old ancestor (*Australopithecus afarensis*), and a modern human. While *A. afarensis* probably lived no longer than a modern chimpanzee, its molar teeth were larger and more complex than either a chimp's or ours. This reflects an adaptation to a highly abrasive diet most likely including grasses, sedges, and roots (Ungar 2004; Sponheimer and Lee-Thorp 1999).

Larger molars tend to have more cusps and fissures, and thus more surface area, than smaller molars. The Mesolithic Nubians had large molars

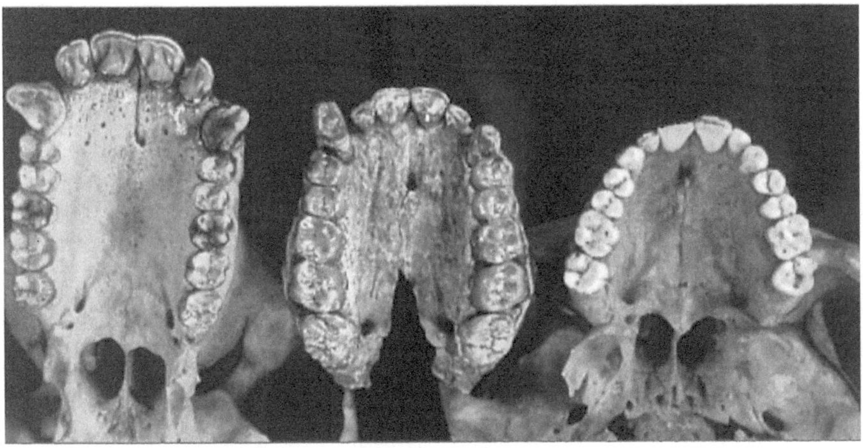

Figure 5.3. Upper jaws, from left to right: chimpanzee, *Australopithecus afarensis*, and modern *Homo sapiens*.

with five or six cusps, while the later Meroitic population had smaller molars, typically with four cusps (figure 5.4). Larger, more complex Mesolithic molars resisted wear well. The smaller, less complex molars of later Nubian populations were less likely to trap food, making them more resistant to caries in a cultural setting characterized by a diet of more processed, higher carbohydrate foods. Any dentist will tell you that all things being equal, molars with more cusps are prone to trap more food particles than molars with fewer cusps.

Tooth wear has a practical side for osteology. Population-specific rates and patterns of wear can provide another tool for age estimation. This can be problematic, however, when patterns of tooth wear are used to age fragmentary remains. You can't always tell whether the tooth in hand had a

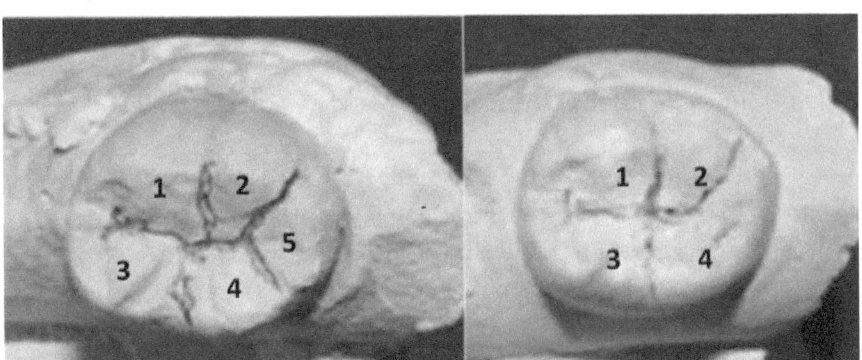

Figure 5.4. Five-cusp and four-cusp human molar patterns.

tooth on the opposite side. That obviously affects rate of wear. It's also important to reemphasize the importance of population specificity. Baseline patterns of population-specific tooth wear have to be established, and this can be difficult to do with small samples.

Abscess

Teeth pay the ultimate price for dental caries and wear. Once the pulp cavity is exposed, bacteria are free to follow the neuro-vascular supply downward through the apex (tip) of the root (Siqueira and Rôças 2009). The result can be an apical abscess (figure 5.1). Accumulating pus eventually bursts the abscess, resulting in drainage either externally into the mouth or internally into the bloodstream. Internal drainage can spread the infection into vital organs such as the heart and brain (DeStefano et el. 1993; Hujoel et al. 2000).

Given our modern diet of highly processed food, wear is no longer a factor in dental disease, and with the advent of modern dentistry, we tend to think of cavities as a painful but relatively minor (and certainly not fatal) inconvenience. Our biggest problem today is periodontal disease, and even this is seldom life-threatening. In contrast, caries, wear, and periodontal diseases were major sources of life-threatening infection and an important force of natural selection in ancient populations.

Dental Pathologies at Wadi Halfa

George's dissertation analysis of dental pathology focused on the relationship between tooth loss, caries, wear, and abscess (Armelagos 1968). As always, his approach was biocultural. I remember reading his dissertation shortly after he had finished it and asking him what he thought turned out best. He gave me a two-word answer—"the percentages." There is no way to appreciate how profound those two words were unless I let George tell the story behind it. So I'll turn the narrative over to George as he told it to me:

As I read the literature, I was consistently frustrated by the paucity of information. I had spent weeks tracking down articles on ancient diseases in Nubia and elsewhere, only to be disappointed. I read with interest the reports from Grafton Elliot Smith and colleagues (Smith 1909a). They had analyzed 10,000 burials, and what did they report? They reported 190 cases of fractured humeri. But they didn't include how many humeri there were. What they had provided was a numerator without a denominator. And without a denominator, I couldn't calculate percent frequencies.

I was determined to correct that problem in my dissertation, but my commitment turned out to be more complex than I anticipated. If I was going to move from ten cases of abscess to "ten percent of 85 crania had an abscess," I had to understand and explain what the 85 crania represented. They had to be a sample of something, and understanding that something was important. I could think of any number of possible samples—sexes, ages, tooth types, or locations on the tooth. Once I opened the door to sampling, I also opened the door to quality control. How good were my samples, and what did they represent? There were problems in that regard that particularly worried me.

Even though each grave was carefully screened for loose teeth, some teeth were inevitably lost in the course of excavation. The problem had the potential to be serious. Teeth with a single root (like the incisors and canines) are more likely to fall out of the mandible or maxilla during excavation and handling than are teeth with multiple roots (like the molars). The problem was compounded because different types of teeth had different likelihoods of disease. For example, molars trap more food on their crown than do incisors. The problem was complicated further by an age effect. All things being equal, older people have more time to develop dental diseases than young people. So, in order for me to compare the Wadi Halfa populations in any meaningful way, I had to make certain that there were no underlying differences in the numbers and kinds of lost teeth or differences in age distribution.

For my first step, I compared the age distributions of my three populations (figure 5.5).

I did this by calculating the cumulative percentage of individuals by age for each of the cultural periods. The Meroitic and X-Group samples were statistically the same, while the Christians weren't. All I could do was eliminate the Christians and focus on a Meroitic–X-Group comparison. I then compared the distribution of tooth types between the Meroitic and X-Group samples (figure 5.6). There were no significant differences between the two.

Once I satisfied myself that I had good samples (I had a total of 1,093 Meroitic and 720 X-Group teeth to examine), I asked two questions. First, did the causes of tooth loss differ between the Meroitic and X-Group populations; and second, could the differences, if found, be understood in biocultural terms? However, before I could begin my analysis there was an additional problem—the problem of causality. While it may seem overly philosophical, the problem involved the difference between proximate and ultimate causes. A proximate cause is the one immediately preceding an effect. Ultimate cause(s) are the "real" causes of an effect. In my case, abscess was the proximate cause of tooth loss. The ultimate causes were

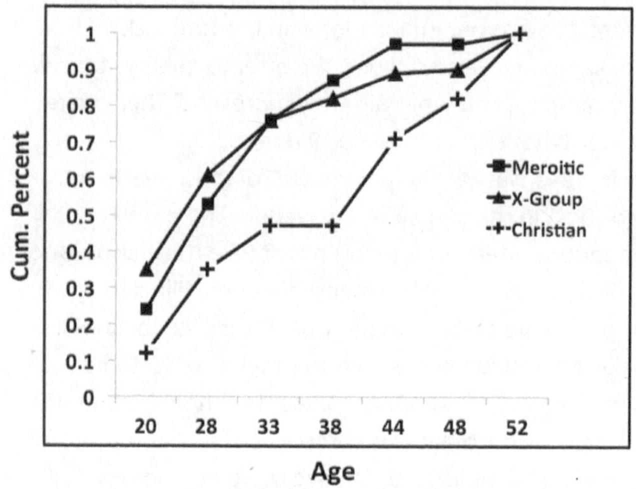

Figure 5.5. Percent adult mortality for the Wadi Halfa Meroitic, X-Group, and Christian samples.

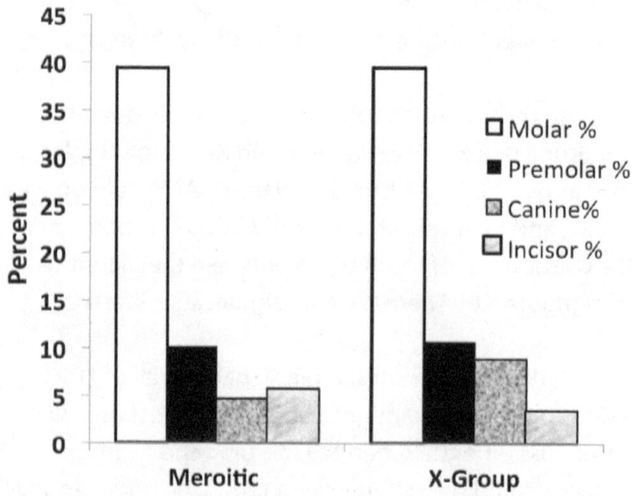

Figure 5.6. Frequencies by tooth type.

the caries and wear that caused abscessing. That distinction structured my analysis. While I could never directly know what abscessed a given tooth, I could analyze the contribution of caries and wear to the abscess that cost the tooth its life.

My analysis proceeded in steps. First I established a criterion to distinguish between antemortem and post-mortem loss. When a tooth is lost prior to death, its socket is gradually resorbed (figure 5.7). I only counted a tooth as lost when there was clear evidence of socket resorption. I then examined the frequency of resorbed sockets and abscesses for my Meroitic and X-Group samples. The X-Group had higher frequencies of both (figure 5.8). This led me to a hypothesis. I hypothesized that the higher frequency of abscess and resorbed sockets during X-Group times

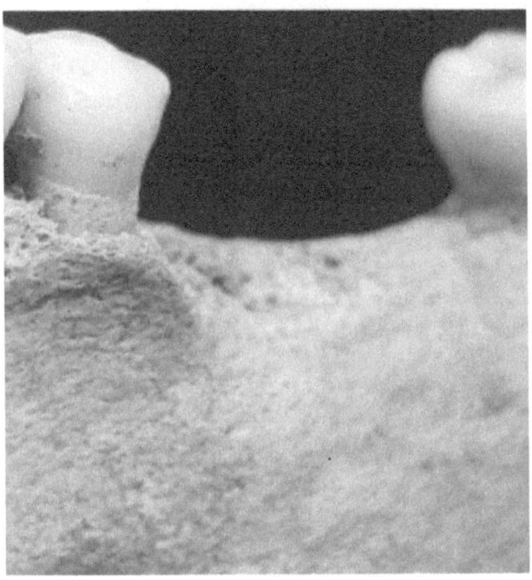

Figure 5.7. Resorbed first mandibular molar socket.

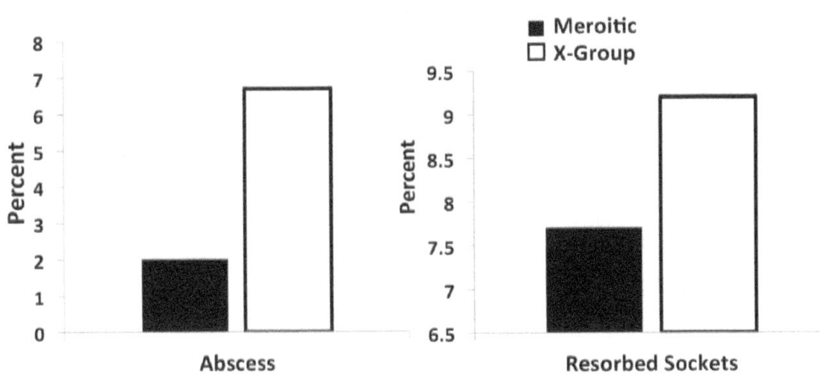

Figure 5.8. Percent frequencies of resorbed sockets and abscesses.

should correspond to higher frequencies of caries and/or wear—the ultimate causes.

I began with caries. The average number of caries per individual (figures 5.9 and 5.10) was remarkably similar between the Meroitic and X-Group samples with one exception. No Meroitics appeared in the highest frequency category for caries. I then shifted my comparison from total tooth involvement to the location involved. It turned out that the X-Group population had a substantially higher frequency of occlusal caries, meaning that the caries occurred on the surface used for chewing (figure 5.11).

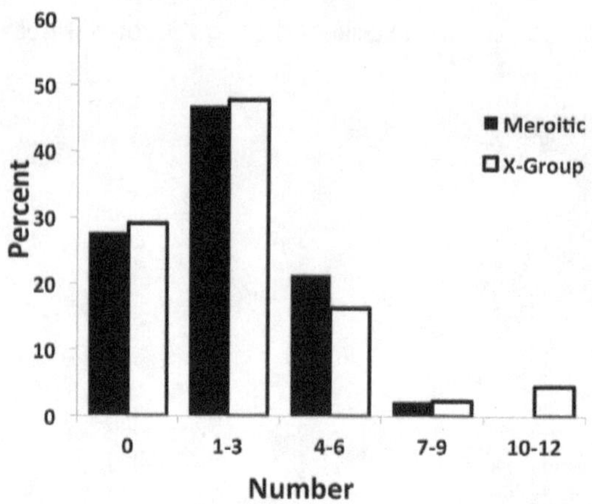

Figure 5.9. Percent frequency of individuals with up to three abscesses and resorbed sockets.

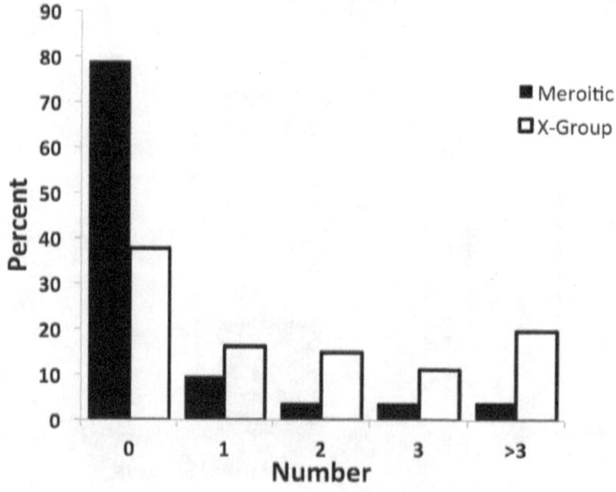

Figure 5.10. Percent frequency of individuals with up to 12 caries in the total dentition.

My next step was to compare wear between the two populations. The X-Group population had six percent fewer individuals with no wear, and six percent more with severe wear (figure 5.12). I asked myself if such a small difference could matter. I concluded that it did, and that the relationship between wear and abscess supported my case. Wear only leads to an abscess when the tooth is severely worn and the pulp cavity is exposed to infection. The tooth remains healthy until that point is reached that the infection breaks through to the pulp cavity. So, while the percentage difference in the severe category appeared to be small, virtually all of the abscesses appeared in the severe category. I concluded that the high rate of abscess during X-Group times could be attributed

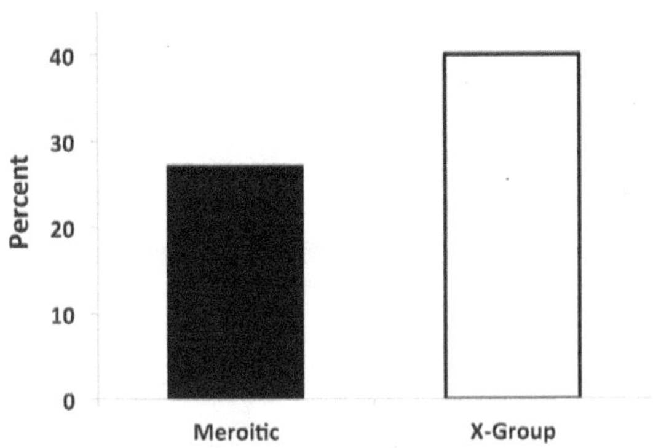

Figure 5.11. Percent frequency of occlusal caries.

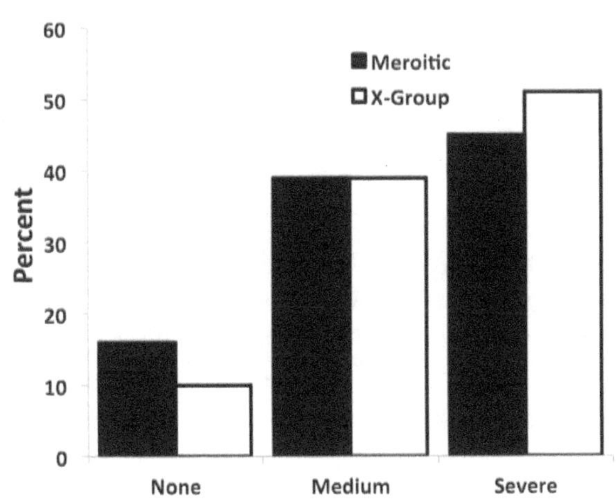

Figure 5.12. Percent frequencies by degree of wear.

primarily to the ultimate causes of increased wear in combination with an increase in occlusal caries. I argued further that this interpretation made sense from a biocultural point of view.

The transition from the Meroitic to the X-Group period represented a shift from an urbanized to a more agrarian lifestyle. Adams characterized it as an emergence of local "hegemony" (Adams 1965:167). There was far less trade, and most material goods (including agricultural products) were produced locally. A new technology was also added to the mix. The saqia (animal-driven waterwheel) made year-round irrigation possible. It also made it possible to irrigate further back from the river. New crops were also introduced, including wheat and pear millet (Edwards 2004). It's interesting that current stable isotope research supports the interpretation I made almost a half century ago. The isotopic data indicates a significant increase in millet production during X-Group times (White and Schwartz 1994). Millet has high levels of selenium (4 parts per million), which is known to be cariogenic. It's particularly satisfying that I had also suggested a link between selenium and caries in my dissertation. Finally, while I had no direct evidence, it seemed likely to me that the cereals and other food products arrived at the X-Group family table less refined than in times past. Less-refined foods would certainly be more abrasive to the teeth.

George loved recounting the story of his dental analysis because it illustrated how simple frequencies revealed interesting patterns that would have remained invisible without them.

Osteoporosis

A second analysis of the adults focused on age-related bone loss, or osteoporosis (Armelagos et al. 1976; Armelagos et al. 1972; Armelagos and Martin 1990). I introduced osteoporosis briefly in chapter 3 as part of the discussion of paleodemography. Bone is a dynamic, living tissue designed to support and protect organs and muscles. It renews itself as it ages and repairs itself when damaged. It can change its shape in response to new mechanical demands, and it stores the minerals necessary for life itself. All of this is made possible by two basic processes. In addition to its roles in support and protection, bone stores and releases minerals vital to virtually every physiological process necessary to sustain life (Arnold 1960). Storage occurs when bone is produced, and minerals are released when bone is resorbed. Ideally the two processes remain in balance, but in reality, there is a shift toward excess resorption as we age. The result is a condition known as osteoporosis or osteopenia.[2] Age-related bone loss is of particular importance to elderly women (Agarwal and Grynpas 1996). While men are less affected, the average woman may lose as much as 40 percent of her bone volume in the years following menopause. Given that the fastest growing age group in the United States is 85+, postmenopausal bone loss has become a household word as more and more elderly women (and some men) break hips and collapse vertebrae due to bone loss. The condition's social cost (Cauley 2013) in pain and suffering, as well as in medical dollars, continues to rise. In 2008, there were 340,000 hip fractures related to osteoporotic bone loss (one every minute) (Kim et al. 2012), with a medical cost approximating $22 billion (Blume and Curtis 2011).

Our interest in osteoporosis was stimulated by a comment made by a physical anthropologist named Saul Jarcho back in 1964 in his book titled *Some Observations on Diseases in Prehistoric North America* (Jarcho 1964). He suggested that osteoporosis had not been demonstrated in prehistoric populations. George realized that the Wadi Halfa skeletons provided excellent skeletal material to evaluate Jarcho's suggestion. The material consisted of the proximal (upper) portion of the femurs, including the head and about one-third of the shaft. The budget only permitted those and a few of the pathological specimens to be shipped back to Colorado. The femurs had been chosen for blood typing as a complement to Greene's genetic analysis of the dentition (Gabora 2006; Greene 1967b, 1972, 1973, 1982). Both the pathologies and the femur sections had followed George to the University of Utah. Many of the pathologies will be presented as cases for the first time in the next chapter. Now back to the first osteoporosis story.

One afternoon, George and I were showing the Wadi Halfa material to Murray Bartley, an M.D. and bone biologist from the University of Utah's medical school. Bartley was, at that time, involved in a large clinical study of osteoporosis. As he examined the femur sections he commented, "This is interesting; they have osteoporosis." George immediately made the connection to Jarcho and over a half century of research into the question of osteoporosis began.

John Dewey took on the first osteoporosis project for his master's thesis. He decided to assess bone loss by measuring cortical thickness at six points (figure 5.13) around the cut surfaces of the femur shafts. His results (Dewey et al. 1969) were exciting (figure 5.14). He found that osteoporosis did occur in antiquity—at least in Nubian antiquity. As was the case with modern

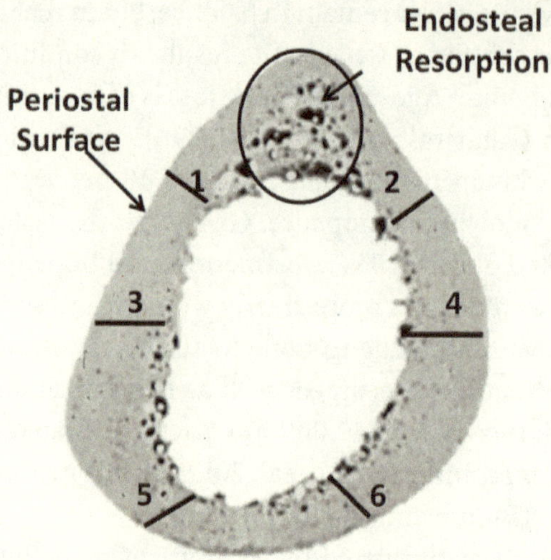

Figure 5.13. Measures of cortical bone thickness.

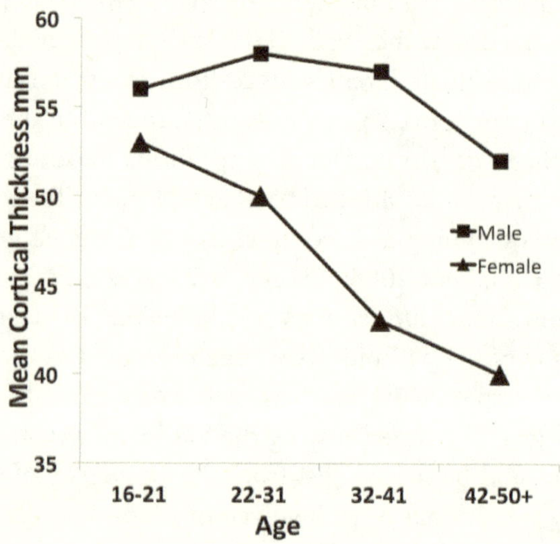

Figure 5.14. Mean cortical thickness in the combined Wadi Halfa samples.

populations, females lost bone with advancing age, while males did not. Indeed, males continued to add bone in their young adult years—probably as a result of their later maturation. There was, however, an intriguing difference among the females. Whereas modern females in the advantaged world do not begin to lose bone until around the fourth decade, with more rapid loss after menopause, the Nubian females began losing bone rapidly as young adults. Like all good research, that discovery led to more research down the road.

John's project also made an important contribution to clinical research. Clinical measures of bone loss had to rely on X-rays. A subject's femur was X-rayed from above, and two measures of cortical thickness were taken directly from the image (figure 5.15) (Smith and Walker 1964). The two measures were then assumed to represent the amount of bone present around the bone's entire circumference. By measuring thickness at six places, John determined that bone loss varied from one area to the next (note the differences in figure 5.13).

As we have done so often, the osteoporosis research begun at Wadi Halfa was extended to Kulubnarti. Age changes in cortical thickness at Kulubnarti (figure 5.16) were strikingly similar to the pattern at Wadi Halfa (Van

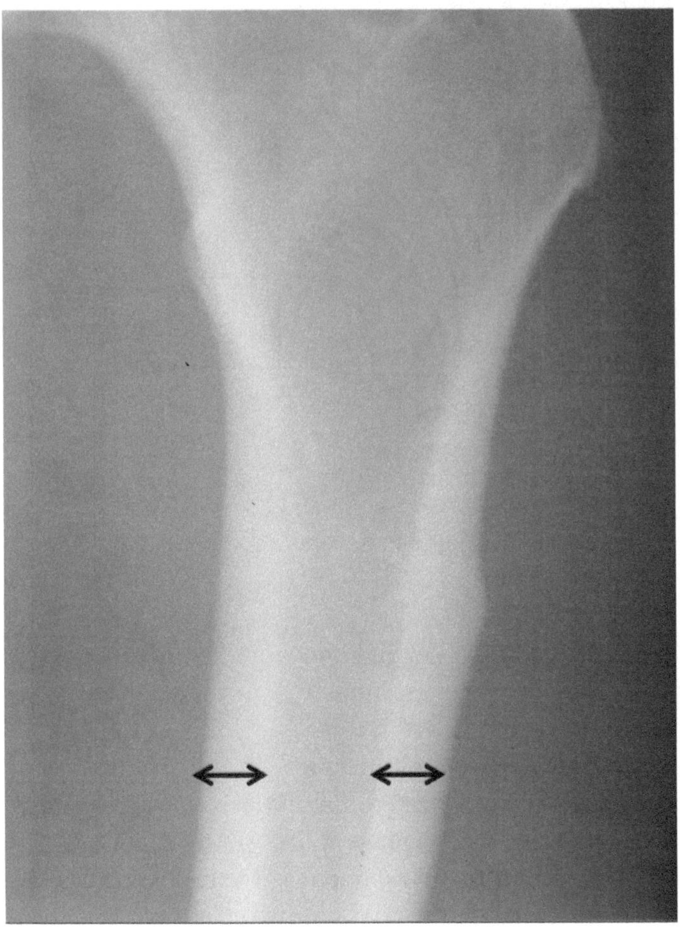

Figure 5.15. Radiographic measures of cortical thickness.

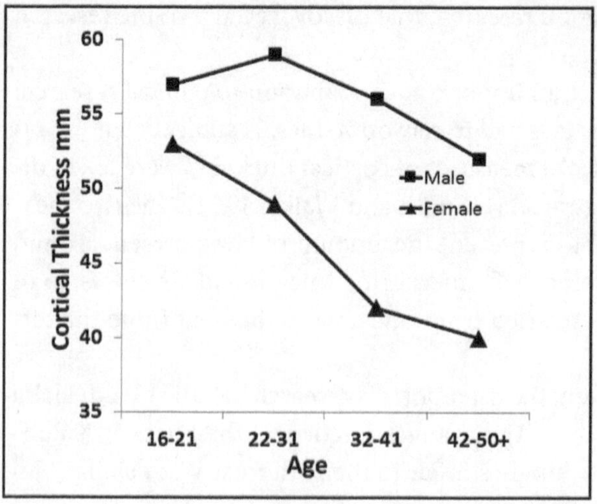

Figure 5.16. Mean cortical thickness for the combined Kulubnarti samples.

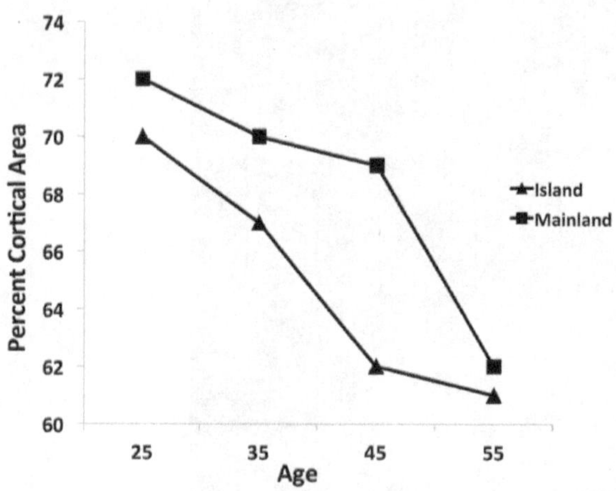

Figure 5.17. Percent cortical area for the Kulubnarti females as they age.

Gerven et al. 1990). Males continued to add bone until their early thirties (ages 22–31), while females began losing bone in their middle teens (ages 16–21).

While it was necessary to use cortical thickness for our comparisons to Wadi Halfa,[3] we compared the Kulubnarti communities to each other using percent cortical area.[4] By using a percentage value, we were able to avoid any body size effect.[5] Because there was no important bone loss among the males, we focused on the females. The community differences in female bone loss were consistent with the health differences observed in the infants and children. The island females started with less bone and lost bone more quickly in their younger years (figure 5.17), and my grandmother knew why. She told me about an old saying that went like this: "Have a baby, lose a tooth." While she had no way to know it, she was describing the mineral cost necessary to supply adequate nutrition to babies in the womb and on the breast.

As our studies of cortical thickness and percent cortical area continued, it became clear that we had to move on. Measuring bone loss at the organ level had told us all it was going to. George began envisioning the next step—moving from the organ to the tissue. We knew that bone loss involved the release of minerals into the body, so measuring the relationship between bone loss and bone mineral content was a logical next step. Before we present the research, we once again need a biological baseline.

The Biological Baseline

Bone consists of two major components. There is the inorganic mineral portion, and there is the organic collagen protein. If bone were entirely mineral it would be brittle and fracture like chalk. On the other hand, if bone had no mineral, it would be rubbery like the cartilage in your ear or at the end of your nose. The combination of mineral and collagen produces a bone that is strong (able to resist stress and strain) without being brittle.

The most abundant minerals in bone are calcium and phosphorus. Together, they constitute 65 percent of bone mass. Ninety-nine percent of the calcium and 85 percent of our body's phosphorus is stored in bone. Half of our body's magnesium is also stored in bone. There are, in addition, minor and trace elements such as boron, copper, fluoride, iron, silicon, zinc, and vanadium. Deposits and withdrawals of minerals are made according to bodily needs.

The Bone Mineral Study

The bone mineral study on the Wadi Halfa femurs was undertaken by a master's student named Kipling Owen. If he were conducting his study today, he would use the bone mineral analyzer discussed in the previous chapter. Without it, he took a series of simple low-tech steps. First, cubes of trabecular bone were removed from the femur head (Armelagos et al. 1972). The cubes were then filled with wax (trabecular bone is extremely

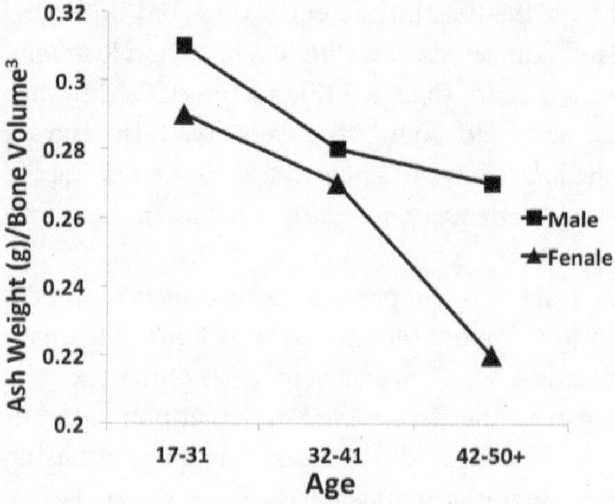

Figure 5.18. Bone mineral content for the combined Wadi Halfa samples.

porous), and their volumes were measured. The wax and bone collagen were then burned away in a kiln, leaving only the mineral ash. Finally, the ash was weighed in grams per unit volume of bone.

His results confirmed what we had inferred for females, but not for males (figure 5.18). Female bone mineral content behaved virtually the same way as females' cortical bone: bone mineral content decreased with age, with a rapid decrease at menopause. Males, on the other hand, behaved differently. Even though they had not lost a significant amount of cortical bone with age, they did lose a significant amount of mineral. It appeared that the males lost bone quality even though they hadn't lost bone quantity at the organ level. Still, relative to their female counterparts, they remained ahead of the game.

The Histology of Bone

The bone mineral study was an important first step in the shift from organ to tissue analysis, but George wanted to take the research a step further. Back in 1965, a biological anthropologist by the name of Ellis Kerley had developed a method for estimating age at death based on microscopic changes in bone tissue (Kerley 1965). George believed that Kerley's approach was limiting. Once microscopic changes were used to estimate age, the changes couldn't be used to study the consequences of aging. George's plan was to estimate age at death using the standard techniques and then investigate age changes in bone tissue at the microscopic level as a complement to

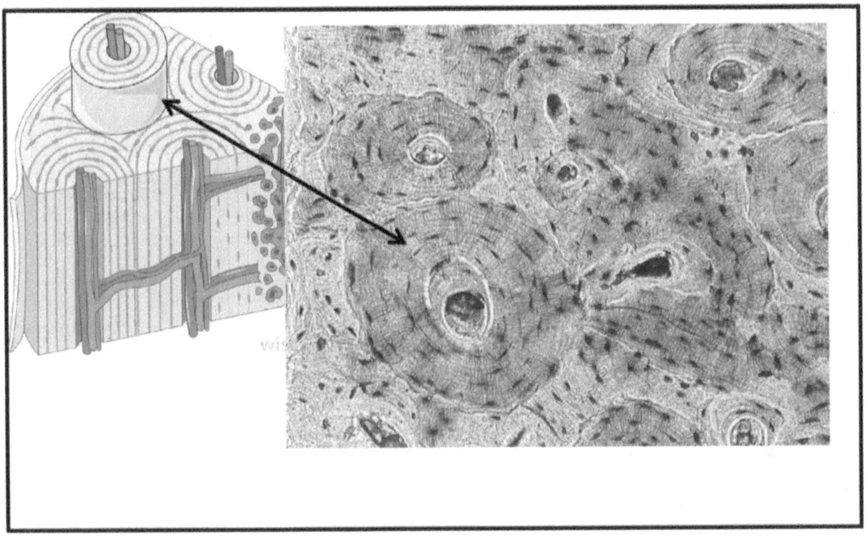

Figure 5.19. Osteons.

the bone mineral study. George's vision once again took the osteoporosis research in a new direction, and once again we need some baseline information to appreciate it.

Let's start with bone as seen through a microscope (figure 5.19). The most predominant features are osteons. Osteons are composed of concentric layers of bone surrounding a central Haversian canal. The canal contains a neuro-vascular bundle consisting of a vein, an artery, and a nerve. The rings are separated by small rice-shaped capsules. Each capsule (called an osteocyte lacuna) contains a cell known as an osteocyte. Osteocytes are the living, cellular components of bone. They were originally the cells that created the layers of bone between which they are embedded. Osteocytes are nourished by way of a network of tiny canals (canaliculi) connecting them to each other and to the vein and artery in the neuro-vascular bundle. Osteons range in size, but generally are about 0.3 millimeters (300 microns) in diameter and 3–5 millimeters in length.

Osteon creation is a two-step process (figure 5.20). Cells known as osteoclasts excavate tunnels spanning the width and length of what will be a new osteon. As the tunnel is advancing at one end, bone-forming cells known as osteoblasts are creating successive layers of new bone at the other. Osteoblasts become osteocytes once they become surrounded in bone. The rate at which new osteons are created varies with the age of the individual.

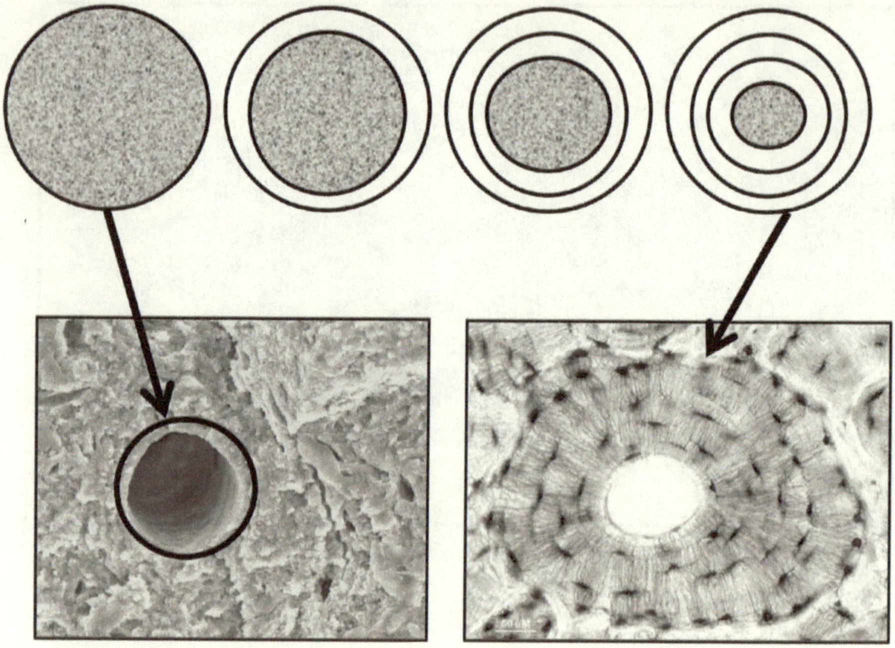

Figure 5.20. Osteon creation.

It takes 46 days for a 10-year-old to produce one, whereas it takes 108 days for a 60-year-old (Lips et al. 1978).

New excavations by osteoclasts inevitably encroach into the spaces occupied by older osteons. The consequence is an ever-increasing accumulation of osteon fragments. You can liken the process to the accumulation of partial footprints as the same ground is repeatedly walked over. The longer the ground is walked over, the more partial footprints there are. A typical cross section also contains forming osteons and resorption spaces excavated in preparation for the construction of new osteons (figure 5.21).

The continuous resorption and formation of osteons (bone turnover) performs three important functions. First, it rejuvenates the skeleton with new tissue. It is estimated that our entire skeleton is replaced about every ten years. As pointed out earlier, bone resorption and formation are also the mechanisms by which minerals move in and out of the skeleton. When mineral needs exceed supply through dietary sources, resorption rates exceed the rates of formation. The result is the loss of the bone tissue observed in the cortical bone studies and the loss of mineral observed in Kipling Owen's study. Bone can be replaced during times of dietary surplus.

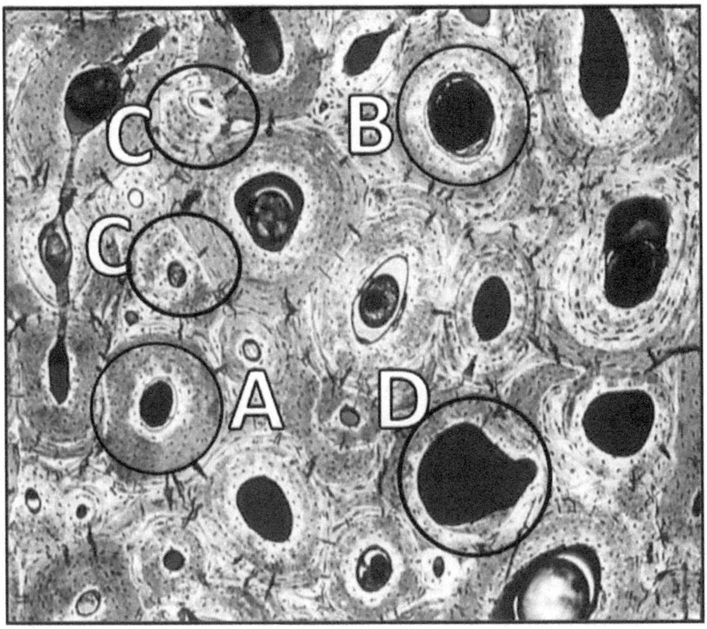

Figure 5.21. Whole osteons (A), forming osteons (B), osteon fragments (C), and resorption spaces (D).

Poor nutrition isn't the only cause of an imbalance between rates of resorption and formation leading to osteoporosis. A decrease in estrogen production in postmenopausal women can result in what is referred to as senile osteoporosis. The clinical use of protein pump inhibitors to treat acid reflux and steroids used to treat inflammatory diseases can also depress bone formation. Diseases such as diabetes and hypothyroidism can also disrupt the balance between formation and resorption. Inactivity is another source of bone loss. Bone requires constant stimulation by bending forces to maintain normal turnover. Without these forces, bone formation is depressed. Astronauts experienced measurable bone loss during periods of weightlessness in the early days of the space program. They now follow an exercise regime during their flights. There are videos showing astronauts riding stationary bicycles while in space.

Beyond their role in mineral transport, osteons also play an important role in the repair of bone tissue. Structural materials of all kinds subjected to frequent stresses and strains develop structural fatigue. Tiny microfractures can accumulate to the point that the material fails. This is a problem for airplane wings and bridge struts. The same is true for bone. The bones in our body are continuously subjected to bending forces resulting in microfractures. If these aren't repaired, a bone can fail. Osteons trap and repair microfractures. An analogy is a crack spreading across the surface of a frozen pond. The crack can run only until it reaches a hole in the ice. The hole traps it. David Burr has studied this process and found that once an osteon has trapped the spread of a microfracture, new osteons are created along the crack to repair it (Burr 1993).

The Bone Histology Studies

Debra Martin took on the problem of measuring microscopic-level age changes in the Wadi Halfa femurs for her Ph.D. dissertation. The necessary thin sections of cortical bone had already been prepared while George was at the University of Utah.[6] Her data included frequency counts of whole osteons, osteon diameters, partially completed osteons, resorption spaces, and osteon fragments.[7] The counts and measurements were made using a microscope fitted with a grid in one eyepiece. The grid superimposed an image over the scope's field of vision and was employed like the grid used in the macroscopic studies. She took her measurements in eight fields,[8] each covering 0.235 square centimeters of surface. The fields were positioned to measure tissue activity at the inner (endosteal) and outer (periosteal) surfaces (figure 5.22).

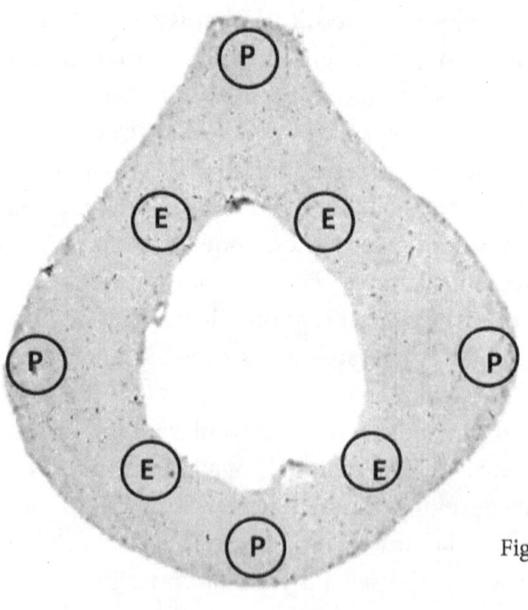

Figure 5.22. Measurement fields.

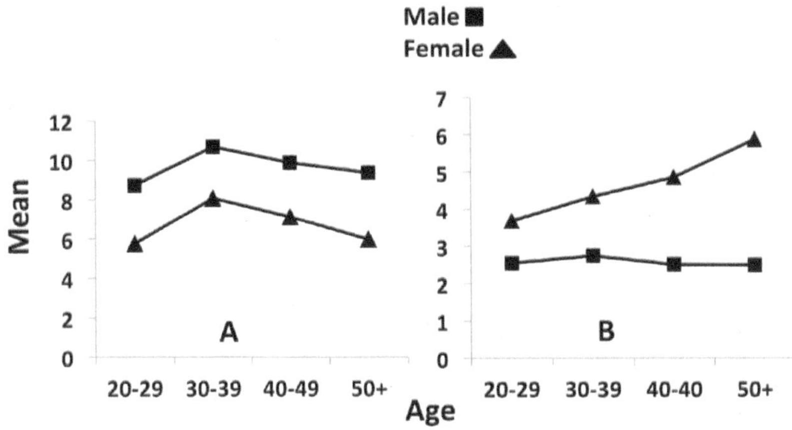

Figure 5.23. Mean number of intact osteons (A) and osteon fragments (B) per square millimeter.

Debra's results corroborated what had been seen macroscopically (figure 5.23). While both sexes showed parallel changes in whole osteon numbers (females consistently had fewer), the number of osteon fragments diverged significantly between the sexes. The number of fragments underwent virtually no changes with age among the males but increased by 37 percent among the females. It was also interesting that just as the youngest females had already begun to lose bone at the organ level, they were accumulating osteon fragments at the microscopic level, just as would be expected. I remember how excited George was to see the way in which Debra's tissue-level analysis corresponded to what John Dewey had seen macroscopically. But this is only one aspect of what Debra was able to accomplish. Debra went on to apply her results to questions of diet and general health (Martin and Armelagos 1985).

Once again, the Wadi Halfa research laid the foundation for microscopic-level analyses at Kulubnarti. Dawn Mulhern conducted a histological analysis of the femurs for her master's thesis and on the ribs for her doctoral thesis (Mulhern and Van Gerven 1997; Mulhern 2000). She is now a professor of anthropology at Fort Lewis College in Durango, Colorado. The results of both analyses were consistent with Martin's results as well as those obtained from other archaeological populations (Martin and Armelagos 1979; Stout 1978). But her work wasn't limited to a repetition of previously done research. There was an aspect of her research that we both found intriguing. Male osteon sizes in the femurs were consistently smaller

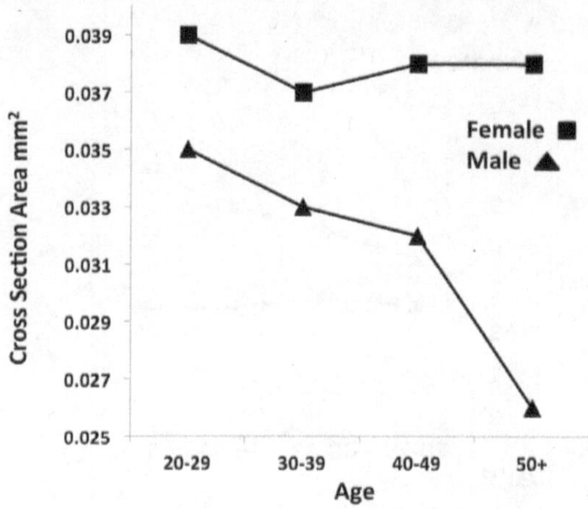

Figure 5.24. Sex differences in osteon size at Kulubnarti.

in comparison to females (figure 5.24). They also decreased in size with age, while female osteon sizes did not.

David Burr had found a similar difference in remains from Pecos Pueblo (Burr et al. 1990). The Pecos males had more intact and smaller osteons. While Dawn was rightly disinclined to propose any explanation with certainty, she cited research suggesting that smaller, more tightly packed osteons, like the ones she observed in the femurs, may enhance the bone's resistance to fatigue (Corondan and Haworth 1986). Could sex differences in the fatigue properties of the femur reflect some sex differences in behavior at Kulubnarti? Could the behavior have been gendered as we discussed earlier? Dawn's rib analysis provided some support for that interpretation. She found no differences in osteon size in the rib—a non-weight-bearing bone.

While there is always some danger in the use of ethnographic analogy, males today are responsible for the heavy work of field preparation, while females tend the fields and livestock. Lynn Kilgore, another of my doctoral students, also found a higher rate of arthritic changes in the lumbar spine among males, suggesting higher frequencies of heavy physical activity. Does this prove the strain hypothesis? No, but it supports a strong inference. It also lays the foundation for future inquiry. Good research always does that.

Oakley Sunglasses in King Tut's Tomb

What if an archaeologist had found a pair of Oakley sunglasses in King Tut's tomb? Something very much like that happened to Debra Martin when she was doing her histology study. The story began one day when she was working in a bone research laboratory at Henry Ford Hospital directed by Harold Frost, a physician and good friend of George's. She was intending to measure the thickness of her bone sections, but a regular light-transmitting scope wasn't available, so she used a microscope that transmitted fluorescent light instead. A microscope transmitting fluorescent light may seem odd, but it had an important function. It was used to measure bone turnover rates in patients after they had been given two doses of an antibiotic called tetracycline.

Tetracycline was developed as an antibacterial "wonder drug" back in the 1950s. It was particularly effective in the treatment of staph infections caused by *Staphylococcus aureus*.

The bacterium has become tetracycline-resistant over time, and today the antibiotic is used to treat acne and periodontal disease. But tetracycline has two important properties critical to measuring bone turnover rates. First, it is attracted to bone, and second, it glows bright yellow under fluorescent light when present in bone tissue.

If you are prescribed tetracycline, you will notice an instruction on the label: *do not take with dairy products*. You see, tetracycline binds to calcium. If you take it with a glass of milk, it binds to the calcium in the milk and goes through your digestive system without being absorbed into your bloodstream. Of course, your bone is full of calcium; so every time you take tetracycline it binds to the calcium in forming osteons. Tetracycline is called a "bone seeker" for that reason. You will occasionally see people with mottled and discolored enamel on their teeth. The damage was caused by taking too much tetracycline when the enamel on their teeth was forming.

This makes tetracycline a wonderful "label" for measuring bone formation rates.[9] A patient is given a dose of tetracycline on day one and then a second dose after a specified number of days. Then, after a second number of days, a biopsy is taken from a rib (ribs heal well after biopsy) and examined under a fluorescent scope (Frost et al. 1960). Two fluorescent bands appear within the osteons that were forming at the time of the dosages. The distance between the bands represents the amount of bone made during the interval between doses.

Many of the osteons in Martin's sections were glowing bright yellow

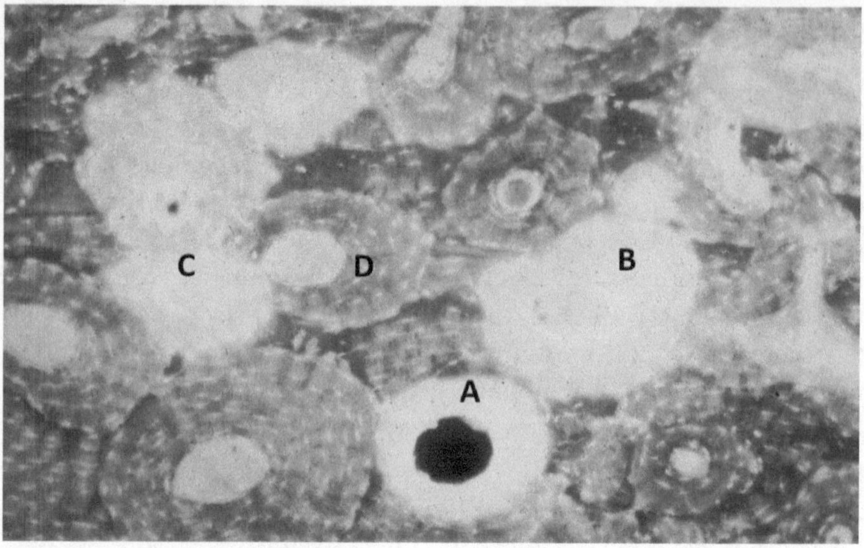

Figure 5.25. Tetracycline labeling.

under her scope's fluorescent light (figure 5.25). It appeared that the Wadi Halfa Nubians were taking tetracycline some 1,500 years before it was "discovered" by modern science. Debra had made an astounding discovery all because a light microscope was being used by another student.

There was one difference between her labels and biopsy specimens. There weren't tetracycline bands within the osteons. The labeling occurred across the entire osteons (figure 5.25a–c) (Bassett et al. 1980). It appeared that the antibiotic was being taken continuously—at least through the time it takes to fill an osteon, which is about 80 days.

As you might imagine, such a surprising discovery did not go unchallenged. Some critics suspected that the bone had been contaminated by invading bacteria producing similar fluorescence (Piepenbrink 1986). Others proposed that the natural processes of decay had produced the fluorescence (Keith and Armelagos 1983, 1988). However, histology supported the tetracycline hypothesis. Labeling occurred within the boundaries of osteons just as it does clinically. Boundaries were maintained even when labeled osteons encroached on those that are unlabeled (figure 5.25c). Such boundaries wouldn't have existed if the substance had been introduced by diffusion. Finally, Mark Nelson and colleagues extracted tetracycline from the Wadi Halfa skeletons. It had the same properties as the modern drug (Nelson et al. 2011). A follow-up study on the Kulubnarti remains found the same labeling with the same properties (Hummert and Van Gerven 1982).

The presence of tetracycline naturally raised an important question. How, and perhaps why, was it being ingested? There were interesting clues. Natural tetracycline is produced by *Streptomycetes* bacteria in soil. The bacteria lived in exactly the kind of dry, hot, alkaline soil found in Nubia. The *Streptomycetes* produce mold that contains tetracycline, much like a bacterium produces penicillin. It initially seemed that consumption of molded grain near the end of the growing season might be the explanation for labeling.

The molded grain hypothesis didn't stand the test of time. It turned out that grain contamination in and of itself would have been insufficient to explain the amount of tetracycline observed in the bone. Something had to be amplifying the bacteria before it was consumed. There was good evidence that the mechanism was beer. Representations in both Egypt and Nubia always show bread production and beer production together. The beer was not the beer of today. It was most likely a food as well as a beverage (Kemp 1989). It was low in alcohol content, with a consistency much like cereal gruel. It has been demonstrated experimentally that beer produced from *Streptomycetes*-molded bread amplifies the bacterium tremendously.

There is also a clue from modern times. Egyptians today use beer as a remedy for various illnesses, and there is similar evidence for a belief in beer's medicinal value going back to ancient times (Darby et al. 1977). Beer was used:

- To treat the gums by rinsing the mouth;
- To strengthen the gums;
- As an enemata;
- As a vaginal douche;
- As a wound dressing;
- To treat disease of the anus using anal fumigant.

There is a final clue supporting the beer hypothesis. Low in alcohol as it was, beer likely had substantial nutritional value for children and adults alike. This may explain the presence of tetracycline labeling across all ages in the Wadi Halfa remains.

There's a last question worth consideration. So what? What value does the discovery of tetracycline in long-dead Nubians have? As difficult as it may be to understand in a practical-minded society, the answer may be simply "because it's interesting." It's another interesting thing that we've learned about the Nubian past. Discoveries with no practical value can be worthwhile. There may also be some practical value that we cannot anticipate today. Armelagos and coworkers found no evidence of bacterial resistance to the antibiotic so commonly observed today (Armelagos et al. 2001). They argued that were resistance occurring, there should be a rise in the frequency of infectious lesions in the bones. No increase was observed. It may be that the disease load was not great enough to create the bacterial competition necessary for the evolution of resistance (Wiener 1996). This may indeed contribute to greater practical understanding of bacterial evolution today. The tetracycline work gave us an additional understanding of how culture and biology interact. In this case, the linkages between bread, beer, tetracycline, and possibly the course of infectious disease connect the ancient and modern world. Modern ethnographic and historical evidence provides concrete evidence for such linkages.

Woody Allen once said that 85 percent of life is showing up. Debra Martin showed up in Frost's lab. She couldn't find the microscope she was looking for, and we ended up knowing a little more about the human condition. We can't create if we don't show up, and if nothing else, the tetracycline work reminds us of that.

Trauma at Kulubnarti

> "You're nobody unless somebody's signed your cast."
>
> Dean Martin, singer and comedian (1917–1995)

It shouldn't come as a surprise that bone fractures "are never a matter of chance." We don't break bones randomly. We do things that cause us to break bones, and the more we do those things, the more likely it is we'll break a bone doing them. I made the point with my students by asking them to guess how the frequency of wrist fractures (called Collie fractures) changed after introduction of the skateboard. Thomas Burger and Erik Trinkhaus examined fractures among Neanderthals and found that the location and kind of fractures found closely resembled those observed among rodeo cowboys (Burger and Trinkhaus 1995). They suggested that this may reflect hunting large animals with a spear (figure 5.26). Hunting with a spear as opposed to a bow and arrow requires close contact. Fracture studies are a major aspect of the study of occupational stress in ancient populations (Lovell 2008; Judd and Roberts 1998; Judd 2002).

We were struck by the high frequency of fractures when we were packing the skeletons (figure 5.27) to ship them back to the States. As high as the frequencies were, the actual numbers in the community were certainly higher. We were only recognizing those with some degree of healing. Those

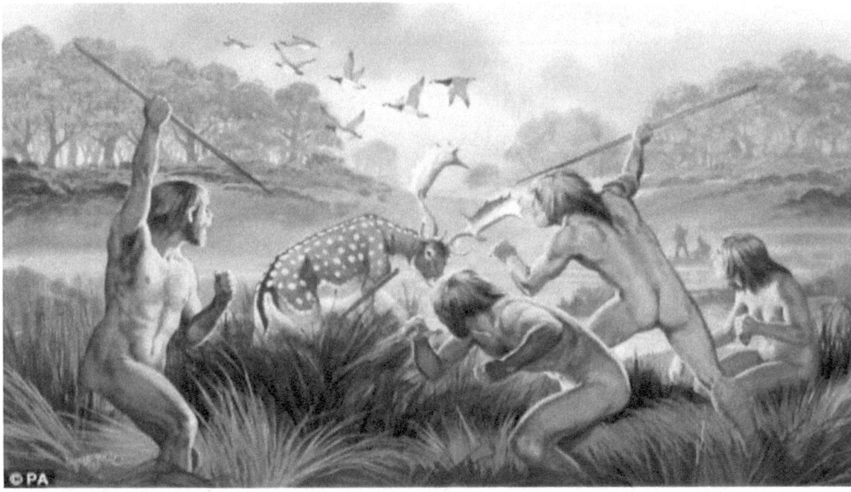

Figure 5.26. Neanderthal hunting.

occurring at or very near the time of death are often impossible to distinguish from postmortem damage. Fortunately, healing begins quite quickly. First, blood clots at the fracture site. Osteons then construct a patch using material from the fracture. The patch is then mineralized into a callus (figure 5.27b, c). A fracture will typically heal completely within 250–300 days. However, if the patch is insufficient to stabilize the fracture, the result can be a non-union fracture (figure 5.27a).

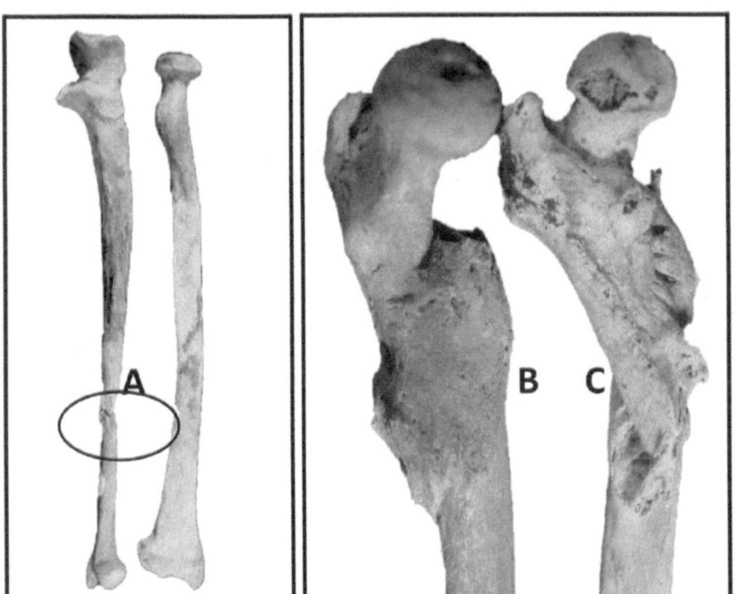

Figure 5.27. Non-union ulna fracture (A) and femur fractures (B, C).

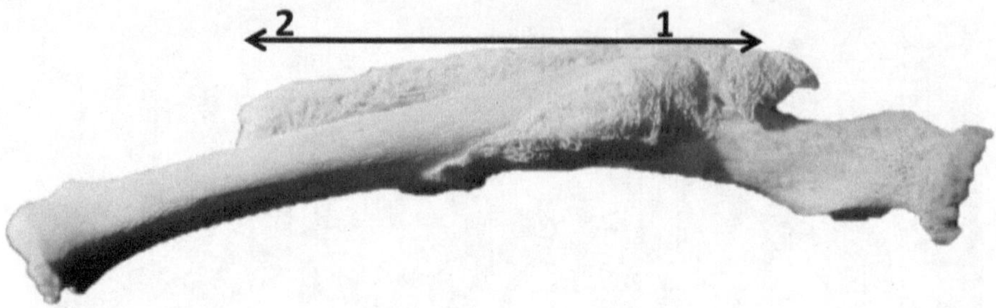

Figure 5.28. A fractured infant femur.

Fractured femurs at Kulubnarti were particularly dramatic. In every case, the two sides of the shaft were pulled apart and then slipped into a side-by-side position (figures 5.27b, c, 5.28). This was likely a result of contraction (spasm) of the powerful quadriceps and biceps muscles at the front and back of the shaft. Treatment was clearly beyond the ability of our Nubians. In fact, there is no evidence of any intervention in any of our fracture cases. There is one other point worth noting. Infants have what are referred to as "soft" bones due to their incomplete mineralization. It is not common for an infant to break a large limb bone without substantial force. If a modern infant appeared in an emergency room with the femur fracture illustrated in figure 5.28, there would be some suspicion of child abuse.

The Fracture Study

Lynn Kilgore (a former Ph.D. advisee and now adjunct professor) and her husband, Robert Jurmain (then a professor of anthropology at San Jose State University in California), analyzed fractures in the Kulubnarti adults in 1997 (Kilgore et al. 1997). Owen Lovejoy had recently completed a study of fractures in skeletons from the site of Libben in Ohio (Lovejoy and Heiple 1981). Because his sample was large, he was able to do an elaborate risk analysis for various skeletal elements. Our sample (66 males and 80 females) was much smaller, making a risk analysis impossible. Nevertheless, by following George's example and placing our faith in simple frequencies, interesting patterns emerged.

The first thing that became apparent was the high frequency of fractures. Thirty-five percent of the island adults and 32 percent of the mainland adults had at least one (figure 5.29). There was only a 2 percent difference by sex (figure 5.30). It appeared that whatever the causes, males and females in both communities shared a similar risk. What appeared extraordinary

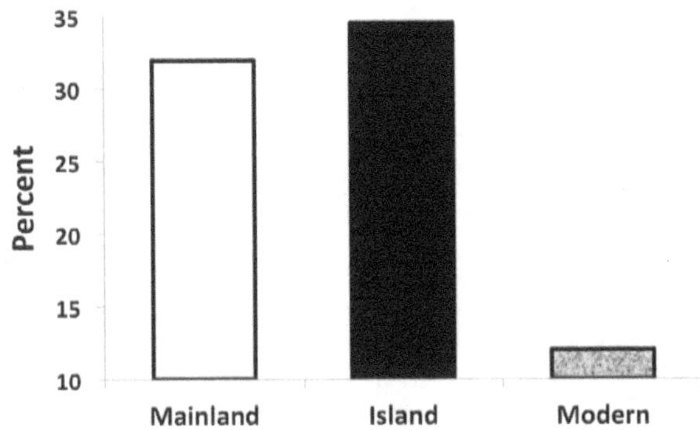

Figure 5.29. Percentage of individuals with at least one fracture.

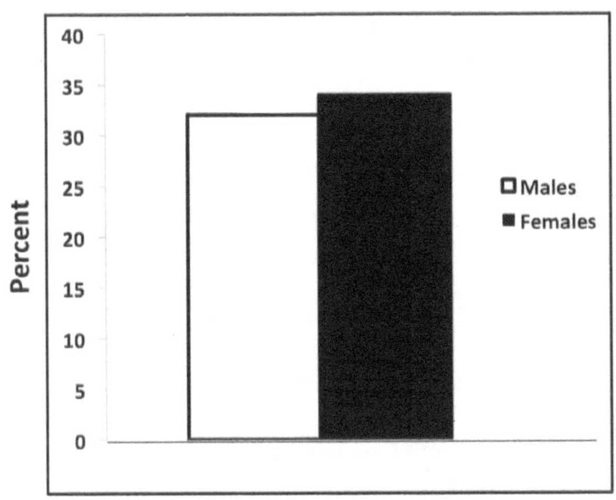

Figure 5.30. Male and female fracture frequencies.

was the frequency of ulna fractures compared to other archaeological populations (figures 5.31, 5.32). When Lynn and Bob compared Kulubnarti to four other archaeological populations, they found that ulna fracture frequencies were more than double the next highest population. In fact, every frequency that exceeded the comparative samples involved a bone of the upper limb (Kilgore et al. 1997). This couldn't be a matter of chance. It reflected the setting in which the Kulubnarti folk lived.

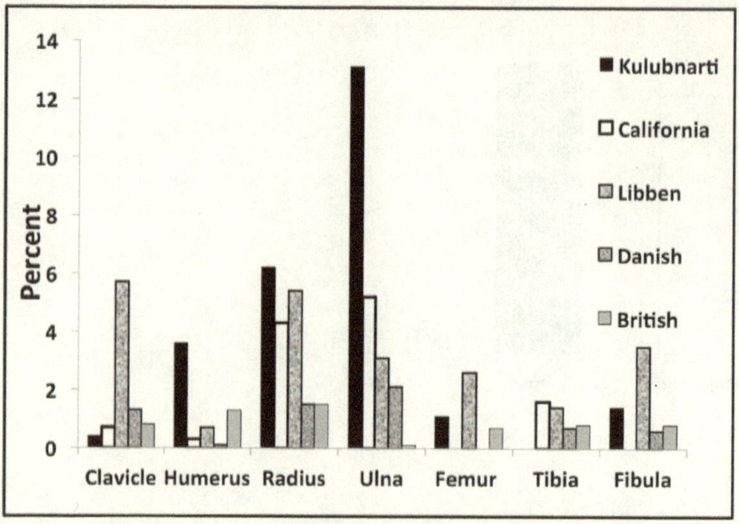

Figure 5.31. Fracture frequencies in five archaeological populations.

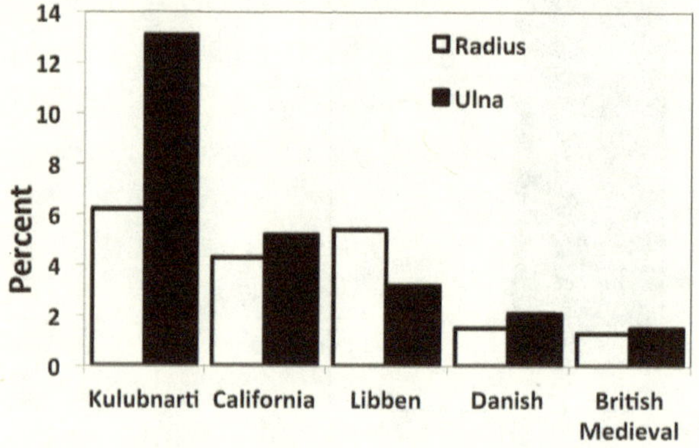

Figure 5.32. Frequency of radius and ulna fractures in five archaeological populations.

Remember, Kulubnarti is located along an 80-mile stretch of river called the *Batn el Hajar* (Belly of Rock). Adams (1977) has referred to the region as lunar. Giant granite boulders dominate the area, extending into the river itself. Agriculture is limited to small patches of alluvial soil deposited at bends in the river, and even then check dams were built in order to trap additional soil. Villages are located high on jebels overlooking the river in order to conserve what little ground is available for fields. As I said in chapter 1, Bill Adams once told me that there wasn't 300 feet of elevation from wadi bottom to jebel top, and not 3 square feet of level ground.[10]

Daily life consisted of a constant walk up the jebel over and around the boulders from village to fields. The natural response to a stumble and fall among the rocks is to break the fall by extending the arm. The bones most likely to break are in the wrist or the forearm, the distal ulna being the most common.

Up to this point, our focus has been on the Nubian communities (populations) of Wadi Halfa and Kulubnarti. We have extolled the virtues of a population approach. But we cannot lose sight of the fact that populations are composed of individuals. No picture of ancient times can be complete without such stories.

6

CASE STUDIES

> In the last analysis, the essential thing is the life of the individual. This alone makes history.
>
> C. G. Jung

Messages

In the years leading up to the Civil War, volumes had been written on the question of slavery, and statistics had been collected and compounded, correlated and tabulated. Antislavery passions ran high in the North, but it wasn't the statistics that raised them. It was a work of fiction. In 1852 Harriet Beecher Stowe penned the novel *Uncle Tom's Cabin*. The story of Tom, Eliza, and the wicked Simon Legree gave slavery a face. The book sold 30,000 copies in its first printing and galvanized the Northern states against slavery. It has been said that Abraham Lincoln referred to her as the little lady who caused the great war.

The Diary of Anne Frank and Elie Wiesel's *Night* gave the horrors of the Holocaust a reality far beyond what statistical analysis could convey. In anthropology, the case of Ishi, the last Yahi Indian, exemplified the wholesale destruction of native cultures around the world (Kroeber 1964). Like Anne Frank, Ishi is relevant to this day. His story was telecast in 1994 on NBC in an award-winning documentary titled *Ishi: The Last Yahi*. Case studies such as these are a time-honored tradition in both literature and the social sciences. Case studies make the abstract concrete.[1] Case studies are messages.

The same can be said for case studies of disease and injury in ancient human populations. Few students of paleontology have missed the case of the one-eyed, one-armed Neanderthal from Shanidar. His case raises important questions regarding Neanderthal mentality and the nature of their society. For example, did he require or receive compassion from his fellows? Or, put more broadly, were Neanderthals capable of compassion? Studies of Neanderthal cranial capacity or facial morphology are far less likely to raise those kinds of questions.

We present a series of case studies in this chapter hoping to raise similar questions for the next and last chapter. Like the cases of Ishi, Uncle Tom, and Anne Frank, our cases send us messages about what life was like for real people afflicted by disease and injury. Their stories are more intimate than our population studies. They are a vital part of our quest for a bioethnography.

We have organized our cases into four categories: neoplastic diseases, congenital defects, diseases of unknown etiology, and infectious diseases. Categories such as these, while useful for organizational purposes, inevitably impose some degree of artificiality. For example, we have placed rheumatoid arthritis (RA) in the category of diseases of unknown etiology (cause). Diseases of unknown etiology involve a host of contributing factors—some are likely to be genetic, and others environmental. It is known that RA is an immune system disease, but it is not known what causes the immune condition. Our case of hydrocephalus is categorized as a congenital defect. However, it can also be caused by an infection of the nervous system and trauma. In creating our categories, we have attempted to strike a balance between practicality and biology.

Neoplastic Diseases

The Biological Baseline

The term "neoplasm" derived from the Greek *neo* (new) and *plasm* (formation). Neoplasms are most often tumors that are either malignant or benign. Benign tumors do not invade other organs and tissues. Malignant (cancerous) tumors do. Hippocrates examined a woman with several lumps on her breast. Each had large blood vessels radiating from it producing a crablike appearance. They had also invaded (metastasized into) other tissues. He called her condition "karkinos," meaning crab in Greek. Karkinos was later translated into the Latin word "cancer."

The rate of spread varies greatly from one cancer to the next. For example, some prostate cancers are aggressive—meaning they metastasize quickly—while others spread slowly. Approximately 200,000 men are diagnosed with prostate cancer each year, and 30,000 will die. Most prostate cancers appear in men 65 or older. As a consequence, men are routinely screened (either by a digital exam or a PSA blood test) beginning in their mid-forties.

The most important question for a man after a positive diagnosis is what to do. Many doctors now recommend "watchful waiting," particularly in elderly men. The idea is to wait and see how the tumor behaves before performing surgery. If the cancer is aggressive, it is apt to spread quickly, often to bone. On the other hand, if the cancer is nonaggressive, an older man may live to die of something else.

Cancer is currently the second highest cause of death in America today, but rare in prehistory. A physical anthropologist by the name of Eugene Strouhal surveyed the literature in 1998 and found 176 reported cases in the Old World (Strouhal 2015). Even if that number has doubled as of today, cancers remain a rarity in the archaeological record. Whether the numbers represent evidence of rarity or a rarity of evidence is a matter of continuing debate. Whichever the case, the Wadi Halfa remains have contributed three cases to the archaeological record, and that is extraordinary.

Cancers metastasize most commonly from soft tissue to bone. Breast, lung, and prostate cancers are more likely to do so than others. There are also cancers that arise in bone. These sarcoma cancers are relatively rare compared to the metastatic types. All bone cancers result in some degree of bone destruction, and the differences among the various tumor types can be subtle. As a result, today's paleopathologists seek to incorporate as many kinds of evidence as possible when making a diagnosis, including evidence from gross morphology, histology, genetics, and X-ray. Because few of the Wadi Halfa remains were brought to the United States for long-term analysis, we were mostly limited to the morphological and photographic information collected in the field. We nevertheless have good confidence in the diagnoses we have made.

The Case of Metastatic Bladder Cancer

Our first case is a metastatic carcinoma. The victim was a middle-age Meroitic male. He had two large erosive (lytic) lesions in his skull at the time of his death. One was located on his frontal bone (figure 6.1a) and the second on his parietal (figure 6.1b). The edges of both were scalloped and porous due to beveling on the inner surface of the vault. This is indicative of an outward-growing mass. There were also internal blood vessel tracks radiating outward from the lesions in the crablike manner observed by Hippocrates.[2] There are four identical lesions on the postcranial skeleton—one on the left ilium (figure 6.2a), one on the fifth lumbar vertebra (figure

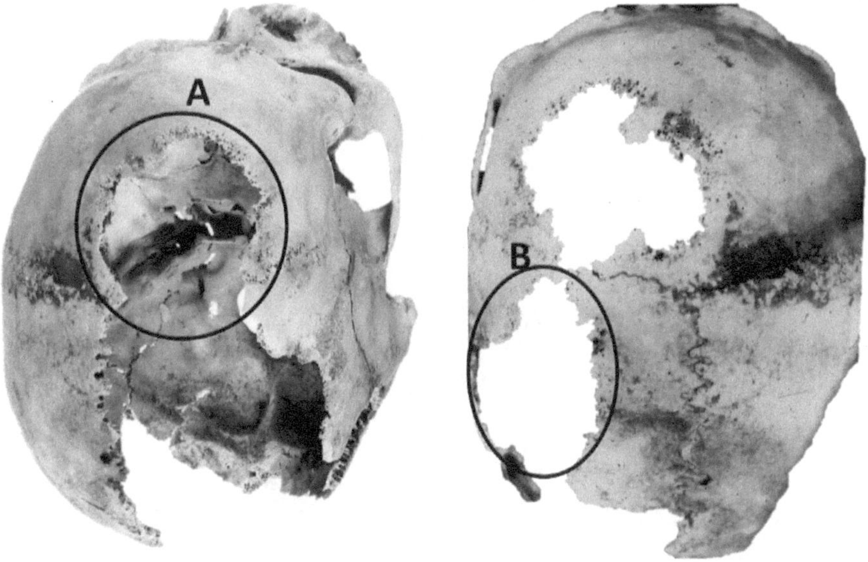

Figure 6.1. Laboratory (*left*) and field (*right*) photographs showing lesions of the frontal (A) and parietal (B) bones.

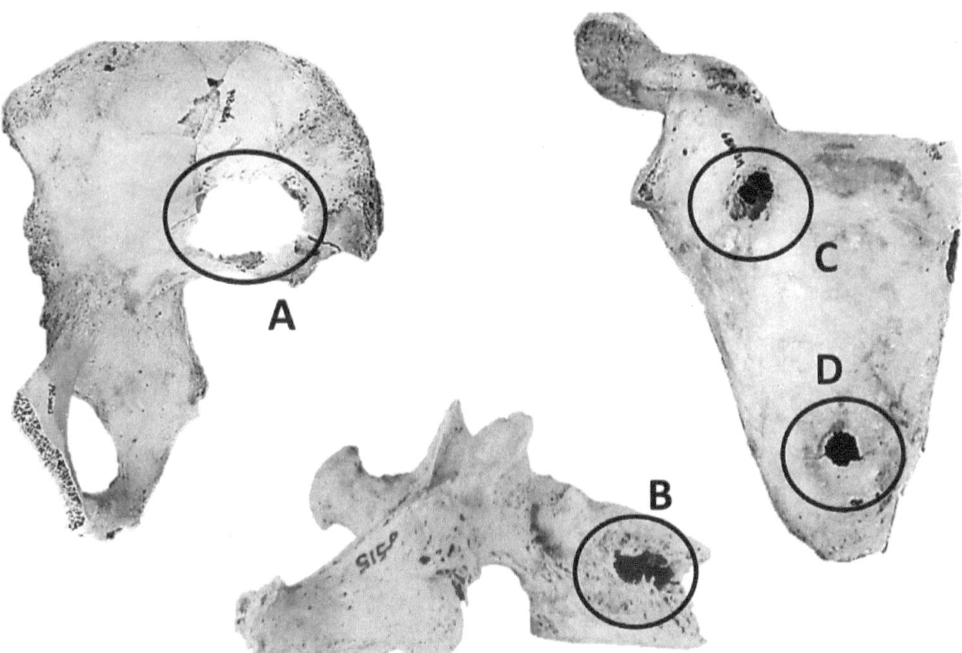

Figure 6.2. Lesions of the ilium (A), lumbar vertebra (B), and scapula (C,D).

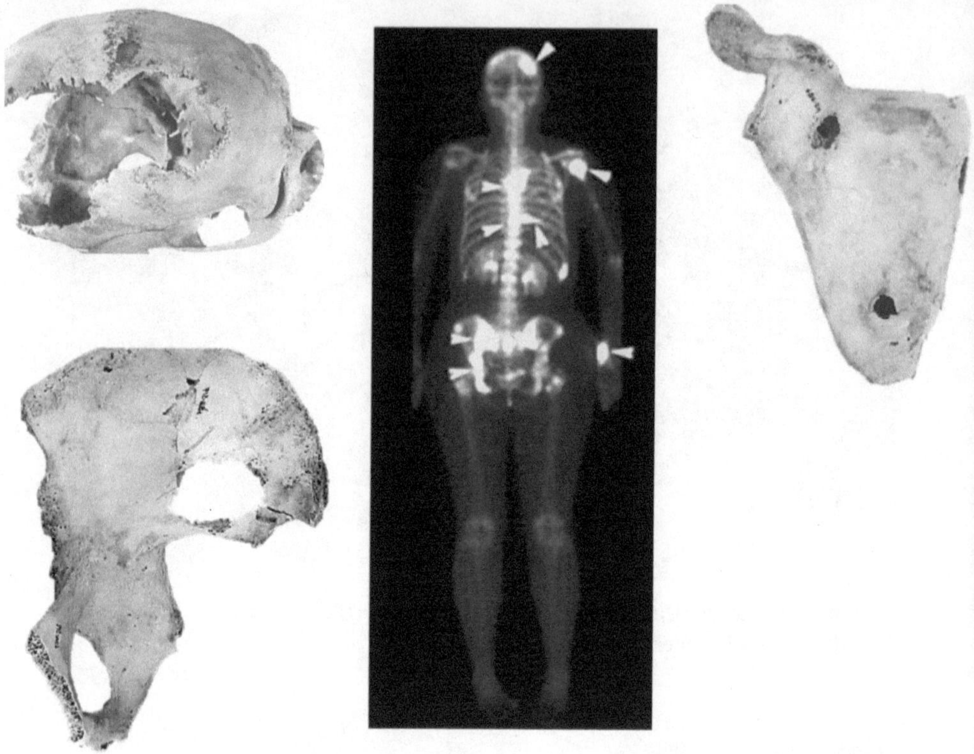

Figure 6.3. Common sites of metastatic carcinoma.

6.2b), and two on the right scapula (figure 6.2c, d). The morphology and distribution of all six lesions meet the criteria for a metastatic carcinoma. The lesions are lytic, well defined, scalloped and pitted at the margins, and variable in size. Lesion distribution also supports our diagnosis (figure 6.3). The skull, scapula, and pelvis are the most common areas affected. With a diagnosis established to our satisfaction, our next step was to place the condition in its biocultural context. What we found was a wonderful example of Wells's observation that diseases are never a matter of chance.

The context at Wadi Halfa and villages throughout Lower Nubia was irrigation agriculture based on an animal-driven waterwheel known as a saqia (figure 6.4). The saqia made it possible to extend agricultural fields farther beyond the river than before, as well as increase the number of crops that could be produced in a season. There was, however, a consequence that the villagers of Wadi Halfa could never have understood any more than slash-and-burn agriculturalists could have understood the connection between their slash-and-burn agriculture and malaria.

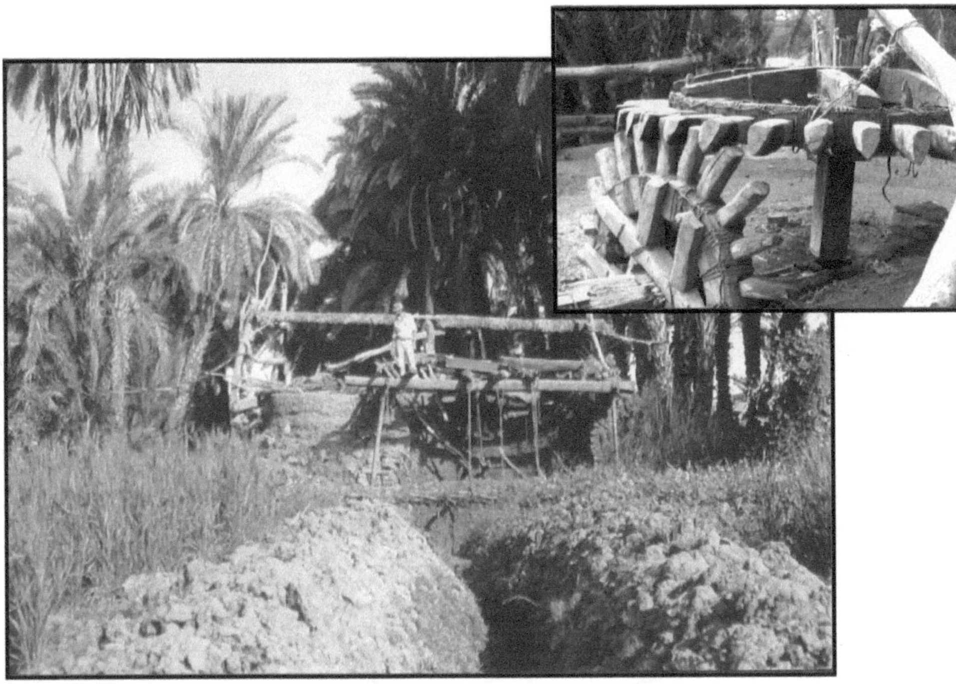

Figure 6.4. A saqia at Kulubnarti.

Ditch water full of organic matter, including human feces, provided an environment conducive to the growth of large populations of freshwater snails carrying a disease known as schistosomiasis. Schistosomiasis is an infectious disease—primarily of the liver—caused by a flatworm named *Schistosoma mansoni.* The human-snail-parasite relationship is cyclical. Infected humans deposit parasite eggs into the ditch by way of their feces. The eggs hatch and develop into a form of parasite capable of infecting snails, and once in the snail, they develop into the worm. Once the worms are released back into the ditch by the snails, they burrow through the skin of a human host tending the ditches, and then migrate to the liver.

Studies of contemporary populations have shown a clear link between contact with canal waters and exposure to schistosomiasis, not only in the Nile Valley but throughout Africa. Studies have also shown that the likelihood of infection increases with time spent cleaning and maintaining irrigation ditches. In settings where one gender spends more time at those tasks than the other, the rates of infection are correspondingly asymmetric. Today, schistosomiasis is endemic in Africa, South America, and the Caribbean, infecting some 200 million people. The disease is considered among

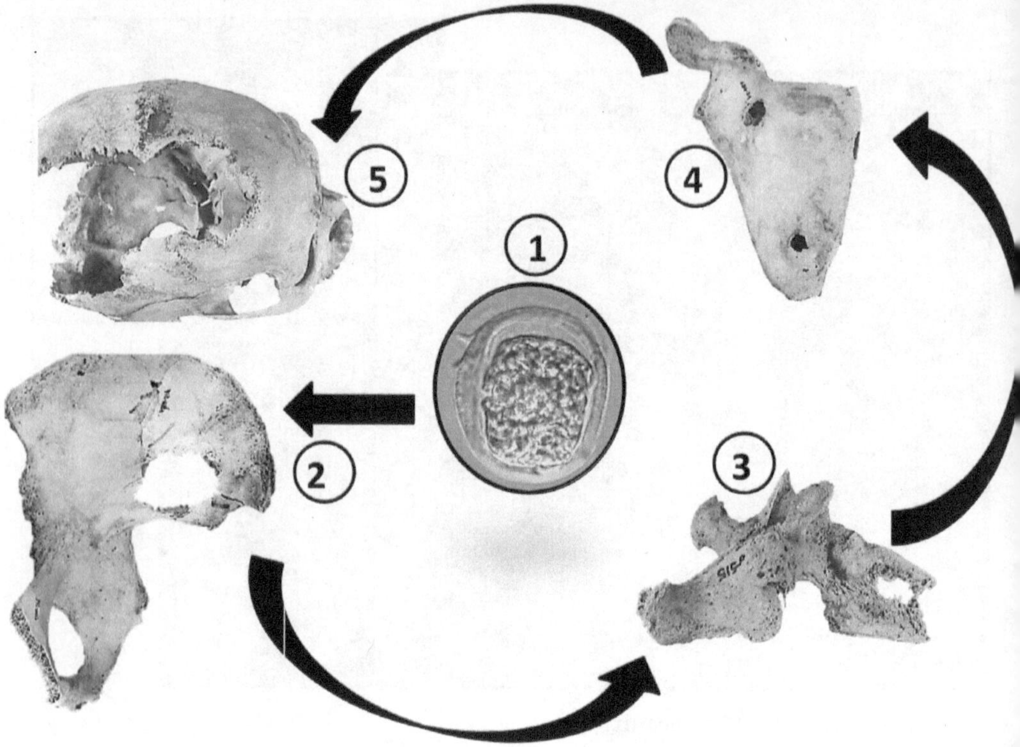

Figure 6.5. A schistosome egg from Kulubnarti and the likely spread of carcinoma.

the most important water diseases on earth from the standpoint of human illness and death.

We hypothesized that schistosomiasis would have been present in the irrigated fields of ancient Nubia just as it is today, but we had no direct proof until Hibbs and coworkers conducted an immunological study using skin samples from Wadi Halfa and Kulubnarti (Hibbs et al. 2011). Using techniques too complex to discuss here, they discovered *Schistosoma mansoni* antigens (proteins produced by the parasite) in both populations. Even more direct evidence emerged following Hibbs and coworkers' study. Schistosome eggs were found in fecal samples from Kulubnarti.

Why is this extended discussion of schistosomiasis relevant to our interpretation of metastatic carcinoma? The answer goes back to the parasite. In addition to infecting the liver, the parasite often infects the urinary tract. In the bladder, the parasites produce N-nitroso compounds known to cause bladder cancer. There is a positive correlation between the frequency of schistosomiasis and the frequency of bladder cancer throughout the Nile Valley.

The association of our metastatic carcinoma, schistosomiasis, and bladder cancer suggests a scenario. Our farmer contracted schistosomiasis while working in an irrigation ditch. He may have been cleaning it or repairing it. The parasite first infected his liver and then spread to his urinary tract—particularly his bladder. He developed a bladder cancer that spread first to his pelvis, then to his spine, his scapula, and eventually his skull. I remember the time that George showed the skeleton to an oncologist. The doctor was astounded, saying he had never seen a cancer spread that far. He told us that today, "we either cure the patient or he dies" long before that.

The Case of Metastatic Prostate Cancer

Our second case is also a middle-age X-Group male who was suffering from a metastatic carcinoma at the time of his death. The cancer in this case had most likely metastasized from the prostate gland.

As we have said, most bone cancers are osteolytic (they cause bone resorption) with some secondary bone formation. Prostate cancer is primarily osteoblastic (bone is added) with a lesser degree of bone loss (Keller and Brown 2004). Some researchers argue that prostate cancer is unique in that regard (Logothetis and Lin 2005). This gave us an important criterion for diagnosing our case. Prostate cancer also produces a characteristic distribution within the skeleton that was useful to our diagnosis. The importance of both morphology and distribution is well illustrated in two previously reported cases—one from Canterbury, England, and the other from Dynastic Egypt.

The medieval-aged Canterbury case was published by Jennifer Wakely and coworkers in 1995 (Wakely et al. 1995). The victim was an elderly male with lesions consisting of rough bony spicules on the visceral side of the pelvis, proximal femur, and rib. Scanning electron microscopy confirmed that they were "predominantly of a bone forming nature" (Wakely et al. 1995:471).

Carlos Prates and his team reported a Ptolemaic dynasty case in 2011 (Prates et al. 2011). The victim was an elderly (60+ years) Egyptian with lesions also typical of metastasized prostate cancer. On X-ray the lesions were found to be denser than the surrounding bone. Both the Egyptian and the Canterbury cases provided an excellent comparative context for our diagnosis.

Our X-Group male had two tumors on his skull—one on the anterior right parietal (figure 6.6a) and one on the temporal bone slightly behind the zygomatic arch (figure 6.6b). There were also tumors on the visceral

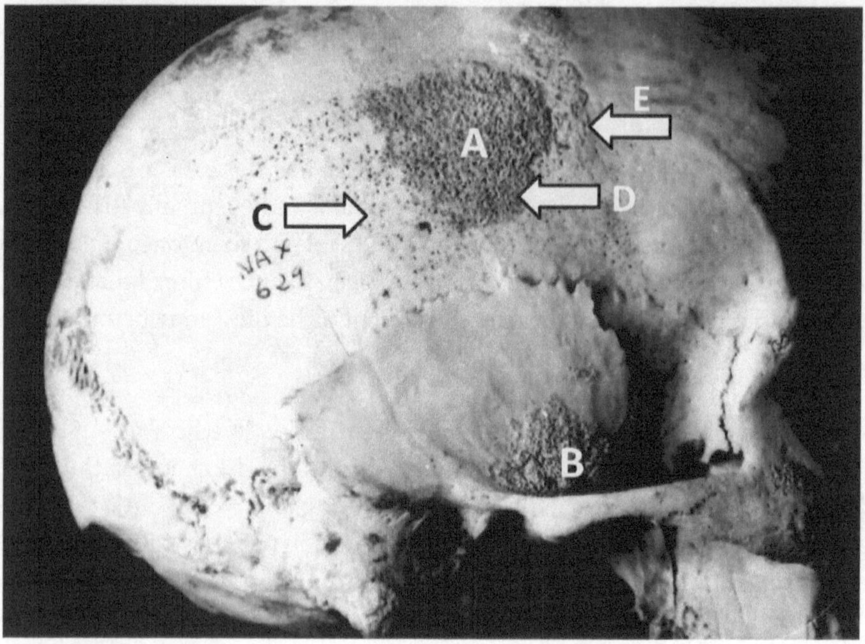

Figure 6.6. Metastatic carcinoma in a middle-age X-Group male from Wadi Halfa.

side of the pelvic cavity.[3] All of the tumors show the same features observed in the Canterbury case (figure 6.6f). There is pitting due to an expanding vascular supply to tumor tissue (figure 6.6c). There is the rough coral-like bone (figure 6.6d) observed in the Canterbury case, as well as the dense bone (figure 6.6e) observed on X-ray in the Egyptian case. Lesion distribution is also consistent with our diagnosis. Tumors within the pelvis were observed during excavation, and metastasis to areas outside of the pelvis, including the skull, is relatively common.

The Case of Chondrosarcoma

Wadi Halfa produced a third bone cancer. The victim this time was a middle-age X-Group male. He had two tumors at the time of his death. The larger was just below the lesser trochanter of his left femur (figure 6.7a). The smaller encompassed his entire left pubic symphysis (figure 6.7b). Both tumors were simultaneously lytic (resorptive) and blastic (formative). The original cortical bone at the tumor sites had been resorbed and subsequently replaced by a mass of disorganized lacelike trabecular bone. The morphology is distinct from our metastatic carcinomas. It does, however, strongly resemble a category of bone tumors known as sarcomas. Unlike

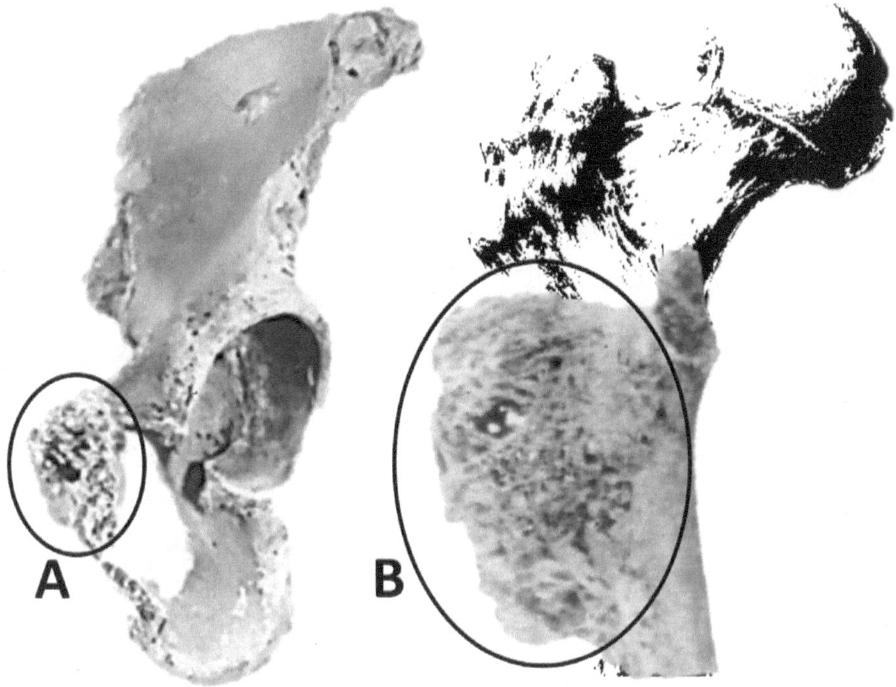

Figure 6.7. Chondrosarcoma of the left pubis (A) and left femur (B).

metastatic cancers, sarcomas originate in bone (Dorfman and Czerniak 1995). They begin in the organic portion of bone or in cartilage—often near the epiphyses of growing bones. Sarcomas make up some 15–20 percent of all cancers in subadults. Long bones are the most vulnerable. Almost half of all sarcomas occur in the femur, followed by the tibia and then the humerus. They are not, however, exclusively long bone tumors. Eight to 10 percent occur in the pelvis.

There are several kinds of sarcomas. The most common are osteosarcoma, Ewing's sarcoma, and chondrosarcoma. In our case, the morphology, distribution, and likely age of onset supported a diagnosis of chondrosarcoma. The morphological similarity to a modern chondrosarcoma was striking (figure 6.8). Both the Nubian and modern show a combination of lytic and blastic changes. The former is apparent in the loss of underlying cortical bone, and the latter by the erratic growth of meshlike trabeculae.

Our diagnosis was also supported by age of onset. Osteosarcoma typically afflicts children and adolescents under the age of 20. The peak age of onset for Ewing's sarcoma is between 10 and 20 years. Chondrosarcoma is the exception. People most commonly develop chondrosarcoma during

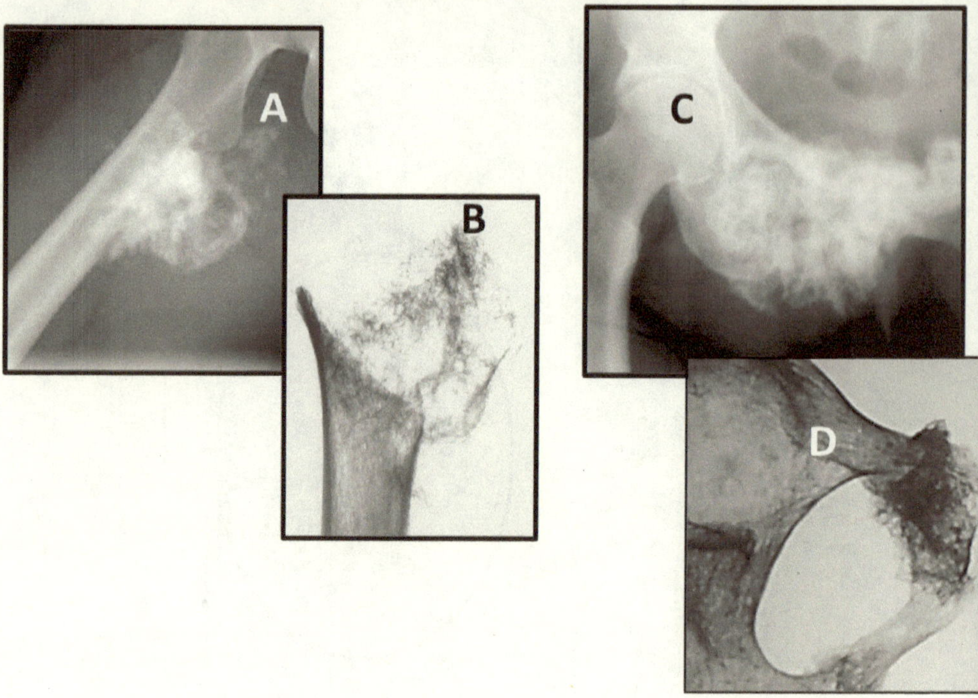

Figure 6.8. X-ray images of four chondrosarcoma: a modern femur (A) (image from Eradiology.bidmc.Harvard.edu), the X-Group femur (B), a modern pubis (C) (image from Learningradiology.com), and an X-Group pubis (D).

their middle years (ages 40–50). Sarcomas are aggressive cancers that metastasize rapidly—commonly to the lung. Our Nubian's cancer would not have been survivable from childhood into middle age.

Lesion distribution also lent support to our diagnosis. Among the sarcomas, chondrosarcoma is the most likely to appear away from long bone growth plates. And finally, there was one additional bit of evidence in support of our chondrosarcoma diagnosis. Chondrosarcomas develop from preexisting benign tumors known as osteochondromas (Dahlin and Beabout 1971), examples of which were found in the Wadi Halfa remains (figure 6.9).

Before we move on to other conditions and cases, let's consider our three neoplasms in a wider context. We have already pointed out that as of 1998, only 176 cases of cancer had been observed in prehistoric human remains (Strouhal 2015), and even if the number has doubled between then and now, cancer is still exceedingly rare in prehistory. Is the low number evidence of absence or an absence of evidence? Clearly, a definitive answer is

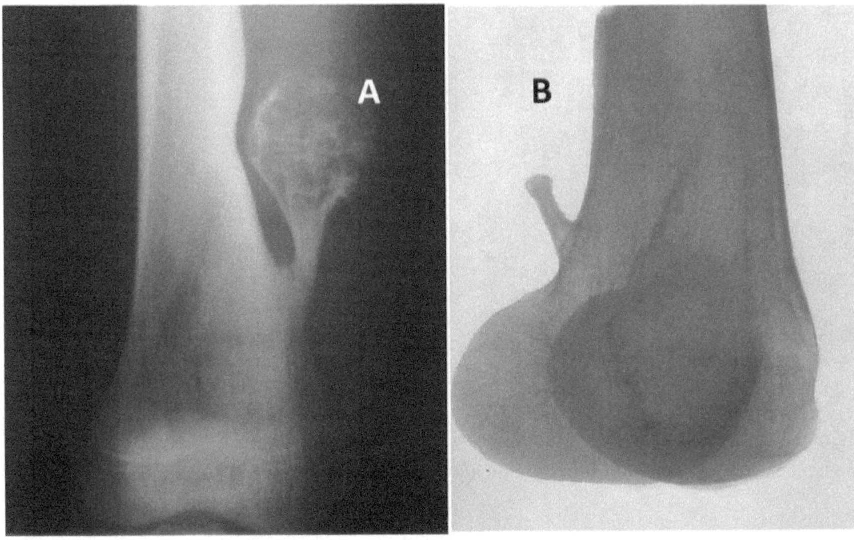

Figure 6.9. X-ray images of a modern (A) and an X-Group (B) osteochondroma of the distal femur.

impossible. However, like many questions with no clear answers, it raises interesting possibilities worth considering.

There is almost certainly a degree of missing evidence. Tumors weaken bone, increasing the likelihood of damage in the ground during burial and during excavation. Lesion edges can easily be mistaken for fragment edges. Differential diagnoses often depend on lesion distributions, and many skeletons are fragmentary. Benign tumors can be difficult to distinguish from malignant ones. There is also a statistical issue. George Johnson, writing for the *New York Times* (Johnson 2010), pointed out that given the likely number of people who have lived since the beginning of the Common Era (about 50 billion) and the number of skeletons excavated (about 100,000), you would probably find one case of cancer for every 10,000 skeletons. By these numbers, finding three cancers at Wadi Halfa was remarkable.

Then there is the other side of the question. Are the low numbers in prehistory partly because cancer was less common in earlier human populations? In addition to the skeletal evidence, this question is informed by the ecology of infectious and degenerative diseases. More specifically, we must examine what has been called the first epidemiological transition. Our Nubian villagers lived during the first epidemiological transition (Armelagos et al. 2004). It began some 10,000 years ago with the shift from foraging to

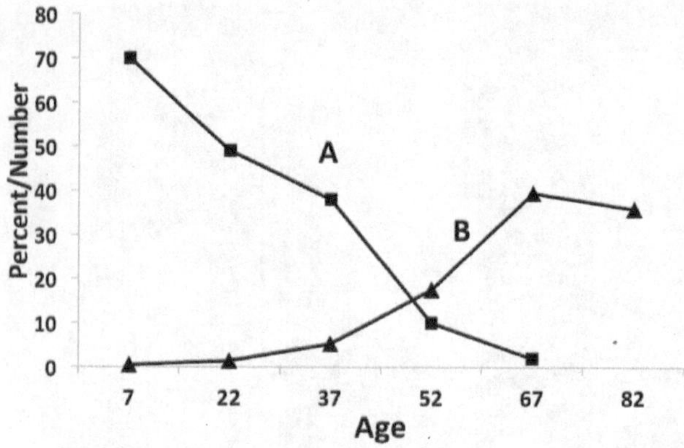

Figure 6.10. Percent of the Kulubnarti population surviving by age (A) and number of cancers diagnosed per 10,000 people by age in Great Britain in 2012 (B).

agriculture. It continued well into the Common Era in areas such as Nubia, where village life and economies remained unchanged for millennia.

Agriculture produced an environmental setting ripe for the emergence of infectious diseases. Population size increased rapidly. Settled villages brought humans and microbes into intimate contact. Domestic animals and their diseases were brought into the village and became a part of village life. The first transition gave birth to the age of the infectious disease and produced human populations characterized by high infant mortality and low life expectancy. These are precisely the conditions we have documented at Wadi Halfa and Kulubnarti. Inasmuch as the likelihood of cancer increases with age, low life expectancies would predict low cancer frequencies (figure 6.10).[4] In other words, cancers were probably less frequent in ancient times partly because people didn't live long enough to develop them.

So is there an absence of evidence or evidence of absence? Is it one or the other, or is it a little of both? There can be no question that cancers have been lost, overlooked, or misdiagnosed in the archaeological record. That said, we can also make a strong inference that cancers were less frequent in the past than they are today.

Congenital Disorders

The Case of Hydrocephalus

Our case of hydrocephalus was that of an 11-year-old X-Group girl (figures 6.11 and 6.12) with what is commonly referred to as "water on the brain." Actually, the common term is wrong, and the medical term is partially wrong. It's not water, so "hydro" is incorrect, and it isn't *on* the brain, it's *in*

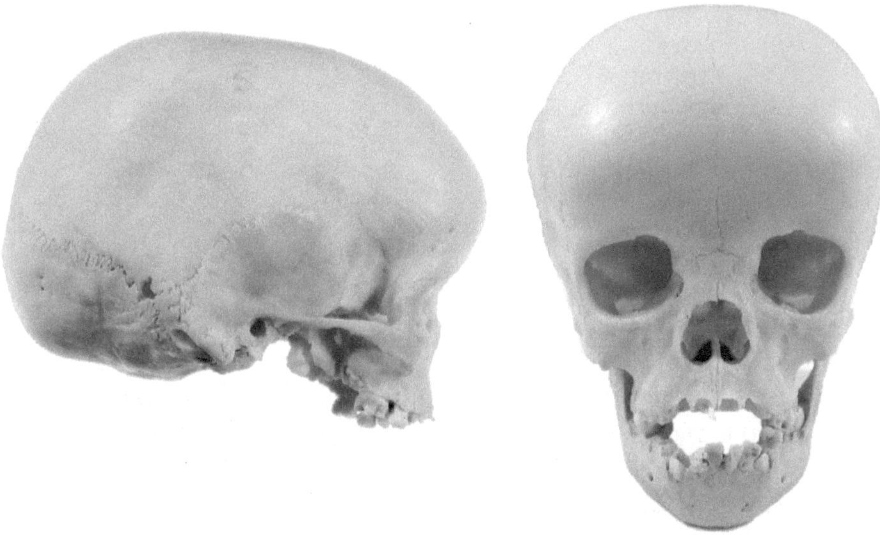

Figure 6.11. Hydrocephalus in an 11-year-old X-Group female (lateral and frontal views).

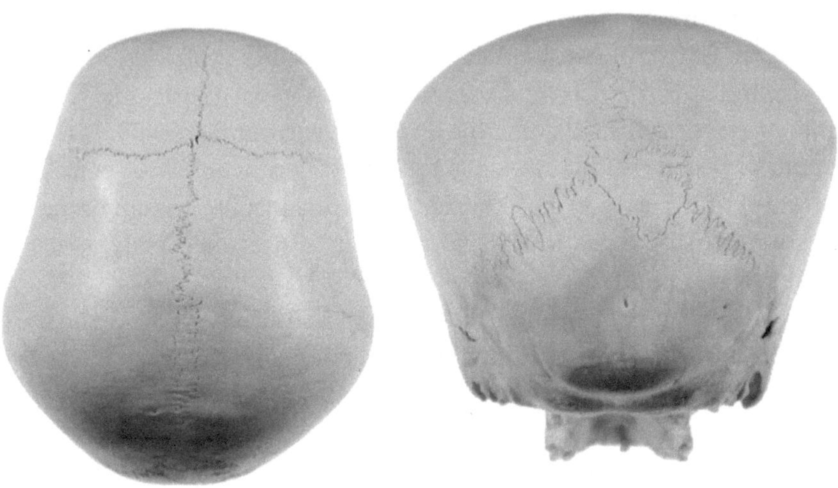

Figure 6.12. Hydrocephalus in an 11-year-old X-Group female (superior and posterior views).

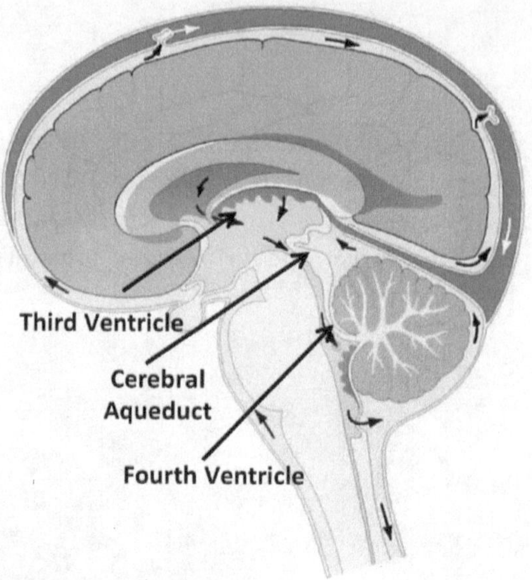

Figure 6.13. The ventricular system and CSF circulation.

the brain. If we wanted to be accurate, we would call it fluid in the brain. These aren't trivial distinctions. Hydrocephalus (Del Bigio 1993) is a condition resulting from an abnormal increase in the volume of cerebral spinal fluid (CSF) within the brain.

CSF is produced in a series of four cavities (ventricles) lying deep within the brain (figure 6.13). This ventricular system also includes the cerebral aqueduct. The aqueduct allows CSF to drain from the third to the fourth ventricle. CSF is in constant circulation out of the ventricles, around the brain, and downward around the spinal cord. One of its principal functions is to provide a buffer between the brain and surrounding skull. It also suspends the brain. The brain weighs about 1,400 grams and is the consistency of wet plaster. Heavy as it is, it would flatten against the bottom of the skull if it weren't suspended in CSF. Suspension reduces its effective weight to about 25 grams.

CSF does more than support the brain; it also cleans it. Metabolic wastes are continuously washed away from the brain by CSF as it circulates from the ventricles, around the brain, around and down the spinal cord, and finally out into the bloodstream. CSF recycles completely four times per day and is replaced at the rate of 500 milliliters per day. It is like a stream of water entering a garden hose from a tap at one end and flowing out the other.

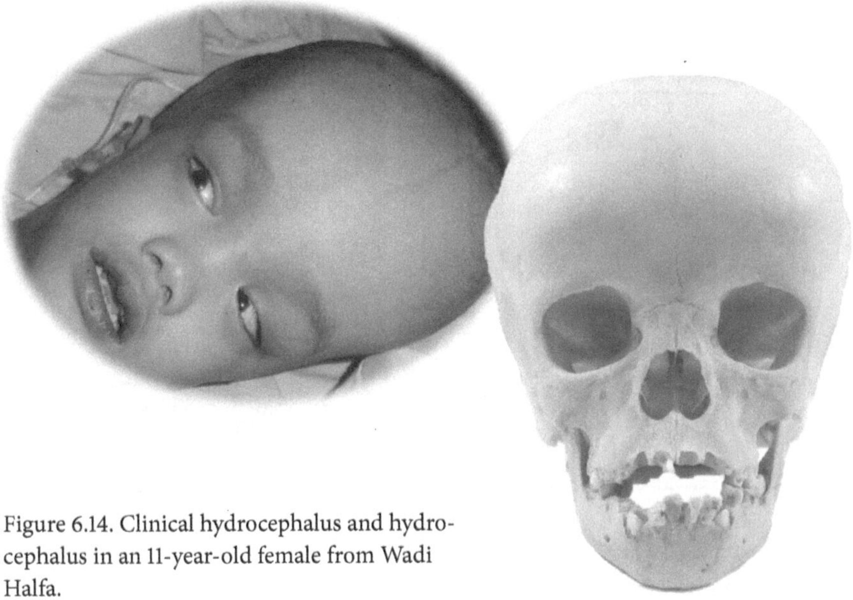

Figure 6.14. Clinical hydrocephalus and hydrocephalus in an 11-year-old female from Wadi Halfa.

The garden hose metaphor is apt for our discussion of hydrocephalus. When a hose running water is kinked, pressure builds, and if the pressure builds enough, the hose develops a bulge behind the kink. A blockage in the cerebral aqueduct in an infant or child[5] is like kinking the hose. Each day, some 500 milliliters of CSF leaves the "tap" with no place to go. CSF builds up, the ventricles expand, pressure rises, and the brain expands, pressing against the underside of the vault. The vault expands, and the brain is compressed. Left to run its course, a point is reached where neither skull nor brain can accommodate the continuing accumulation of CSF. At this point, the child will most likely die. Advantaged children in today's world needn't die. As soon as the condition is diagnosed, shunts can be surgically implanted providing normal CSF drainage.

Our X-Group child appeared strikingly like known clinical cases (figure 6.14). At 1,880 cubic centimeters, her cranial volume was 61 percent larger than a matched age group (1,165 cubic centimeters). The vault was bulbous with a high protruding forehead. The vault also had a triangular appearance due to bossing (bulging) at its parietal and frontal corners. From a diagnostic perspective, we felt that the case was made. However, George and I both agreed that stopping at a diagnosis would waste an opportunity to explore the wider anatomical and behavioral consequences of the condition.

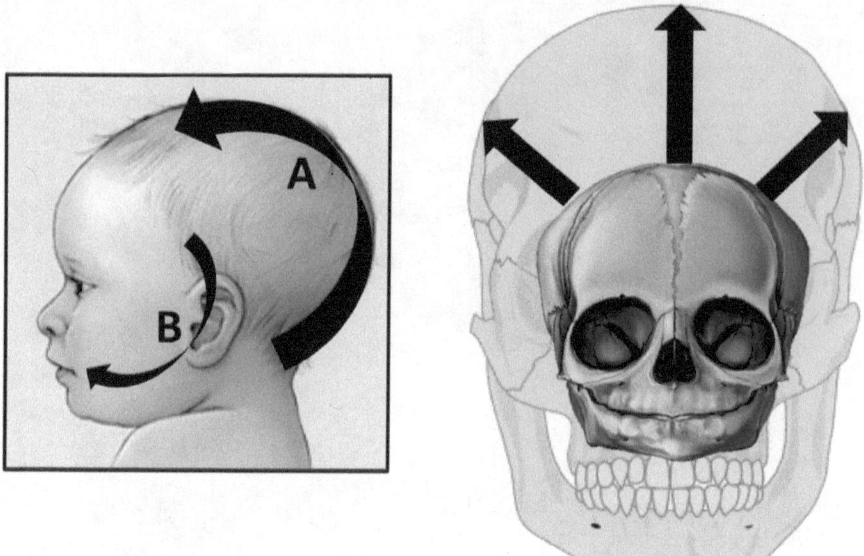

Figure 6.15. Growth of the cranial vault and face.

Our analysis of the anatomical consequences to the skull was informed by a classic paper titled "A Functional Approach to Craniology" written by Melvin Moss and Richard Young (Moss and Young 1960; Moss 1972). In their view, cranial bones don't *grow*; instead, they are *grown* in a functional matrix of organs and tissues. The matrices are then organized by growth and development into functional components. For example, the bones of the vault grow and develop in a matrix consisting of the expanding brain on their inner surfaces and the muscles of mastication on their outer surfaces. The vault itself is a functional component of the skull, whose principal function is to protect the brain and provide attachment for various muscle groups.

Cranial morphology is determined by the trajectories, velocities, and durations of component growth (figure 6.15). Beginning in fetal development, the brain is the fastest growing organ in the body. The bones of the vault are grown as they are carried away from one another on the cerebral surface. Their relative position to each other is maintained by growth at their edges (figure 6.16b) as the expanding neural mass carries them away from each other (figure 6.16a). The dynamics change during childhood and adolescence. Brain growth comes to a virtual stop by age eight. The bones of the vault then grow together and remain separated only by sutures. At the same time the vault is reaching its final dimensions, growth

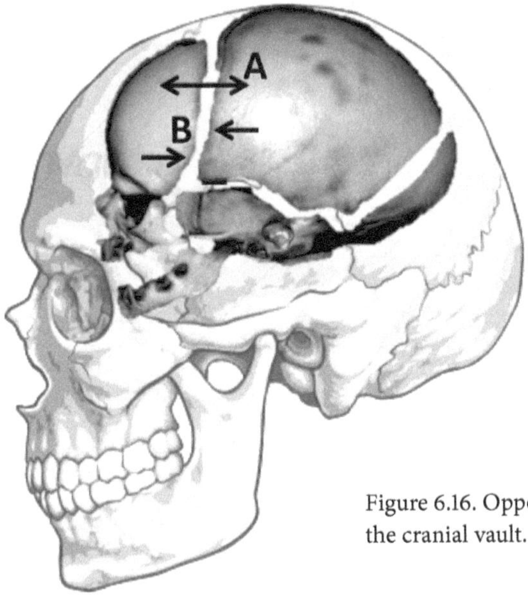

Figure 6.16. Opposing forces during growth of the cranial vault.

of the masticatory component begins to accelerate. As a result, we go from our cute baby faces to our awkward adolescent faces, which hopefully get straightened out by our adult faces.

The principle is illustrated in the evolution (figure 6.17) of the cartoon character Mickey Mouse (Gould 2008). The 1930s Mickey looked a lot like an adult mouse. The cranial vault was small in proportion to the face. People had a hard time relating to him because he looked like an adult mouse. He lacked the large vault and tiny face of a baby. Mickey was transformed by the 1950s. His vault became larger and more rounded, while his face became smaller and remained tucked beneath the vault. Mickey had become a lovable infant.

Moss and Young developed a more sophisticated demonstration by asking a question: why do Neanderthals have a brow ridge while we don't? They argued that the answer lay with the frontal bone. The frontal grows in two functional matrices. One matrix involves protection and support of the eyes, and the other protects and supports the frontal portion of the brain. Neanderthals grew large faces and dentitions. Moderns grow a smaller face and dentition. The larger archaic face grew well ahead of the brain, carrying the eyes and lower portion of the frontal with it. The modern face, with its smaller dentition and masticatory apparatus, remains tucked beneath the frontal lobes of the brain. Neanderthals have a brow ridge because the

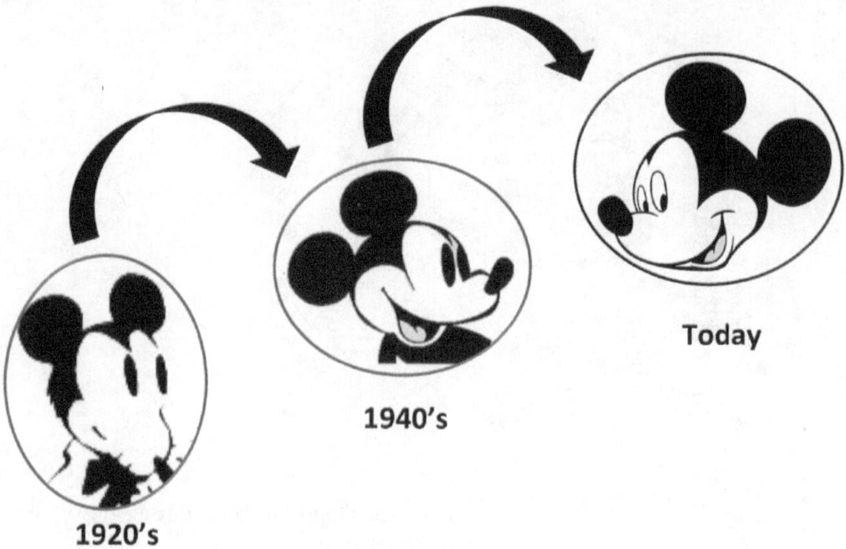

Figure 6.17. The evolution of Mickey Mouse from 1928 to 1990.

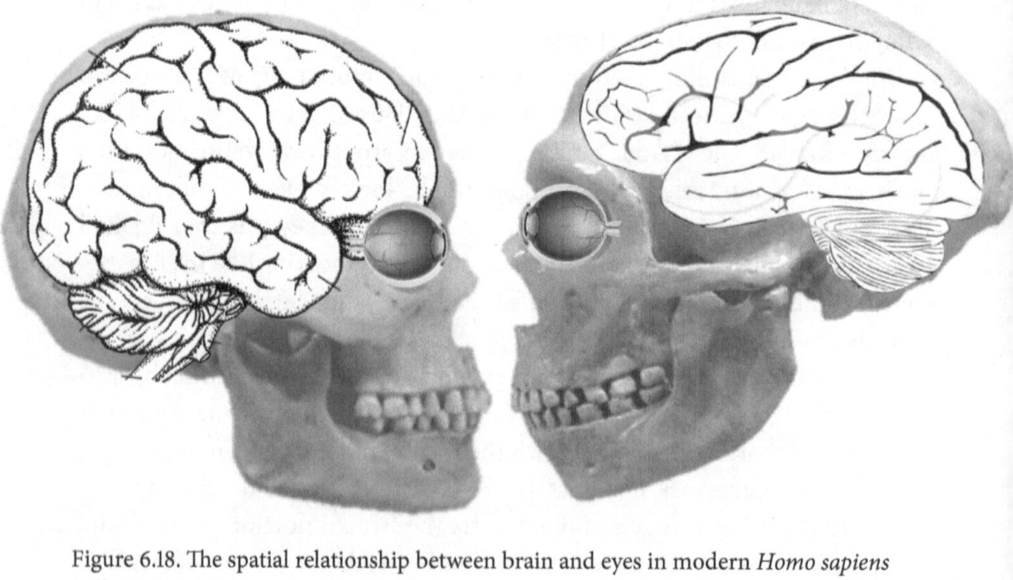

Figure 6.18. The spatial relationship between brain and eyes in modern *Homo sapiens* and Neanderthals.

lower and upper parts of the frontal bone perform their different tasks in different places. Protection for the brain and the eyes occurs in the same place among modern humans (figure 6.18). These relationships don't just apply to humans: think of the difference between the head of a puppy compared to an adult dog. Puppy brains are much larger compared to their face at birth, and that is what gives them their cute, puppylike appearance.

Moss and Young used the Neanderthal-modern comparison to demonstrate their approach using different functional designs—Neanderthal and modern. Our hydrocephalic gave us an opportunity to analyze the consequences of a catastrophic neuro-cranial disease on the growth and development within the same (modern human) functional design. The rapidly increasing volume of CSF within the ventricles of our girl's brain altered the functional matrix of her vault, resulting in two changes. The first involved her cranial sutures, and the second involved the shape of the vault itself.

The Cranial Sutures

Our child had developed Wormian bones at her posterior fontanelle. Fontanelles feel like "soft spots" on the newborn's skull. They're membranous tissue bridging gaps between adjacent bones allowing them to move and mold during rapid brain growth (figure 6.19). The most noticeable one is the anterior fontanelle at the top of the baby's head, though there is also a posterior fontanelle.

Wormian bones are detached "islands" of bone that develop within fontanelles (Bennett 1965). They subsequently become incorporated into the vault by their own network of surrounding sutures. They have been

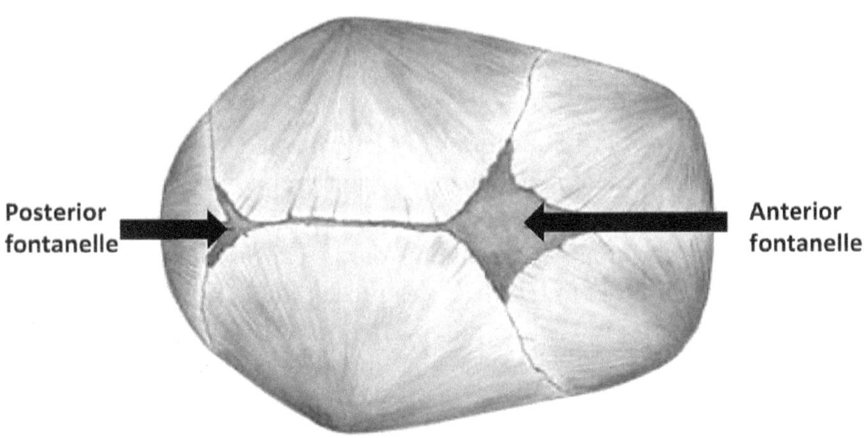

Figure 6.19. Fontanelles of the infant skull.

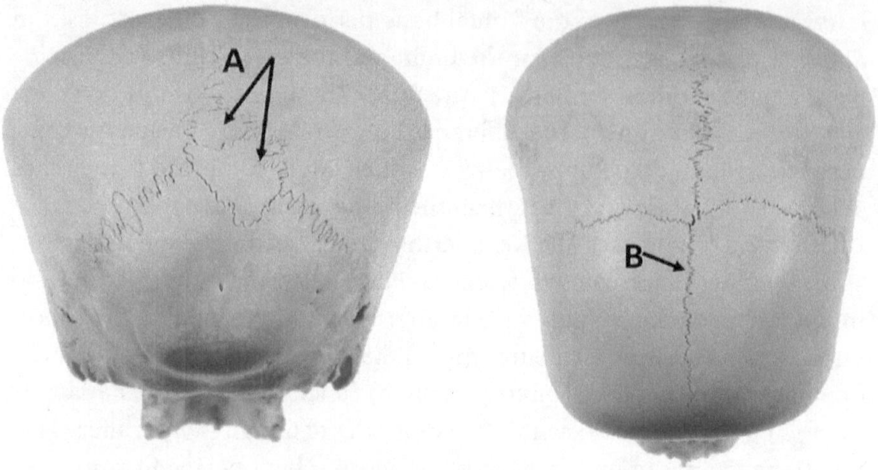

Figure 6.20. Wormian bones (A) and metopism (B).

associated with an insufficient rate of suture closure (Barberini et al. 2008), which is particularly germane to our case. Our Nubian child had developed Wormian bones at her posterior fontanelle (figure 6.20a). What would be a sufficient rate of closure during normal growth would have been insufficient in the presence of an abnormally rapid expansion of the cranial mass resulting in the development of these extra cranial bones. She also had nonclosure of her metopic suture (figure 6.20b). This suture separates left and right halves of the frontal bone during infancy. It typically closes by about age two and disappears within the next few years. It occasionally persists into later childhood and even into the adult years. The persistence of the metopic suture is referred to as metopism. The frequency of metopism is probably around 10 percent and is rare enough to be occasionally misdiagnosed as a fracture (Bademci et al. 2007). Metopism has been associated with hydrocephalus (Chakravarthi and Venumadhav 2012).

The child's Wormian bones and her metopism were likely due to a change in the functional matrix in which her cranial bones were grown. The dura mater (the outer membrane covering the brain) and the bone overlying it are essentially a continuous tissue. Current research suggests that dural cells respond to tensile forces produced by cerebral expansion, which in turn has an impact on the spacing of the overlying bones (Scarr 2008). The result could be nonclosure of the metopic suture.

Vault Morphology

Although 11 years old, our child's vault had remained strikingly infantile (figure 6.21). Like an infant's, the vault is constricted at its base with pronounced bossing (bulging) at the upper parietal and frontal corners. As with her metopism, this infantile morphology is a likely result of alterations in the functional matrix of her vault.

In the course of normal growth, the cranial base is grown as a part of both the vault and facial components. The child retained her infantile appearance largely because vault growth had outpaced normal facial growth. Not all matrix changes were internal. Muscle attachments on the outer surface also played their part. In a normally proportioned 11-year-old, the temporalis muscle would have migrated up the side of the vault almost to the adult position. Due to the enlarged size of the child's vault, the attachment remained lower in a more infantile position (figure 6.22). Without a doubt, this contributed to the infantile morphology of her skull.

The Behavioral Consequences

To this point we had focused on the anatomical aspects of our child's condition. Our question then became whether we could extend our analysis further into the behavioral consequences. In pursuing this line of investigation, we came to two strong inferences. First, she was quadriplegic and had been for several years; and second, she was severely mentally retarded.

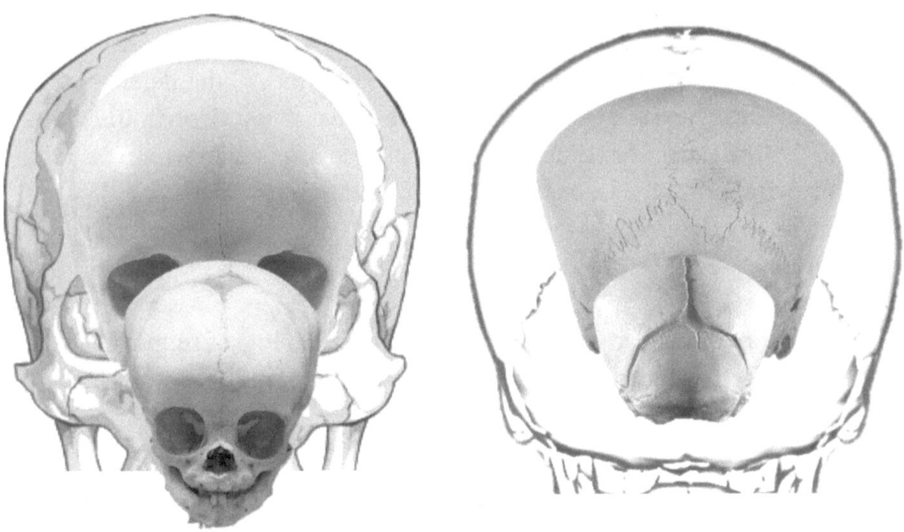

Figure 6.21. Cranial vault expansion.

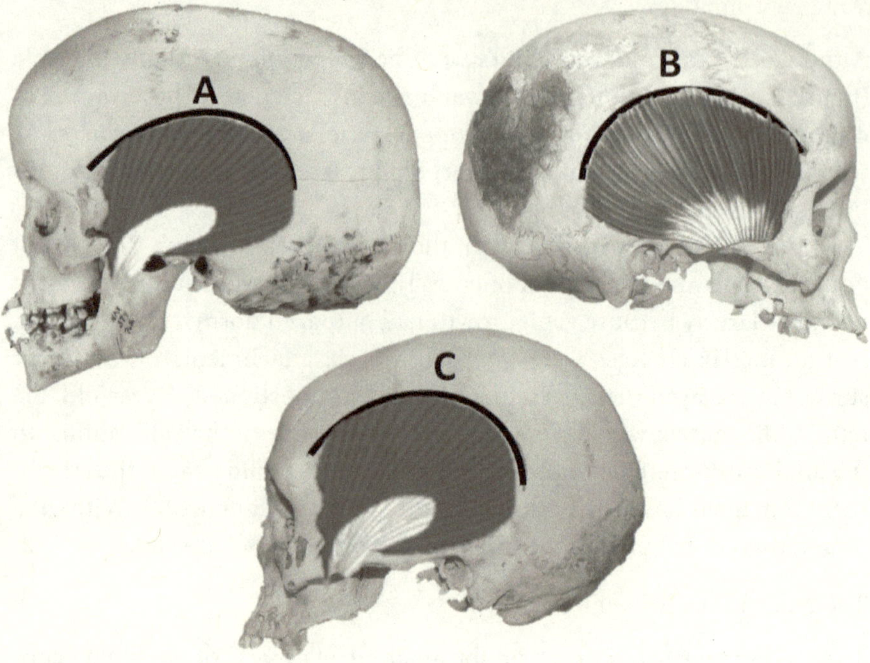

Figure 6.22. Position of the temporalis muscle in the Wadi Halfa hydrocephalic (A), an 11-year-old normal (B), and an adult (C) from Kulubnarti.

The case for quadriplegia is supported by two lines of evidence—one skeletal and the other dental. Based on long bone length, her stature was normal (figure 6.23), but the anterior posterior (AP) and medial lateral (ML) diameters of the long bones—particularly her AP diameters—were retarded. This is to be expected in the case of paralysis. Growth in length is less dependent on bending forces than is growth in diameter. It is also not surprising that the legs were more affected than the arms and that the AP diameters were more affected than the ML diameters, because the AP diameters experience greater bending forces during walking than do the ML diameters.

Evidence from neuro-anatomy provides a second line of support. Nerve fibers connecting motor and sensory areas of the brain become stretched as the ventricles expand. The fibers, however, are inelastic, and stretching can damage their myelin covering. It can even cause them to rupture (Del Bigio 1993; Yakovlev 1947). The likelihood of simultaneous paralysis of the arms and hands is enhanced by their adjacent position on the motor cortex of the brain.

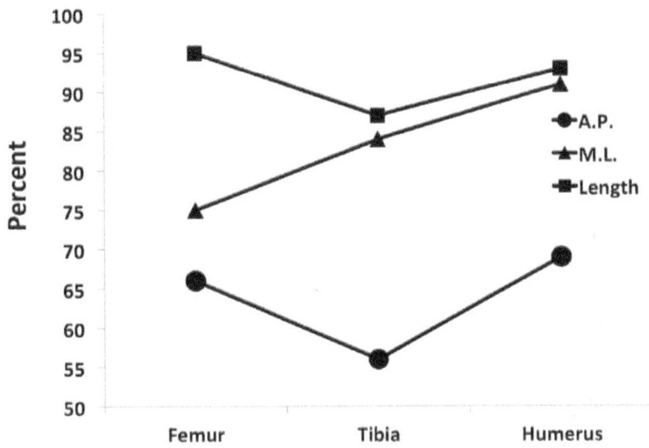

Figure 6.23. Limb dimensions percent of normal.

The dental evidence indicates that she was a tongue thruster and a bruxer. Both have been associated with severe mental retardation. Tongue thrusting is also referred to as "reverse swallowing." It occurs when the tongue is pushed forward between the front teeth as an aid to swallowing. It appears to be a continuation of the infantile suckling response beyond infancy in cases of severe mental retardation (Yokochi 1996). The forward projection of our child's upper and lower incisors (figure 6.24a) is precisely the pattern associated with tongue thrusting. Tongue thrusting also explains the unusual build up of tartar (figure 6.24b) on the lingual side of the lower incisors. Tongue thrusters accumulate excessive amounts of saliva, leading to drooling while they eat. They also propel food forward out of the front of their mouth (Yokochi 1996). Without proper cleaning, accumulations of saliva and incompletely processed food led to tartar behind the lower front teeth.

She was also a bruxer. Bruxing refers to habitual tooth grinding. Tooth grinding is common in children, and usually begins at about ten months (Mindell and Owens 2003). Excessive bruxing associated with physical consequences, such as unusual tooth wear, is commonly connected to severe mental retardation (Mindell and Owens 2003). Our child possesses two features suggestive of bruxing. The first is dental wear. The first permanent molar shows an unusual degree of wear for an 11-year-old. The tooth is sufficiently worn to expose dentin (figure 6.25a) and partially obliterate fissures (figure 6.25b). There is also a large wear facet on the second deciduous molar (figure 6.25c).

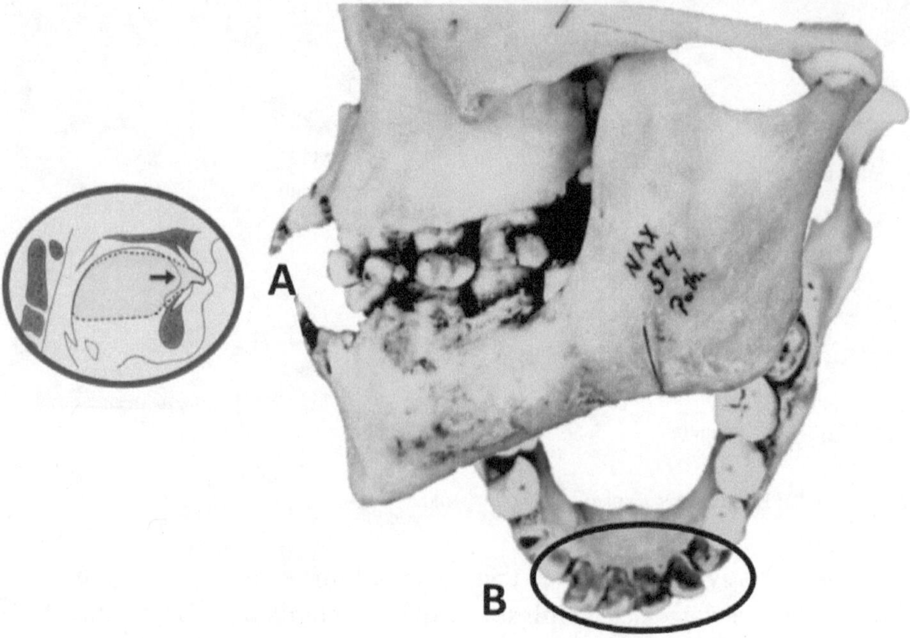

Figure 6.24. Tongue thrusting, malocclusion (A), and tartar (B).

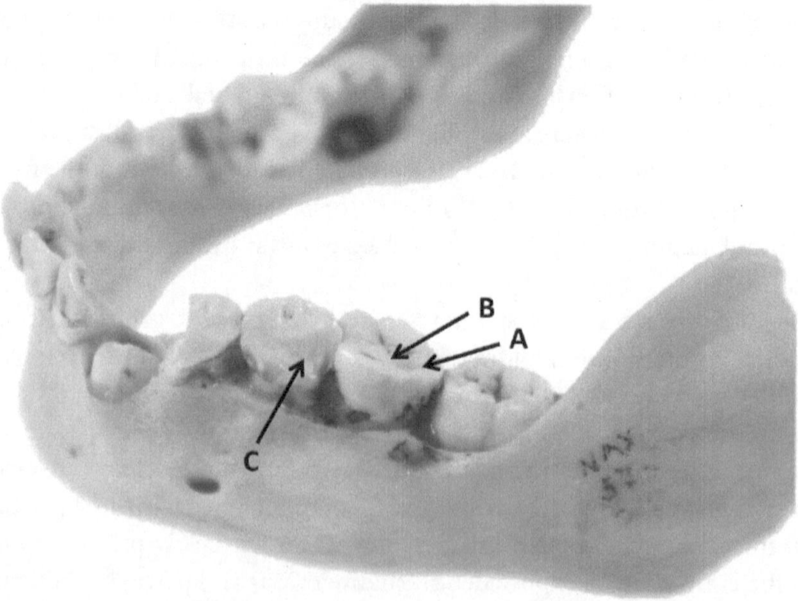

Figure 6.25. Excessive tooth wear.

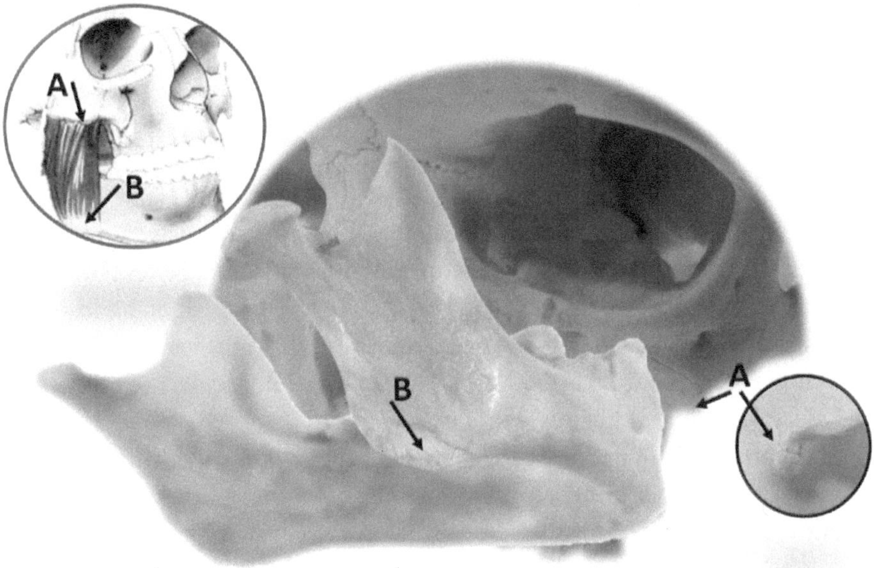

Figure 6.26. Masseter attachment origin (A) and insertion (B).

The second line of evidence involves development of the masseter muscle (figure 6.26). The masseter originates at the zygomatic arch and inserts on the inferior edge of the mandible, particularly at the angle between the mandibular body and the ascending ramus. It is one of the two major chewing muscles, the other being the temporalis (figure 6.26). The masseter's role is to produce grinding force over the molar teeth. As with all muscles, heavy development leads to large bony impressions or crests at points of attachment. The pronounced bony spine marking the anterior-most point of the masseter's attachment on the zygomatic arch (figure 6.26a) and the pronounced crest on the angle of the mandible (figure 6.26b) are highly abnormal in a person this young. This suggests a degree of molar chewing far beyond the normal range.

Interpretive Summary

In summary, our analysis led us to a series of strong inferences regarding this 11-year-old X-Group girl. She suffered from hydrocephalus beginning at birth. As a result, she experienced a series of neurological and cognitive consequences as the condition progressed. She became paralyzed in both arms and legs. She suffered brain damage sufficient to impair swallowing. This damage was sufficient to induce habitual behaviors, such as tooth grinding. Think about the kind of social support a child like this would need—not for days, weeks, or months—but years. We discuss that aspect in the next chapter.

The Case of Scoliosis

Our next case of a developmental defect is congenital scoliosis (figure 6.27) afflicting a mid-20-year-old male from Kulubnarti Island. Several thoracic vertebrae were collapsed and fused, producing a sharp right-hand bend. The spine was also twisted forward. It was one of the most visually dramatic specimens that I had excavated, and it became a standard part of my osteology lectures and public presentations.

I originally presented the case as that of *tuberculosis spondylitis*, or Pott's disease. Pott's disease develops when the tuberculosis infection spreads from the lungs or even the kidneys to the vertebral column. The results

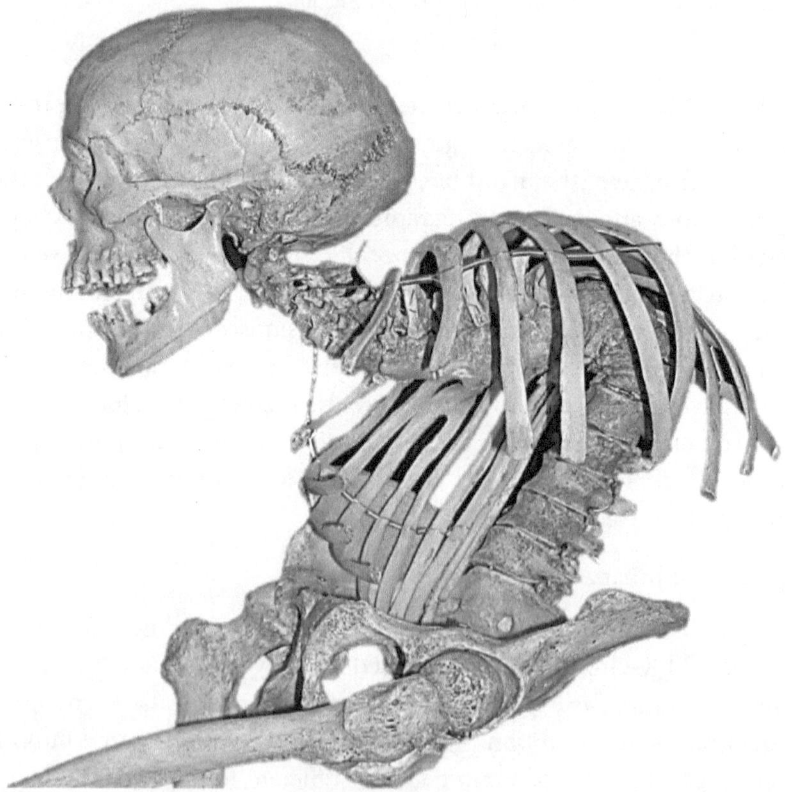

Figure 6.27. Scoliosis in a Kulubnarti island male.

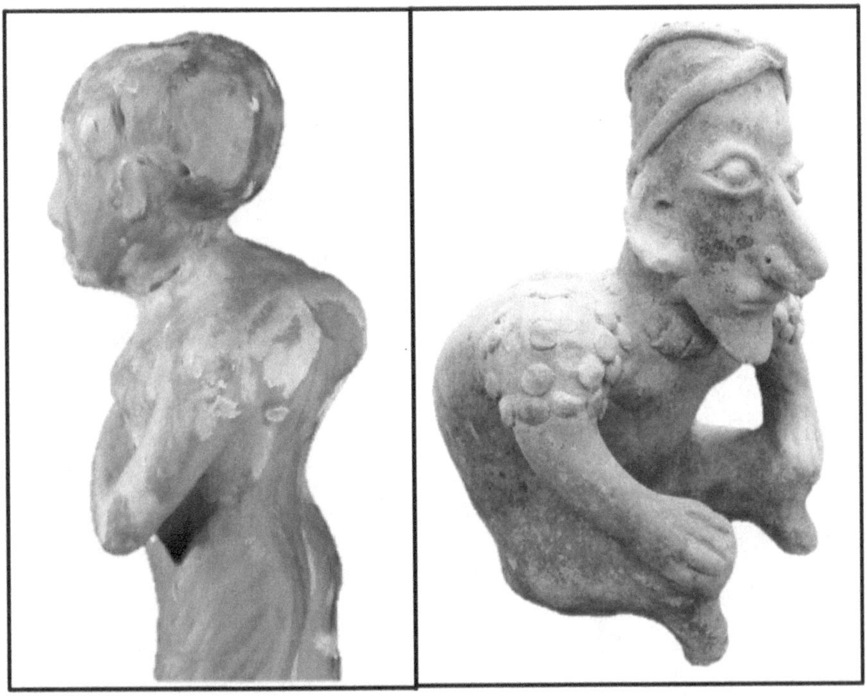

Figure 6.28. Possible Pott's disease in Egypt, 2000–1000 BCE, (*left*) (image from Science-museum.org.uk) and Greece, 100–200 BCE (*right*) (image from c1.liveauctioneers.com).

can be extremely destructive to the spine. Vertebrae become riddled with pus-filled abscesses. The vertebrae become weak and then collapse into a twisted bony mass. Entire segments of the vertebral column can be affected. There is evidence for Pott's disease throughout antiquity. Pott's-like lesions have been found in an Egyptian mummy dated to 2400 BCE (Global Tuberculosis Institute, New Jersey Medical School), and the condition even appears in ancient art (figure 6.28).

The Kulubnarti case was not, however, a classic example. There were no signs of abscessing in the affected vertebrae. This aroused Lynn Kilgore's curiosity back in the mid-1980s when she was studying osteoarthritis for her doctoral dissertation. She was one of the most tenacious students I have ever had. She examined the skeleton and became puzzled. In addition to the absence of abscessing, she noticed a peculiarity that I and any number of colleagues and students had missed completely. There were more transverse processes on one side of the segment of fused vertebrae than on the other. This could mean only one thing. Parts of some vertebrae were missing on one side. Tuberculosis doesn't cause that, but congenital scoliosis

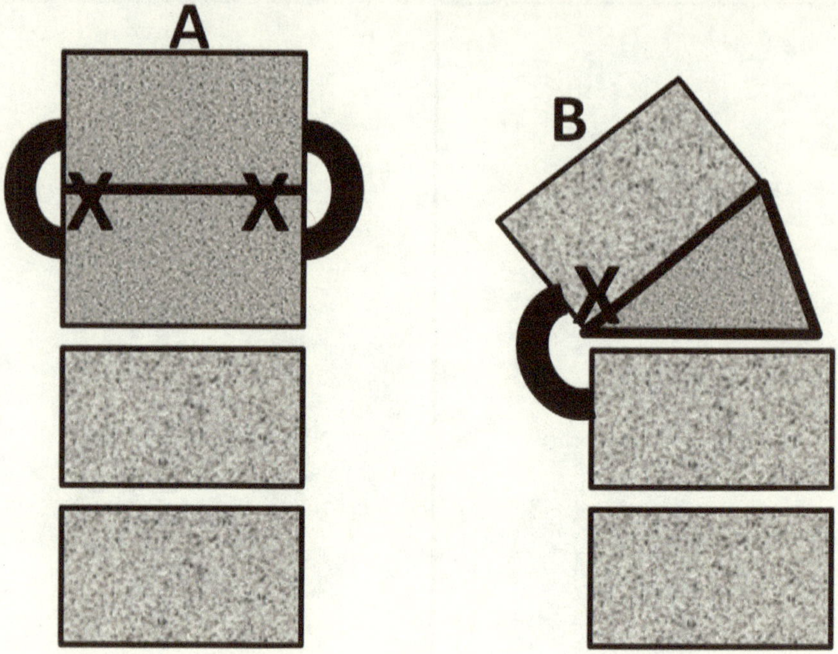

Figure 6.29. Complete (A) and partial (B) segmentation failure.

does. She made a discovery that I had missed for over a decade (Kilgore and Van Gerven 2010).

Congenital scoliosis is a relatively rare condition affecting from 0.5 to 1.0 percent of the living population. It is the result of a developmental error. Developing vertebral bodies become separated from each other during the fourth and sixth gestational weeks through a process known as segmentation. Segmentation is a complex process involving a lot of other structures and tissues. It is sufficient for our purposes to understand that it can fail—either completely or partially. In the case of a partial failure (figure 6.29b), separation between adjacent vertebrae occurs on one side only. The other side remains unsegmented and is subsequently bridged by an overgrowth of bone tissue. The segmented side then grows normally while the unsegmented side cannot. This leads to progressive tipping toward the unsegmented side.

A complete segmentation failure (figure 6.29b) results in a block of completely fused vertebrae. There is no bending of the vertebral column. Lynn found both complete (figure 6.30d, e) and partial (figure 6.30a, b, c) segmentation failures. As expected, the partials had produced the pronounced

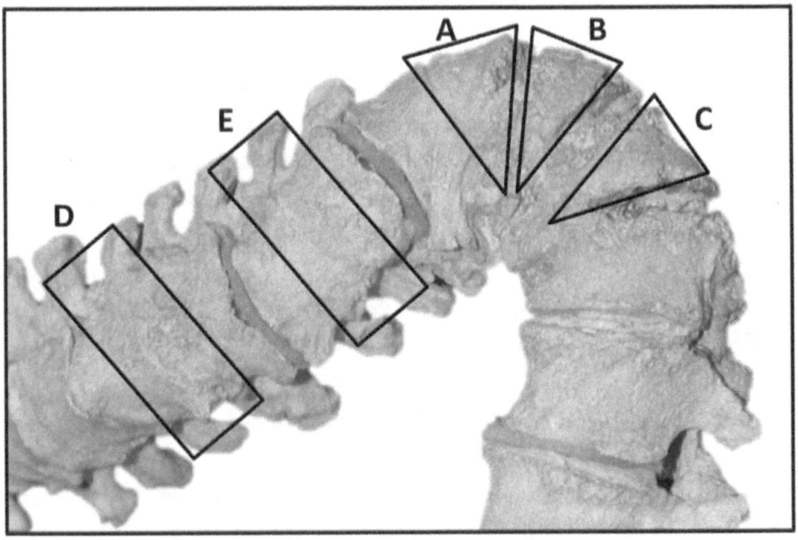

Figure 6.30. Complete (D, E) and partial (A, B, C) segmentation failure.

curvature, while the complete segmentations had not. There were also a series of malformed ribs. The head ends were fused (figure 6.31a), and their bodies were abnormally thin (figure 6.31b). Lynn interpreted this as a second aspect of segmentation failure. Ribs can fail to segment just as the vertebrae can. The abnormal thinning of the ribs was most likely due to their confinement within the pelvic cavity.

Lynn went beyond the evidence for her diagnosis to a consideration of the behavioral consequences. She analyzed cortical bone quality in the femoral shafts and found no evidence of disuse atrophy. There was, however,

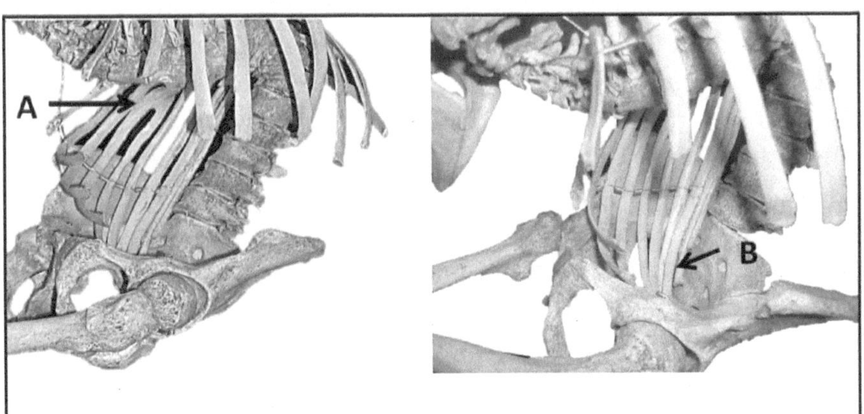

Figure 6.31. Rib fusion (A) and deformation (B).

evidence that his mobility was compromised. Lynn observed that the linea aspera on the right femur was underdeveloped. This feature provides attachment for the adductor muscles—the muscles on the inner thigh used, for example, in horseback riding. This suggests that the muscles were at least compromised, if not paralyzed. The adductor muscles are part of a complex that keeps the pelvis level as we step off one leg and then the other. As a result, his entire weight had to be shifted over his right hip with each step onto his left leg as he walked. His gait would have had a pronounced rocking motion. Lynn also noted wearing on the upper rim of the right acetabulum consistent with rotating the femur head to a greater degree than normal.

There was a likelihood of other organ involvement not evidenced in bone. These would have included cardiovascular anomalies, as well as neurological and gastrointestinal problems. Impaired breathing is also common with this condition. The position of the right ribs within the pelvic cavity supported that interpretation. And yet, with all of those challenges, he survived longer than 74 percent of this community. Lynn and I agreed that he must have had a great deal of social support.

Diseases of Unknown Etiology

The Case of Proportional Dwarfism

Our first case of disease of unknown etiology is an 18–20-year-old male from the mainland community (figures 6.32–6.34). His stature (based on White et al. 2011) was between 4'4" and 5', making him 12" below average for a male in his community. His upper and lower limbs were proportionately reduced, with an intermembral index (percentage of upper limb length to lower) of 70 percent, compared to 72 percent for his community. His limbs were more greatly reduced than his skull (figure 6.35).

Dwarfism is defined as an adult height of 4'10" (147 centimeters) or less. If some parts of the body are small, and others are of average size or above, the condition is referred to as disproportionate dwarfism. If all parts of the body are small to the same degree, the dwarfism is proportionate. The most common cause of proportionate dwarfism is insufficient production of growth hormone by the pituitary gland. About 1 in 3,500 children in the United States are affected.

In addition to his small size, our case had craniosynostosis (Wilkie 1997) of his sagittal suture (figure 6.36). Craniosynostosis is premature closure

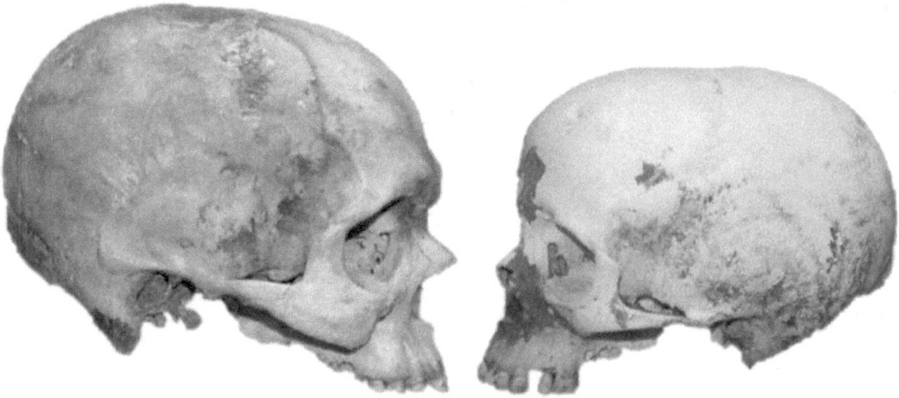

Figure 6.32. Kulubnarti island dwarf and typical male from Kulubnarti island.

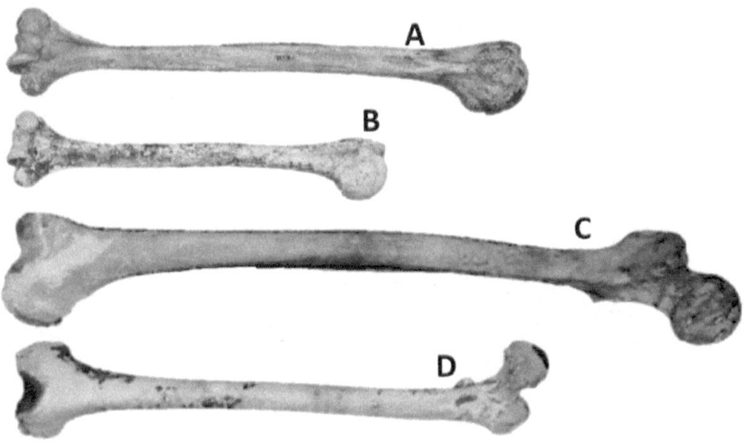

Figure 6.33. Typical (A, C) and dwarf (B, D) femora and humeri.

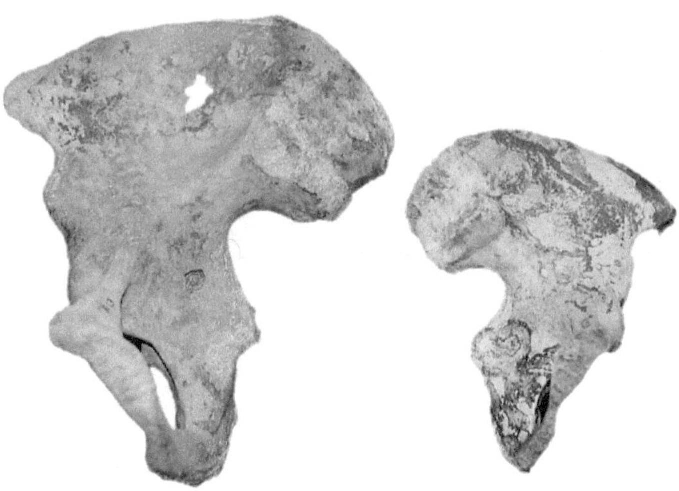

Figure 6.34. Typical and dwarf os coxae.

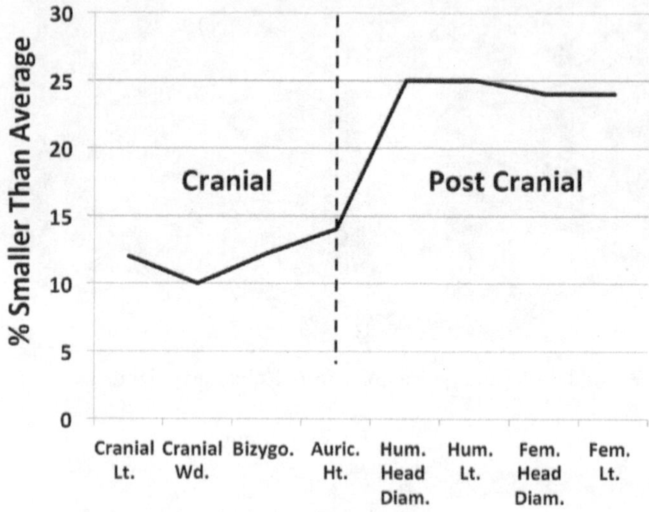

Figure 6.35. Cranial vs. postcranial size reduction.

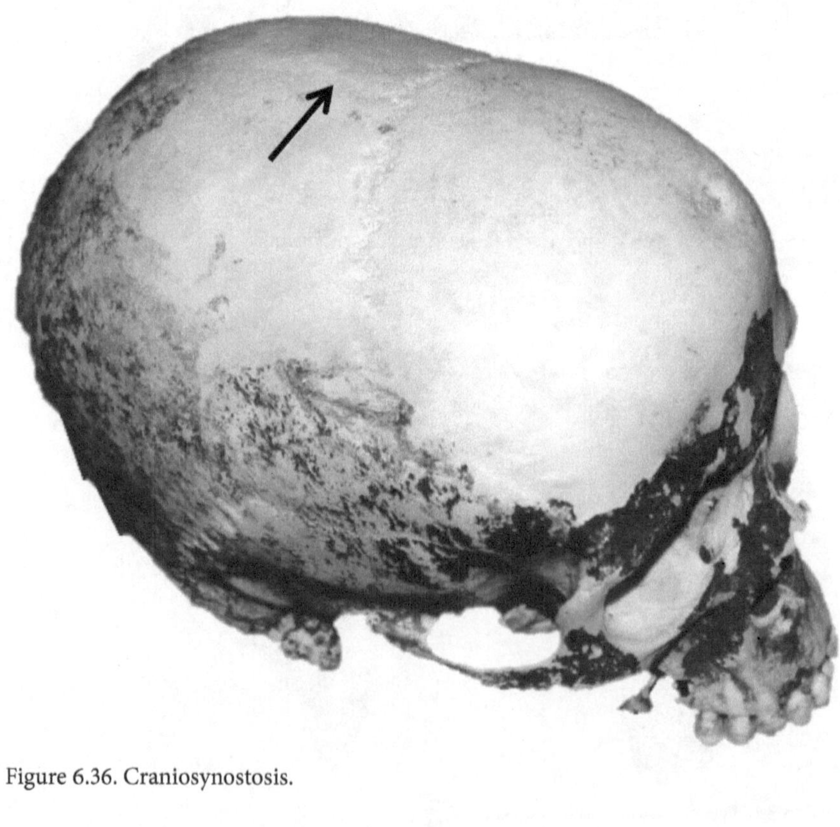

Figure 6.36. Craniosynostosis.

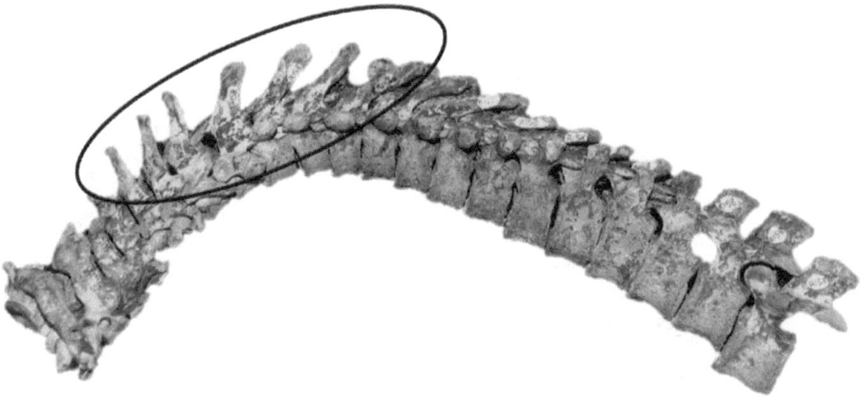

Figure 6.37. Thoracic kyphosis.

of a suture. As a result, lateral (side-to-side) expansion of the brain was constrained, causing his vault to develop a long, narrow shape. This kind of redirected growth would have had no negative impact on normal cognitive function. He also had severe kyphosis (forward bending) of his thoracic spine (figure 6.37).

The craniosynostosis and kyphosis intrigued us. Could they be related to the dwarfism? A clinical case published in 1993 may have held the answer (Kozlowski et al. 1993). The subject was a 12-year-old girl with what the authors described as "a unique short stature, mental retardation, multiple skeletal anomalies syndrome" (Kozlowski et al. 1993:442). Her distinctive skeletal anomalies included short stature, craniosynostosis, and kyphosis of the upper thoracic spine. This unique clinical case was strikingly similar to ours, but not a perfect match. The little girl had fusion of the hamate and capitate bones in her hand while ours doesn't. It still left us wondering if we had an ancient case of a clinically unique (as of 1997) syndrome.

Diffuse Idiopathic Skeletal Hyperostosis

Our next disease of unknown etiology is diffuse idiopathic skeletal hyperostosis, or DISH (figure 6.38). It occurs most frequently in men over age 50 (Sarzi-Puttini and Atzeni 2004). Somewhere between 10 percent and 35 percent of our population has DISH to varying degrees. These numbers are likely an underestimate because less-severe cases are asymptomatic and go undiagnosed. However, severe cases, as in ours, can cause a decreased range of motion, stiffness, pain, and, in some cases, compression of the spinal cord. Although DISH is likely associated with certain metabolic disorders, such as Type II diabetes, its etiology is complex and not fully known.

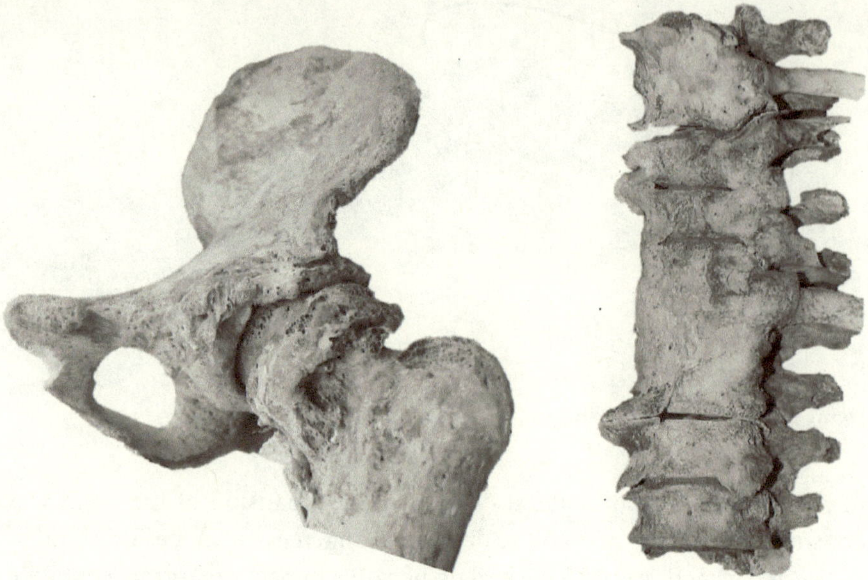

Figure 6.38. Diffuse idiopathic skeletal hyperostosis.

DISH is found as far back as the middle Paleolithic (Crubézy and Trinkaus 1992), and numerous cases have been reported in the literature (Oxenham et al. 2006). It reaches a frequency of 13 percent (Arriaza et al. 1993) at the Meroitic site of Semna located some 15 miles south of Wadi Halfa. Anatomically, DISH is often confused with a similar appearing condition known as ankylosing spondylitis (AS) (Linden et al. 1984). Both involve fusion of vertebrae by bony bridges that look a lot like each other. In fact, I had believed it to be a case of AS until a doctoral student in my osteology class did a more thorough analysis.

A lot of the difference between DISH and AS has to do with the bony bridges between vertebrae. In the case of AS, bridges are formed across intervertebral discs, producing segmental rings much like bamboo (figure 6.39). DISH, on the other hand, is characterized by the hyperproduction of coarse-flowing osteophytes (figure 6.39), which cause an ossification of the lateral anterior ligament of the spine, producing a flowing candle wax appearance (Resnick and Niwayama 1976). DISH is also characterized by the fusion of four or more contiguous vertebrae in the lower thoracic spine with no spinal distortion (forward bending).

Marni LaFleur and Paul Sandberg, two graduate students taking my osteology course, found that our male meets all of the criteria to merit a diagnosis of DISH (LaFleur et al. 2010). There are nine contiguous thoracic

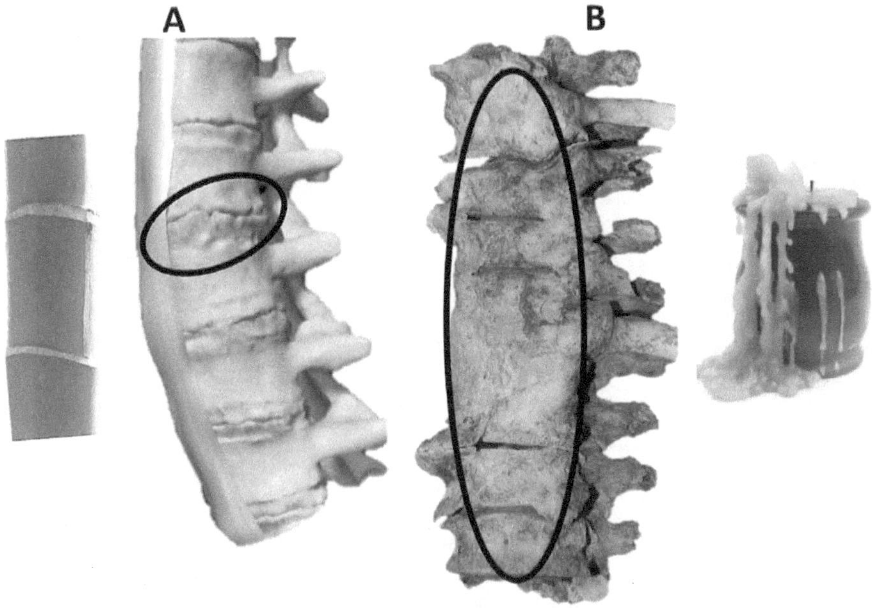

Figure 6.39. Ankylosing spondylitis (A) and Kulubnarti DISH (B).

and three contiguous cervical vertebrae fused by a waxlike bony extrusion. The fusion is along the anterior spinal ligaments, and there is no forward bending distortion of the spine. DISH can also involve areas beyond the spinal column, including peripheral joints such as the hip's acetabular rim (Fahrer et al. 1989). Here again, the Kulubnarti case met the clinical criteria. Marni and Paul made a solid case for DISH.

Rheumatoid Arthritis

The discovery of a likely case of RA in a 50+-year-old female from the mainland cemetery was, like the case of scoliosis, due to the sharp eye of Lynn Kilgore. RA occurs when the immune system attacks the membranes that surround synovial joints.[6] The resulting inflammation can eventually destroy the cartilage and bone within the joint. The tendons and ligaments that hold the joint together weaken and stretch. Gradually, the joint loses its shape and alignment. While it is understood that RA is a condition of the immune system, the cause(s) of the immune response isn't understood.

RA is often confused with osteoarthritis (OA). OA is primarily caused by simple wear and tear. Almost everyone develops some degree of it as they age. Typical changes involve bony formations (beading) around the rim of the joint (figure 6.40a) and erosion of the joint surface (figure 6.40b).

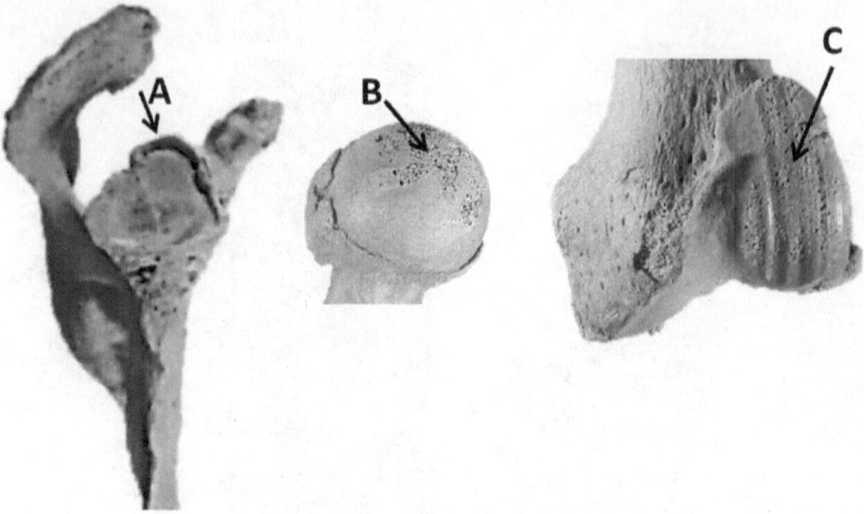

Figure 6.40. Osteoarthritic beading (A), erosion (B), and eburnation (C).

Cartilage loss may also result in bone-on-bone contact between the two sides of the joint. This can cause polishing and grooving on the surface of the bone, known as eburnation (figure 6.40c). Patterns of OA often reveal habitual activities during life (figure 6.41).

RA looks (figure 6.42) and behaves differently. It is primarily a disease of the small joints in the hands and feet. It is also erosive—bone within the

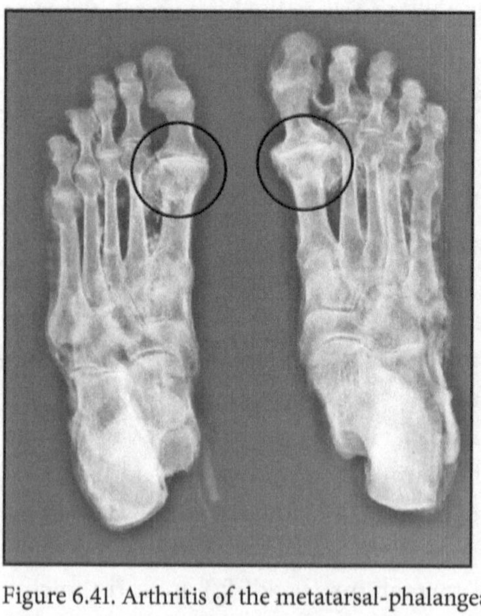

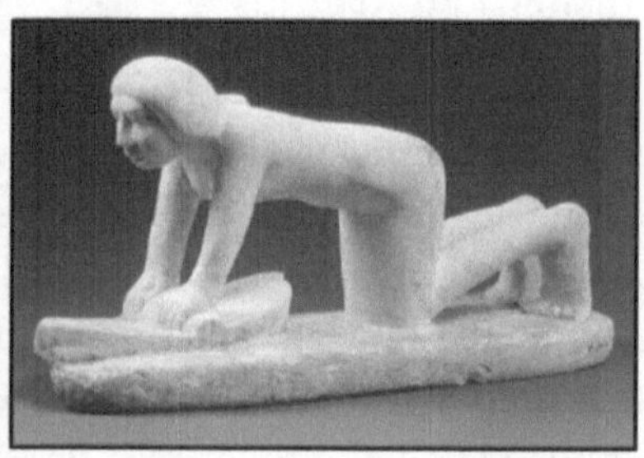

Figure 6.41. Arthritis of the metatarsal-phalangeal joint at Kulubnarti and a figurine from Egypt depicting grain grinding.

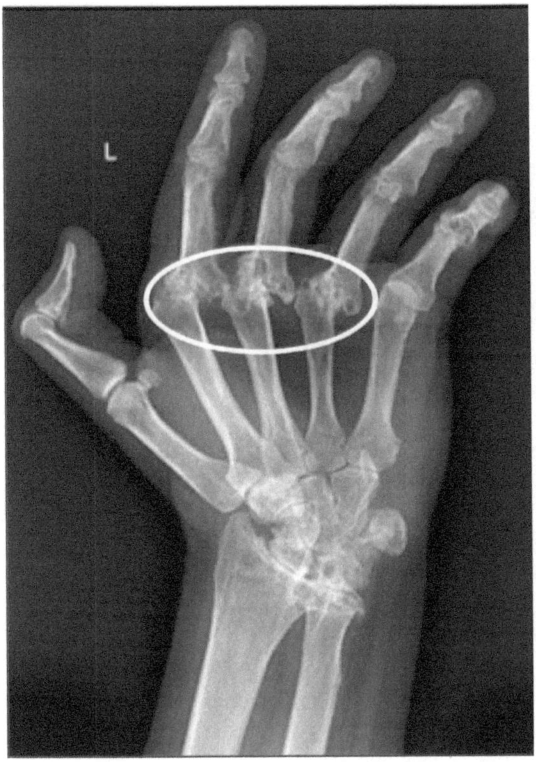

Figure 6.42. Clinical rheumatoid arthritis showing joint erosion and ulnar deviation of the digits (courtesy of Lynn Kilgore).

joint is lost rather than deposited in the manner of typical OA. Surrounding support tissues, such as tendons and ligaments, also become inflamed and weakened. Weakening leads to partial dislocation (figure 6.42b) of affected joints.

Lynn came across the Kulubnarti case while collecting data for her Ph.D. thesis on OA. The skeleton had severe OA in most joints. It was also osteoporotic. Neither of these was surprising, and it seemed as though it would take her only a quick analysis before moving on to the next skeleton. But the joints of the hands (figure 6.43) and feet didn't resemble OA. They appeared much like RA. Her discovery, if true, was indeed surprising. Researchers, including anthropologists and rheumatologists, continue to debate the antiquity of RA. A great deal of research in the 1970s suggested that it didn't appear in Europe until the seventeenth century. The recent origins hypothesis was challenged by several investigations a decade later. A thirteenth-century skeleton with apparent RA was found on Kodiak Island. There were also apparent cases from Europe, including written accounts of RA during the reign of Constantine IX (c. 980–1055). Perhaps the oldest

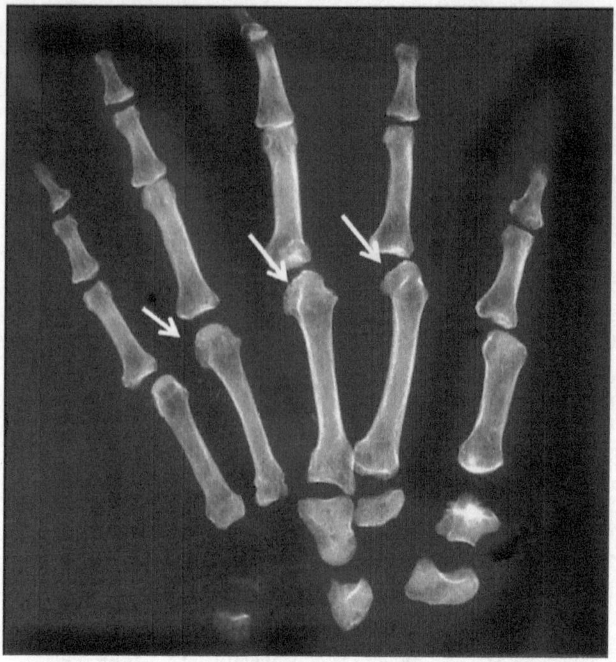

Figure 6.43. Erosive changes in the Kulubnarti case (courtesy of Lynn Kilgore).

example came from a 3rd dynasty Egyptian mummy dated to 2980–2900 BCE. Still, the number of cases was (and is today) few and far between. Indeed, some researchers continue to doubt the presence of RA before the seventeenth century.

The Kulubnarti case conformed to the RA pattern. The changes were clearly erosive (figure 6.43) and involved the joints between the metacarpals and phalanges, as is typical in RA. There was beveling on all of the

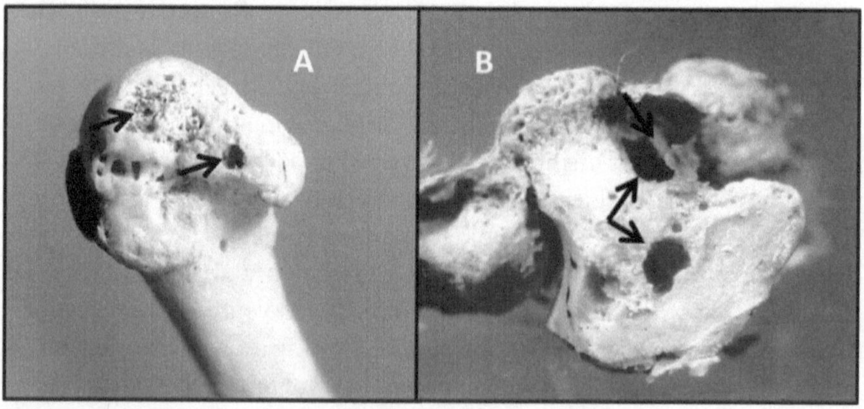

Figure 6.44. Lytic lesions of the right third metacarpal (A) and right hamate (B) in the Kulubnarti case.

metacarpals, and the distal end of the third metacarpal was completely eroded away. There was also trabecular bone loss beneath the cartilage of the affected joints—also characteristic of RA. There were additional changes typical of RA. These included classic circular erosive (lytic) lesions on the right third metacarpal (figure 6.43a) and right hamate (figure 6.44a, b) (Kilgore 1989).

In Lynn's view, the case for RA was strong but not definitive. Other conditions, such as Lupus and even some bacterial infections, can cause similar lesions. Her case, like all of our cases, was circumstantial. There were no attending physicians, and only part of the diagnostic evidence was available. Nevertheless, the evidence supported a strong inference for RA. This included:

1. Involvement of those skeletal elements most frequently associated with RA.
2. Lytic (large circular) lesions on articular surfaces.
3. Osteoporotic bone loss beneath the joint cartilage.
4. Lateral deviation of the digits.

Legg-Calve-Perthes Disease

Legg-Calve-Perthes disease, or avascular necrosis, is commonly referred to in the vernacular as "mushroom-head femur." The condition develops in children when a growth plate loses its blood supply—hence the term "avascular." Lacking nutrition and oxygen, the cartilage and bone tissues die (become necrotic), and the femur head eventually collapses. Doctors describe the condition as self-limiting in children. Young children (six years or younger) resorb the damaged epiphysis and replace it with a new normal one. The chances of a normal recovery go down, however, with advancing age.

The condition is rare in the archaeological record but has been reported in various populations. Two cases were reported in Czech archaeological remains. One of these was a 50-year-old late fifth-century male excavated from a cemetery in Moravia. The second was a tenth-century skeleton from Brandýsek (Bohemia) (Smrcka et al. 2009). A case has also been recently reported from Argentina (Ponce and Novellino 2014). The causes of the condition are mysterious, even in modern clinical cases. Epidemiological studies in Great Britain have shown higher frequencies among poor children as well as children living in inner cities. It is less frequent in children of African and Asian ancestry (Barker and Hall 1986).

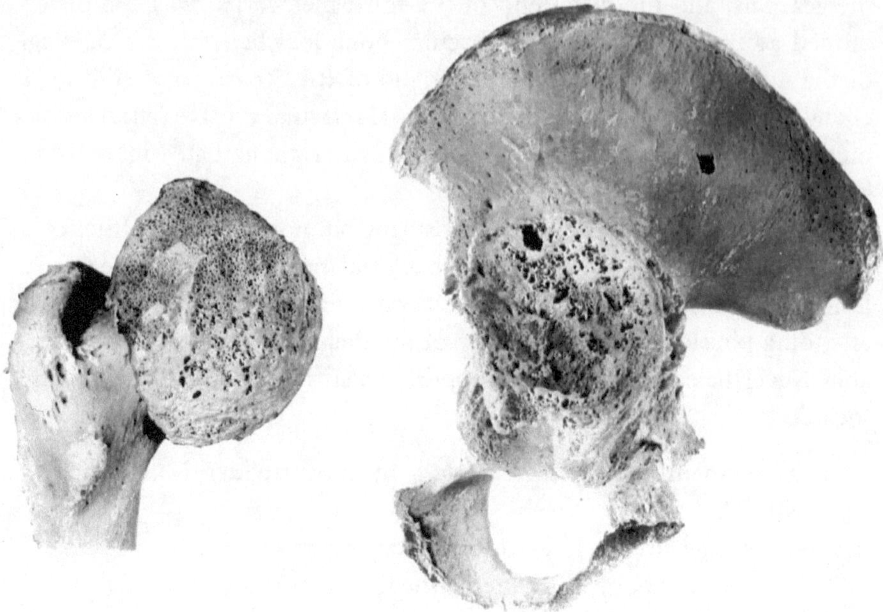

Figure 6.45. Avascular necrosis, or "mushroom head," femur from Wadi Halfa.

Our case is that of a 41-year-old X-Group female (figure 6.45). The condition is well described by the vernacular mushroom head. The femur head appears as though it has been compressed backward against the femoral neck and spread outward at the same time.

This makes it look very much like the cap of a mushroom. The acetabulum has become broadened to accommodate the misshapen femur head. In addition to the malformation, there is considerable evidence for OA, including the kind of polishing (ebernation) associated with OA. This would have compounded the impairment of the joint. Other facts support the inference that joint impairment had a severe impact on mobility. ML shaft diameters at 25 percent, 50 percent, and 75 percent of the proximal-to-distal diaphyseal length are 18 percent, 21 percent, and 25 percent smaller for the affected femur. Femur lengths, on the other hand (taken from the greater trochanter to the inferior lateral condyle), are virtually identical. This is reminiscent of our hydrocephalic child, with limbs of normal length but with dramatically reduced diameters. That said, the presence of eburnation within the joint indicates that while limb function was impaired, the limb wasn't paralyzed.

Infectious Diseases

A Possible Case of *Herpes Zoster*

A common sign of systemic (generalized) infection in skeletal remains is periosteal reaction (figure 6.46). It is most commonly caused by a bacteria known as *Staphylococcus.* The bacteria normally lives on our skin but can become pathogenic when it enters the body by way of a wound or a trauma, such as a broken bone. Perhaps most important for our interests, it can become pathogenic when an individual's immune system is compromised by stressors such as illness or poor nutrition. Staph, as it is commonly known, can infect bone marrow and also the bone surface around and under the fibrous membrane (the periosteum) surrounding the bone. The body's reaction to infection under the periosteal membrane produces a raised scab-like lesion on the bone's surface.

Lesion frequencies have been used extensively by paleopathologists as a measure of systemic infections in populations. They provided important evidence for the decline in health during the transition from foraging to agriculture. A classic early analysis was conducted on human remains from Dickson Mounds, Illinois (950–1300 CE) by A. H. Goodman and coworkers (1984). A paleopathologist named Donald Ortner (1998) surveyed four archaeological sites and found frequencies ranging from 3 percent to 24 percent.[7] The frequency at Wadi Halfa was 1.7 percent and less than 1 percent at Kulubnarti. George has argued that the low frequencies may be due to the ingestion of tetracycline (see our discussion in the previous chapter).

There is, however, one possible case of infection at Kulubnarti that is interesting. It's *Herpes zoster.* The infection is a second manifestation of chicken pox. Chicken pox is an infectious disease caused by the virus *Varicella zoster.* Chicken pox was a common infectious disease as recently as the

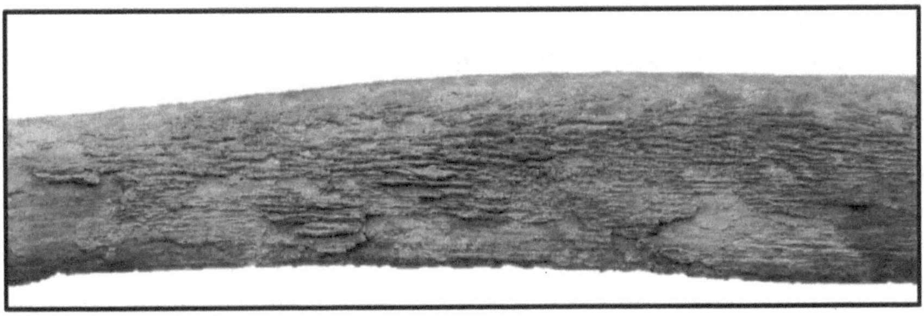

Figure 6.46. Periosteal infection of the tibia.

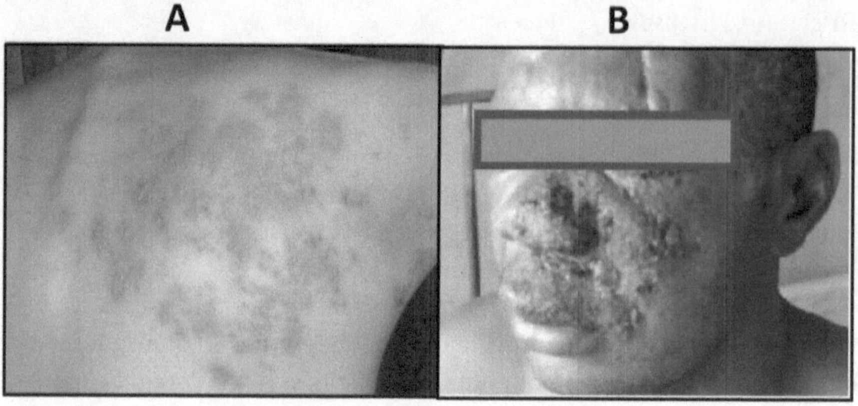

Figure 6.47. *Herpes zoster* infection on the back (A) and face (B).

1990s. Some four million Americans were infected each year, some 12,000 were hospitalized, and between 100 and 150 died. A chicken pox vaccine was introduced in 1995, and the frequency of infection dropped dramatically, with a decline of 82 percent between 2000 and 2010.

Recovery from chicken pox doesn't mean an absence of infection. The symptoms disappear, but the virus remains in our bodies for the rest of our lives, and some 4–10 percent of us will experience a reawakening of the virus in our later lives. The result is a very different condition known as *Herpes zoster*, or shingles. Shingles appears as a painful blistering rash (figure 6.47a) produced as the activated virus travels along cutaneous (skin) nerves. While the rash commonly appears on the chest, back, and arms, it occasionally spreads to the face and mouth (figure 6.47b) by way of the trigeminal nerve (figure 6.48). The trigeminal nerve separates into three branches, forming the maxillary sensory, mandibular sensory, and ophthalmic sensory nerves that serve the face. The infection can lead to necrosis (death) of alveolar bone supporting the teeth (Mendieta et al. 2005) that is far more extensive than the kind of tooth loss we discussed earlier.

It's the oral-facial aspect of *Herpes zoster* infection that we found intriguing in the case of a middle-age X-Group female with alveolar bone loss so severe that George initially interpreted it as resulting from a malignancy. Our subsequent examination suggested the possibility of alveolar necrosis resulting from a herpes infection.

The possibility is based on two areas of infection. The first is the maxilla. Bone loss extends almost to the nasal openings (figure 6.49a) and through the hard palate into the maxillary sinuses in several places (figure 6.49b).

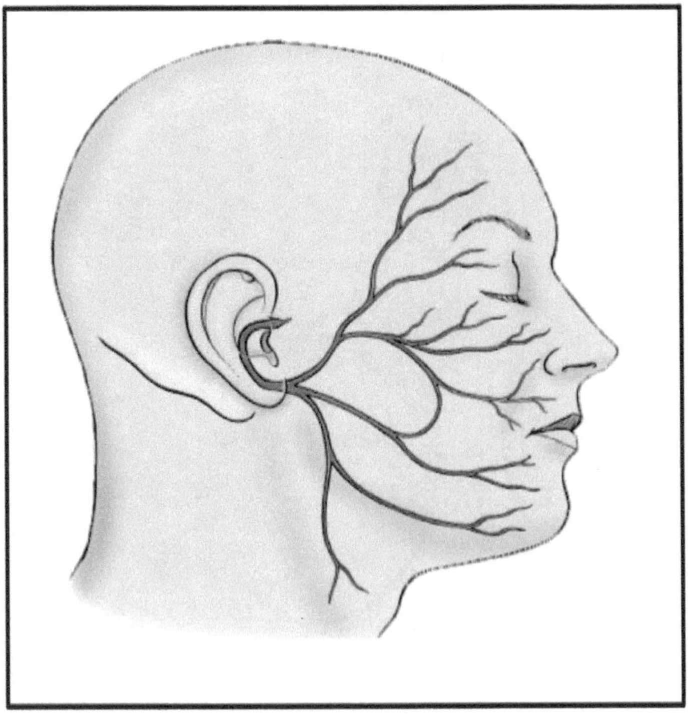

Figure 6.48. Branches of the trigeminal nerve.

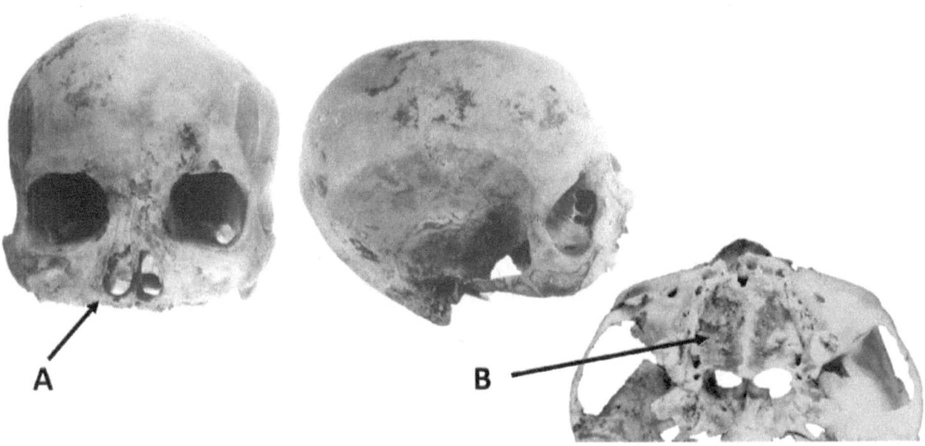

Figure 6.49. Alveolar resorption in an X-Group female.

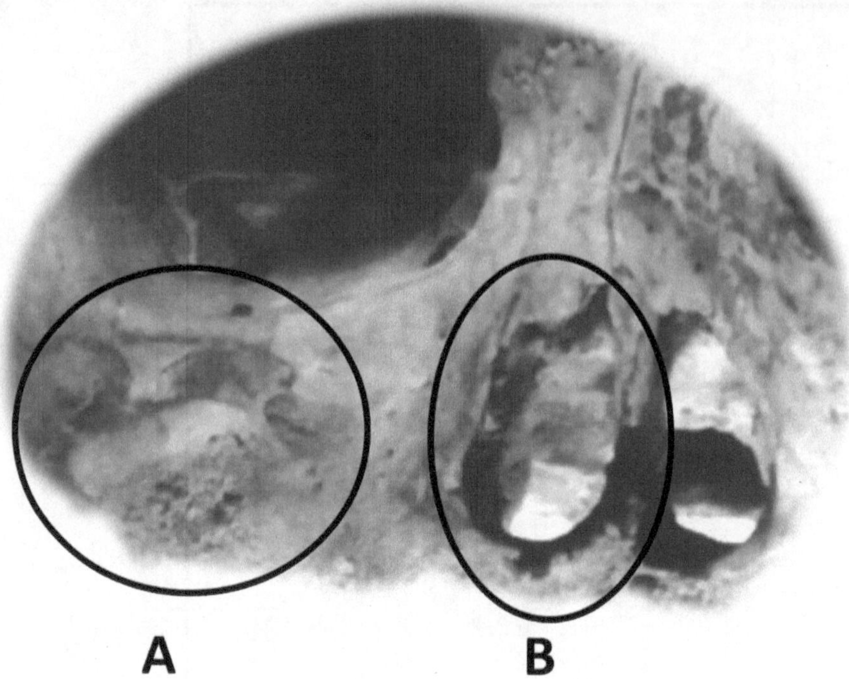

Figure 6.50. Infraorbital foramen infection (A) and nasal infection (B).

The second area is less obvious but also intriguing. There appear to be signs of infection surrounding the opening (foramen) for the right trigeminal nerve (figure 6.50a) and the right nasal opening (figure 6.50b). As we mentioned, the virus typically invades the face by way of the trigeminal nerve and often involves the nasal opening.

The presence of extreme maxillary bone loss and possible infection of the trigeminal nerve suggest an interesting possibility of *Herpes zoster*, but there are weaknesses to the argument. The virus typically infects one side of the face only. That is consistent with what we observed in the trigeminal and nasal lesions, but not with the alveolus. That left us with two possible interpretations that could not be resolved with the evidence at hand. This may have been an atypical case of *Herpes zoster* that affected both sides of the mouth, possibly due to a secondary infection, or we had an extreme case of alveolar resorption resulting from tooth loss. We found the *zoster* hypothesis intriguing, but not as strong as our other cases.

This concludes our case studies. It seemed remarkable to us to have such a wide variety of interesting and relatively rare conditions. Were the Wadi

Halfa and Kulubnarti populations unusual in this regard? It's possible, but not necessarily so. The remains were remarkably well preserved at both Wadi Halfa and Kulubnarti. This had to have increased the likelihood of discovering such a wide range of conditions with multiple lines of evidence, both osteological and archaeological. Our last chapter will attempt to create a narrative of life and death in our Nubian communities. What must life have been like for the sick and dying in communities with none of the medical science we rely on today? And just as important, what was life like for the community—particularly for those who loved and cared for the sick and dying? Does our evidence even allow us to ask such questions? Limited as we are, can we even speak to questions of love and compassion? George and I believed that these are important questions to be considered. We believed that elusive as they may be, they are at the very heart of what we have come to think of as our bioethnography. This brings us to our last chapter.

7

A BIOETHNOGRAPHY

> Anthropology is the most humanistic of the sciences and the most scientific of the humanities.
>
> Eric Wolf

In Retrospect

The best way to appreciate how far you have come is to look back to where you started. That has certainly been the case for George and me. "Bones are like old books in strange languages. Learn how to read them and they have wonderful tales to tell"—the epigraph for the first chapter. That's where our story began. George and I have spent over a half century reading the bones. The discipline has changed a lot in that time.

Some years ago, Jack Kelso,[1] a colleague, friend, and George's thesis adviser, made an interesting observation relevant to the changes we have seen. He pointed out that anthropology's view of the connection between biology and culture has gone through three stages. In the first stage, anthropologists envisioned biology (race) as the determining cause of cultural achievement. In the second stage, race and culture were divorced. Franz Boas, considered to be the founder of anthropology in the United States,[2] led the critical reaction to the racial determinism, arguing for the independence of race, language, and culture (Boas 1940). Stage three emerged with a shift in focus toward the importance of the cultural environment to the evolution of human populations. Stage three, of course, gave rise to a biocultural approach.

You have seen how each has played its part in the history of anthropology in the Nile Valley. Remains from the First Archaeological Survey were viewed almost entirely from a racial determinist perspective. By the second survey, scholars such as Ahmed Batrawi had divorced race from cultural achievement—arguing that the two were independent. And finally, the UNESCO Campaign gave birth to the biocultural approach that has guided our research.

As George's and my interest in the cultural context grew, we began to see parallels between what we were trying to achieve and ethnography. Ethnographers study systems of food production; we studied nutritional diseases. Ethnographers study kinship systems; we studied genetic relationships. Ethnographers study politics; we studied the biological costs of social and economic inequality. The idea of describing our work as a bioethnography came to me while preparing a paper for a Wenner-Gren conference back in 1987. I decided to title the paper "Nutrition, Disease, and the Human Life Cycle: A Bioethnography of a Medieval Nubian Community" (Van Gerven et al. 1990).

I recognized at the time that our bioethnography was not an ethnography in a literal sense. We had dug graves, but we hadn't attended funerals. We had studied growth retardation and various nutritional conditions, but we hadn't witnessed the social cost of poverty and inequality. We had studied cases of grievous disease, but the fear of the afflicted or the pain of their loved ones had elluded us. Our limitations were clear, but had we learned enough to cross the line dividing the material and immaterial sides of our Nubians' lives? What tales had the bones told us? Answering that question seemed a fitting way to look back retrospectively on our six decades of work together. To begin, we needed a way to organize our information. A paleontology course taught by a colleague provided us what we needed.

When Bert Covert teaches paleontology, he organizes his lectures into three categories of information. The categories are these: certainly true, probably true, and possibly true. Some facts are certainly true about the Nubians. We are certain that mummification occurred naturally. We are certain that some of the coprolites contained schistosome eggs. We are certain that at least three individuals from Wadi Halfa had a neoplasm. We are certain that one individual had Legg-Calve-Perthes disease.

The "probables" are more dependent on strong inference. One of the neoplasms was most probably a metastatic carcinoma, and another was probably a chondrosarcoma. The individual with the schistosome eggs in his feces probably had a urinary tract infection. The cancer victims probably died of their disease. It's possibly true that our cancer victims died of something else, and it's possible (but highly unlikely) that our Perthes victim walked with hardly any limp at all. It's possible that the health differences between the island and mainland communities at Kulubnarti had nothing to with class or economic conditions.

If we were laying odds on the distinctions we have made, the certainties are our sure bets. The probables are short odds bets, and the possibles are longer odds. The long odds are always best argued when they can be linked to one or more certainties. Here are some linkages. We excavated five fetuses, each of which was approximately seven gestational months. Each of the five was placed in a jar or urn before interment. We excavated a grave with one newborn, two children (six years old and ten years old), and one teenager (age 14) buried atop each other in the same grave. It was certainly a single grave. There was absolutely no evidence that the grave was opened more than once (the walls were smooth and continuous), and there was no evidence of intrusion. We are certain that the four were buried together, just as we're certain that the fetuses were buried in pots or jars.

Let's now consider a probability and a possibility for each. Our Nubians probably had sufficient experience to recognize premature births, and it's possible that they had symbolically placed the fetuses back in a "womb." There is a probability that the four children were buried together because they shared some culturally defined relationship of importance. Perhaps they were siblings or close relatives. Perhaps they were close friends. Let's do one last interpretation before we move on. An eight-year-old girl was buried with her hair braided into cornrows (figure 7.1). She is one of several with that hairstyle—all girls, and all children. There is a real possibility that it was done for aesthetic reasons. It is possible that it is a gendered style. It's a certainty that whatever the reason, it took a lot of effort to do.

K. A. Dettwyler has argued that paleopathology's focus on physical traits "as the *sole* measure of productive ability" (Dettwyler 1991:375, emphasis ours) leaves us unjustified in drawing conclusions about the quality of life of people with disabilities or the motives and attitudes toward them of the people among whom they lived. In other words, any discussion of what we call probabilities and possibilities is mere conjecture. Conjecture folk such as Dettwyler argue that no conjecture is worth considering because none are more worthy of consideration than the others. And, most important, the anatomical evidence *alone* provides no way of choosing among them. For example, according to Dettwyler, the physical evidence provides us no way to exclude the possibility that someone braided the little girl's hair to shame and humiliate her. Likewise, the physical evidence *alone* cannot resolve whether the four children were buried together because of a social attachment or because having died together it was convenient to bury them in one grave.

Dettwyler is correct in both cases, but her argument is flawed. In debate, there is a strategy known as the straw man argument. The tactic is to

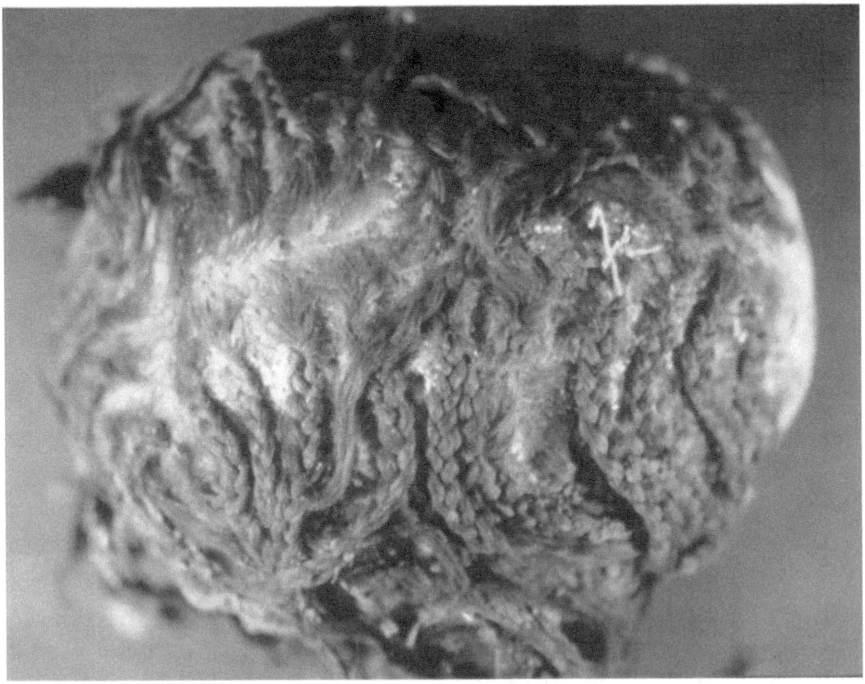

Figure 7.1. Eight-year-old mainland girl with cornrow braids.

create a false position that is easy to argue against. That is what Dettwyler has done. She constructs her argument as though all inferences regarding the conduct of ancient people are based on the physical traits only. That's certainly not true in our case. Done well, inferences regarding the values, attitudes, and conduct of ancient peoples are as bioculturally based as any other aspect of osteological analysis.

This is an important issue for us, particularly at the end of our story. Our intention has been to go beyond data analysis to some kind of ethnographic-like understanding of the Nubians as people. We have hoped to make them more than objects of inquiry. We've wanted to put some flesh on their bones. If we accept the argument that any reach beyond the certain is little more than pointless speculation, we shouldn't even try. We should abandon all hope for a bioethnography. So let's look beyond the data and see what we can see. We'll begin with our little eleven-year-old girl as she lay dying of hydrocephalus.

She was almost certainly bedridden. Remember, her limbs had the diameter of those of a two-year-old. It is a certainty that she didn't lose the diameters; instead, she never gained them. Atrophy would have thinned her bones from the inside. She had probably been immobile, if not vegetative, for years. The morphology of her masseter attachments and dentition indicates that she was almost certainly a bruxer and tongue thruster—both signs of severe mental retardation. The tartar behind her lower incisors suggests that her chewing and swallowing had been seriously impaired for a long time. She was almost certainly bedridden in a persistent vegetative state at the time of her death.

Is it reasonable to infer that she was treated with compassion? This child wasn't sick for days, weeks, or even months. We're talking years—possibly to some degree since birth.

Think about what had to be done, if only to keep her alive that long. Context: the child had to be fed; her urine and feces had to be disposed of. Her bedding had to be changed and washed. These are horribly unpleasant tasks, even on a short-term basis. But they are bedrock necessities. People die of bedsores when forced to lie in their own excrement. They can die of bedsores by simply not being turned. We'll say again, she lived to be eleven years old! Let's push the boundaries of the possible farther. We think it's reasonable to believe that the little girl was loved as well as cared for. We think it's highly probable, given the challenges necessary to keep her alive, that her loved ones grieved for her when she died. We think it is reasonable to make that inference.

Let's revisit another of our cases. A middle-age man developed a metastatic carcinoma, probably in his pelvis and possibly secondary to a schistosome infection in his bladder. The cancer probably spread upward through his vertebral column, into his shoulder and finally into his skull, where it produced two large erosive lesions. We can construct opposing scenarios for the circumstances of the victim's life that the facts alone cannot resolve.

He may have been ignored because a lot of people in the community were as sick as he was. His illness may have been disregarded by his kin because they gave his life little value, and had no sense of moral rightness in his regard. It is conceivable that the hemorrhages in his bladder and the blood clots in his urine were of no particular interest to his family. Bone cancer is extremely painful, but it's possible that the pain provoked no sympathy at all. Perhaps he was just one among many sufferers with no call upon anyone's sympathy.

For the cancer to have progressed as far as it did, he had to have been sick—very sick—for a very long time. You will recall that an oncologist observing the skeleton remarked that he had never seen this kind of cancer advanced this far. He pointed out that patients today are either cured or die of the disease before it reaches that stage. The progression and extent of the disease are relevant to resolving our opposing interpretations. To survive as he did, it is far more likely that he was fed, washed, and cared for than ignored and left to his fate. While recourse to ethnography is often overused, it is relevant to ask for a single ethnographic example of a society with so little sense of moral rightness or value for a kinsman's life as to abandon him. In that context alone it would seem far more reasonable to infer a community of family and friends supported him out of some sense of moral rightness and some sense of basic human empathy.

Thinking about ethnographic analogies got George and me thinking about uniformitarianism. Uniformitarianism "is the principle or assumption that the same natural laws and processes that operate in the universe now have always operated in the universe in the past and apply everywhere in the universe" (Gould 1965). It's the concept of uniformitarianism. The assumption is essential to all of the sciences. What if the law of physics observed in the universe today didn't apply in the past? How would we hope to understand the evolution of the cosmos? What if the action of muscles and bones observed in animals today didn't operate in the same way in the past? How could we begin to interpret the fossil record? What would become of paleopathology and all of archaeology for that matter? What if the laws of human conduct observed throughout the ethnographic record were not in force in the past? Archaeology would amount to so many artifacts and osteology to so many bones, all giving no hope of understanding. It's important to recognize that the assumption of uniformitarianism is as important to the historical-behavioral sciences as the natural sciences. It has been argued that the universal prohibition against sibling– and parent–child incest is due at least in part to selection against the behavior in the past. But what if the relationship between genetics and inbreeding didn't operate in the past?

As with inbreeding, many of the alternative scenarios constructed by conjecture folk employ behaviors that could have no possible adaptive value. It's interesting that Charles Darwin railed against the "tooth and claw" characterization of natural selection. He argued that the most noble and altruistic of human behaviors would be as valuable, and therefore selected, as the most aggressive and violent.

As for the laws of social conduct in operation today that might reasonably be applied to our understanding of the past, George and I both found

Robert Redfield's characterization of small-scale or folk societies particularly revealing. According to Redfield:

> Behavior is personal, not impersonal. A "person" may be defined as that social object which I feel to respond to situations as I do, with all the sentiments and interests which I feel to be my own; a person is myself in another form, his qualities and values are inherent within him, and his significance for me is not merely one of utility. A "thing" on the other hand, is a social object which has no claim upon my sympathies, which responds to me . . . mechanically; its value for me exists only in so far as it serves my end. In a folk society, all human beings admitted to the society are treated as persons; one does not deal impersonally ("thing fashion") with any other participant in the little world of that society. (Redfield 1947)

All of our cases don't have to be as dramatic as cancer and hydrocephalus to make our point. Our case of scoliosis is certainly diagnosed correctly. Still we think the victim probably had a reasonably productive life. Our analysis of his femurs indicated that he most likely got around quite well with the use of some sort of support—perhaps a staff. He may have been able to do a lot of useful things for himself and others. It's unlikely that he was a major drain on his community. The anatomical facts can't tell us if he was teased and emotionally abused. The physical evidence doesn't reveal if he was revered or an object of ridicule. We do know, however, that his disability began in the womb and he became so bent that his right ribs were in his pelvis. It's likely that a trek to the river would have been extremely difficult and possibly required some help negotiating the rocks and boulders. The facts by themselves may not reveal the quality of his social support, but one fact is telling: he lived as long as might be expected today without major medical intervention. That's an important context. Then there are the far more minor cases of broken legs and arms and such. Would such injuries by themselves make the case for compassion and a strong case for a sense of moral rightness in the community? Probably not, but even they were disabling in the short run and required some level of social support. Dettwyler asks whether paleopathology can find evidence of compassion. The answer is yes and no. The anatomical evidence alone can tell us little or nothing, but in context the evidence is intriguing and worthy of analysis.

Last Reflections

As we discussed early on, our discipline isn't an experimental science. We tease out patterns of causality using points of comparison. These are natural experiments. Our Nubian populations have given us a treasure trove of opportunities. Meinarti provided us some 17 centuries of political and economic stability and change. Kulubnarti provided a snapshot of two communities spanning little more than two generations. And of course, both provided opportunities for the fundamental comparisons of age and sex.

Strong inference is a theme common to all of the research presented in this volume. What inferences can we take with us at the end of our story? Most are reaffirmations of the human condition. Some 85 percent of the people living today along the course of the Nile suffer from iron deficiency anemia. It's estimated that 40,000 of the world's children die of weanling diarrhea each day. Thirty-five percent of infants at Meinarti developed cribra orbitalia, and virtually 100 percent developed the lesion at Kulubnarti. Every child at Kulubnarti developed at least one hypoplasia, and over 20 percent of the enamel they produced was hypoplastic. Cribra orbitalia, hypoplasias, and microdefects all peak together near the time of weaning when the probability of dying is highest also. The children of Meinarti and Kulubnarti were dying of anemia and weanling diarrhea as surely as children in the world today.

Our research also confirms that the two laws of social success in force today operated in the past. Law #1: "How you do depends on who you are." The people with enough status to warrant a tomb at Meinarti had the best chance of seeing old age. Law #2: "Where you are is the companion of who you are." All the children of Kulubnarti were worse off by every measure we have taken than their kinsmen to the north. They weren't bad children. They didn't deserve to be sick. As Vonnegut would have said, they simply landed on earth in the wrong place. The children of the itinerant laborers living on the island were worse off yet—they were victims of both laws. They were born in the wrong place to the wrong people. The consequences of social disadvantage within and between communities ran as true in the past as they do today.

There is an old saying that goes something like this: "The sins of the fathers are visited on the children." We'll change it to the ills of the mothers are visited on the children. Among the Kulubnarti women, poor nutrition resulted in poor growth in their children. Poor growth constricted the little girl's pelves. Constricted pelves advantaged small babies at birth who were

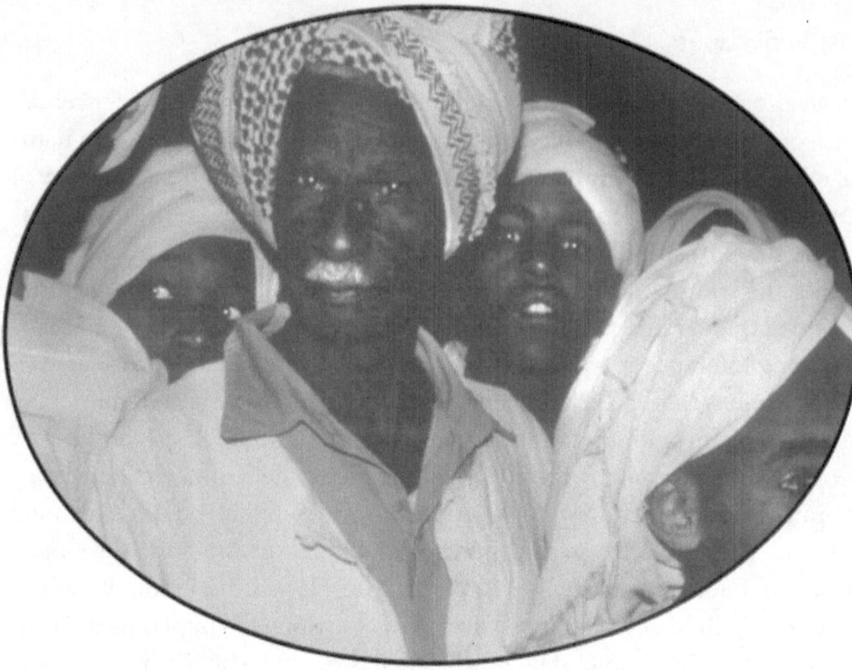

Figure 7.2. Abdul Salam at a wedding.

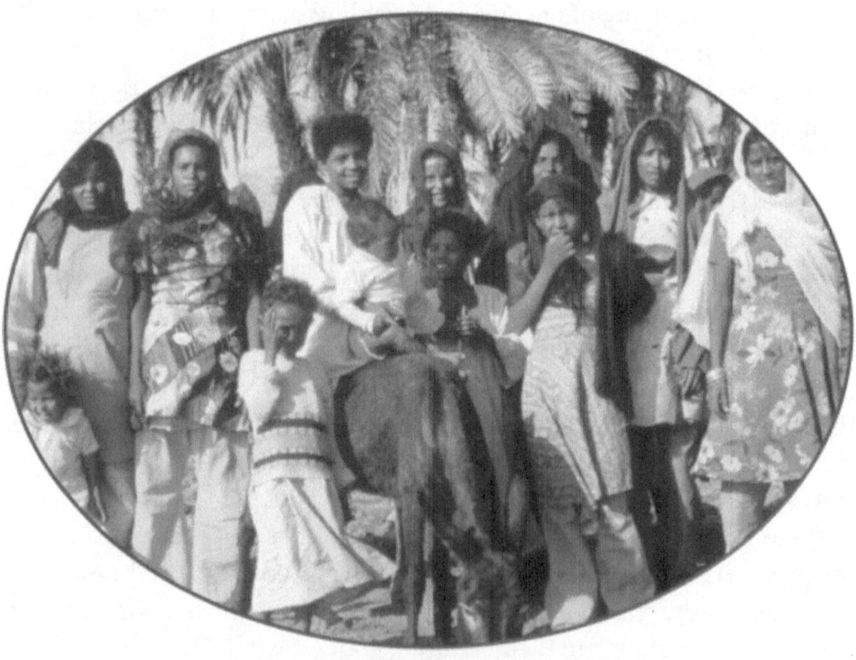

Figure 7.3. Kulb women and children seeing off a sister.

disadvantaged when they were challenged by the stresses of infancy and childhood. Those disadvantages reverberated through the adult years, and the cycle began again. Not all of the challenges were faced by infants and children. It is unlikely that the birth rate in the island population could have kept up with the high rate of infant mortality. The rate would have been nearly maxed out on the mainland.

We mentioned back in chapter 5 the old saying that my grandmother taught me: "Have a baby, lose a tooth." We also pointed out that even in the harshest environments, babies will not be malnourished in the womb or on the breast as long as mothers have bodily resources to provide. The women of Kulubnarti had to have been pregnant or lactating virtually all of their reproductive lives. The women of Kulubnarti island lost more bone than their mainland counterparts.

Then there is the notion of cultural achievement and success. Periods of cultural florescence and decline have often been measured in Nubia and elsewhere in terms of artistic and architectural achievements. Our analyses have suggested that such assessments have too often been made without due regard for the well-being of the populations involved. The X-Group folk lived poorer lives (in a material sense) compared to the Meroitic folk that preceded them, and yet they were, in many ways, healthier and more robust than their Meroitic ancestors.

Finally, we won't shrink from what we assert as strong inferences regarding our case studies. Recall how Karl Pearson (the famous statistician) talked about measurement by appreciation. He was describing those things that can't be measured with calipers. They have to be appreciated by judgment of the eye. We can well appreciate the care and devotion, *and* compassion, that supported our eleven-year-old girl with hydrocephalus or our cancer victims. The same can be said for our victims of DISH and scoliosis. Even the fractures and abscessed teeth would have been challenging without a modicum of help from others.

We can't forget a context common to them all. They were all confronted without the advantages of even rudimentary (by modern standards) technologies of medical intervention and support. In that context alone we challenge any proposition that ancient people such as our Nubians reacted to the pain and suffering of kin and neighbors any differently than we do today. We'll say once again because it bears repeating: all the possibilities of human conduct aren't equally likely simply because they can be imagined. There is a quote from Albert Einstein that is worth keeping in mind for all scientists: "To raise new questions, new possibilities, to regard old problems from a new angle, requires creative imagination and marks real advance in science" (Einstein and Field 1932:92).

People often ask what our Nubians looked like. The answer is quite simple. Look at them today. The Nubian people today are a living testimony to biological and cultural continuity. We should never forget that for all of their seeming poverty, they are the sons and daughters of pharaohs.

AFTERWORD

The future depends on what you do today.
Mahatma Gandhi

When David Greene, Bill Adams, and I proposed the Kulubnarti project to the National Science Foundation (NSF) back in 1978, we requested funds to bring the remains back to Colorado rather than leave the skeletons behind after conducting our analysis there. Our rationale was to create a collection that would support future research employing technologies yet to be invented.

The tremendous success George was having with little more than pieces of femur supported our argument. The NSF decision to support our proposal has paid off with a greater abundance of new science than we ever expected. One of the questions I am frequently asked after a public presentation is when we will be finished. It pleases me to say never, or at least not in the foreseeable future.

When I think about the future and all of the research we have accomplished in the past, I'm reminded of how prophetic George was. He never lost sight of his commitment to biocultural synthesis, but he also saw the potential of emerging technologies—many of them from medical research. I suspect his early training in medical school had a lot to do with that. George saw an exciting future in which traditional organ-level analyses would delve deeper to the tissue and chemical levels as was being done in biomedical research. John Dewey did the cortical thickness work. Kip Owen did the bone mineral content analysis, and Debra Martin did one of the early analyses of the histology.[1] Then there was Debra's discovery of tetracycline.

The Kulubnarti remains opened a new chapter for David, George, and me. David analyzed the genetic relationship between the island and mainland populations using the discrete dental traits he had applied to population relationships at Wadi Halfa. This time he applied new multivariate statistical techniques not available when he did his Wadi Halfa analysis. David, George, and I also conducted an analysis of Kulubnarti demographics using a life table technique that wasn't being applied to ancient human populations at the time of the Meinarti research. B. L. Turner and coresearchers performed isotopic analyses of the Kulubnarti populations supporting our evidence for nutritional privation in the island community compared to their mainland counterparts. Once again, the technology was unheard of when we returned the Kulubnarti skeletons. The list could go on, but my point is made; Kulubnarti has continued to be a rich source of research using emerging technologies.

Here are two examples from two extraordinary students. Paul Sandberg is conducting an isotopic analysis of infant and childhood diet using a recently developed high-resolution technique. Where isotope amounts are typically measured from enamel or dentine taken from an entire tooth crown, Paul is able to sample slices of dentine along the length of a tooth crown in six-month intervals. Because the relative amounts of carbon and nitrogen isotopes change at weaning,[2] Paul has been able to measure the actual age of weaning in the Kulubnarti children.

Where in the past we defined the age of weaning as two years and made our comparisons on that basis, Paul's data has revealed a weaning process varying from child to child and playing out over many months or even a year or more. This is giving us a whole new perspective on childhood stressors such as weanling diarrhea.

Kendra Serak was George's last doctoral student, and since George's death I have had the privilege of serving as her co-advisor. George was committed to extending our analyses of the Nubian remains from the morphological to the microscopic levels. Kendra is taking the analysis one step further to the molecular level, or more precisely the level of DNA. Up until now our analyses of genetic relationships among the Wadi Halfa and Kulubnarti populations have been based on imperfectly understood discrete and metric features of the skull and dentition. We have talked about these.

Kendra's work promises to change all of that.

Kendra's analysis of DNA extracted from the Kulubnarti remains promises to accomplish two important goals. First, it will deepen our understanding of the genetic relationships between the two Kulubnarti communities. We have referred to the island folk as itinerant workers traveling about as opportunities for work dictated. But how closely were they related to the farmers for whom they worked? David Greene's analysis of discrete dental characters found little difference between the communities, but that was using evidence one step removed from the actual genes. Kendra will be looking at single nucleotide polymorphisms, or SNPs, sites of within- and between-population variation in DNA sequence, to explore the genetic relationships to address the question.

It's been 52 years since George and his fellow graduate students went to Wadi Halfa and 40 years since I went to Kulubnarti—almost a century of combined research. Amazingly, the handful of femur sections that George brought back are still generating research, and the Kulubnarti remains continue to attract researchers from around the world. I am proud of what George, I, and our many students have accomplished. We hope you have enjoyed our story.

THE END

NOTES

Chapter 1. Life and Death on the Nile

Epigraph: This quote arose in a conversation between the authors. If you have information about this quote, please contact the University Press of Florida.

1. "Narti" means island in Arabic; hence "Kulubnarti" means island of Kulb.
2. This was before Armelagos's arrival to Emory University when he switched his allegiance to Coca Cola.
3. Meinarti will provide the cultural context for all of the remains to be discussed in this volume.
4. For the remainder of the volume, site 21-S-46 will be referred to as the island community and 21-R-2 as the mainland community.

Chapter 2. Skulls, Races, and Evolution

1. Technically it is the standard error, but that is unimportant to our discussion.
2. The debate as to the quality of archaeological samples is beyond our discussion.
3. There are statistical tables that provide the likelihood of Student's *t* values.
4. The values 1.7, 1.4, 1.8, 1.7 are Z-scores calculated for each skull from its original measurements.
5. We discuss the technology in chapters 5 and 6.
6. The term used to describe skulls with large projecting faces is "prognathic."
7. David argued this in his dissertation prior to our Mesolithic project.

Chapter 3. Health and Disease: The Children

1. Harris lines are no longer considered evidence of growth disruption.
2. There are a number of excellent readings on the subject, including an article titled "The Five Sexes" written by Anne Fausto-Sterling back in 1993. She published a second titled "The Five Sexes, Revisited" in 2000.
3. You will note that in some of our subsequent analysis individuals are represented in whole years. Some statistics require a single number for each case. In that case all individuals were assigned the category's middle value.
4. Survivorship is computed by starting with 100 percent of individuals in the first age category and then calculating the percentage remaining in each successive category.
5. Refinements in the timing of crown development and defect formation have been made since my work. I chose to present the methods applied to my measurements.

Chapter 4. Growth and Development

1. The chair of the department refused to serve on Paul's thesis committee, saying that he thought the analysis was meaningless.

2. The periods were combined in order to increase sample size.

3. *Indian Pediatr Suppl* (2009):46:S12–S19.

4. Mummified sex organs aren't as easy to diagnose as you might think. But it can often be done.

5. He used his femur data for the Wadi Halfa comparisons because that was the only data available for Wadi Halfa.

Chapter 5. Health and Disease: The Adults

1. Periodontal disease is a fourth, but I will not be presenting it in this chapter.

2. Technically, bone loss is referred to as osteopenia until there is a loss-related fracture.

3. Only thickness was available for Wadi Halfa.

4. Percent cortical area was measured using the grid technique discussed in chapter 3.

5. A large individual with osteoporosis may have a thicker cortex than a small individual without. Using percent cortical area solves that problem.

6. My wife, Claudia, and I spent the summer prior to our move to Massachusetts with George preparing the sections.

7. Other data was collected, but is unnecessary for our discussion.

8. It was impossible to analyze the entire cross sections.

9. This is what we couldn't do for the Nubians and why Frost developed his algorithm.

10. He said it tongue in cheek, but he made the point.

Chapter 6. Case Studies

1. We include images in the category of cases. Consider the power of the images of the Holocaust victims.

2. These were observed on the interior surface of the vault at the time of excavation.

3. There are no photographs available for the pelvic tumors.

4. Great Britain cancer frequencies come from Cancer Research UK, Office for National Cancer Statistics: Registration Series MB1.

5. Hydrocephalus can also develop in adults. It can be the result of several factors, including head injury, cranial surgery, hemorrhage, stroke, and tumors.

6. Synovial joints are the most common and most movable joints. There are also less movable cartilaginous joints between vertebrea, and immovable joints between the cranial sutures.

7. We averaged male and female frequencies.

Chapter 7. A Bioethnography

1. Jack Kelso founded the biological anthropology program at the University of Colorado in the late 1950s and was a friend, mentor, and adviser to George much as George had been my friend, mentor, and adviser.

2. Boas created the first Ph.D. program at Columbia University.

Afterword

1. What made Martin's research unique was her application of an algorithm for calculating bone turnover rates. The algorithm was created by Herold Frost at Henry Ford Hospital. She made the tetracycline discovery in his lab.

2. While nursing, infants subsist entirely on the mother's body (milk) and have isotope amounts of a pure carnivore. The amounts become like the mother's after weaning.

LITERATURE CITED

Adams, W. Y. 1965. Post-pharaonic Nubia in light of archaeology II. *Journal of Egyptian Archaeology* 51:160–178.

Adams, W. Y. 1966. The Nubia campaign: Retrospect and prospect. In *Mélanges Oferts á Kazimierz Michalowski*. Warsaw: Panstowowe Wydawnictow Naukowe.

Adams, W. Y. 1967. Continuity and change in Nubian culture history. *Sudan Notes and Records* 48:1–32.

Adams, W. Y. 1977. *Nubia: Corridor to Africa*. Princeton, N.J.: Princeton University Press.

Adams, W. Y. 2004. Peasant archaeology in Nubia, Azania. *Archaeological Research in Africa* 39:111–124.

Adams, W. Y., and N. K. Adams. 2006–2007. The Kulubnarti underclass. In *Cahiers de recherches de l'Institut de Papyrologie et d'Egyptologie de Lille*, ed. Brigette Gratien. Cripael 26.

Adams, W. Y., and H. A. Nordstrom. 1963. The archaeological survey on the west bank of the Nile: Third season, 1961–1962. *Kush* 11:10–46.

Agarwal, S. C., and M. D. Grynpas. 1996. Bone quantity and quality in past populations. *Anatomical Record* 246:423–432.

Albert, A. M., and D. L. Greene. 1999. Bilateral asymmetry in skeletal growth and maturation as an indicator of environmental stress. *Am J Phys Anthrop* 110:341–349.

Allison, A. C. 1954. The distribution of the sickle-cell trait in East Africa and elsewhere, and its apparent relationship to the incidence of subtertian malaria. *Trans R Soc Trop Med Hyg* 48:312–318.

Almagro, M. F. 1963. Preliminary report on the Spanish excavations in the Sudan. *Kush* 11:175–195.

Anderson, D. L., G. W. Thompson, and F. Popovich. 1975. Evolutionary dental changes. *Am J Phys Anthrop* 43:95–102.

Armelagos, G. J. 1964. A fossilized mandible from near Wadi Halfa, Sudan. *Man* 64:12–13.

Armelagos, G. J. 1968. Paleopathology of three archaeological populations from Sudanese Nubia. *Dissertation Abstracts* 29(4):124B. University Microfilms, No. 5814. University of Colorado, Boulder.

Armelagos, G. J. 1969. Disease in ancient Nubia. *Science* 163:55–259.

Armelagos, G. J. 1994. *The concept of race, racism and anthropology*. Paper presented at annual meeting of the American Association of Physical Anthropologists, Denver.

Armelagos, G. J. 1997. Smith, (Sir) Grafton Elliot (1875–1937). In *History of Physical Anthropology: An Encyclopedia*, ed. F. Spencer. New York: Garland.

Armelagos, G. J. 2013. Reading the bones. *Science* 342:1291.

Armelagos, G. J., K. C. Barnes, and J. Lin. 2004. Disease in human evolution: The re-emergence of infectious disease in the third epidemiological transition. In *Understanding Humankind: The Best of Smithsonian AnthroNotes*, ed. R. O. Selig and M. R. London, chapter 8. Washington, D.C.: Smithsonian Institution Press.

Armelagos, G. J., D. S. Carlson, and D. P. Van Gerven. 1976. Patterns of age-related cortical bone loss (osteoporosis) within the femoral diaphysis. *Hum Biol* 42:295–314.

Armelagos, G. J., G. H. Ewing, and D. L. Greene. 1968. Physical anthropology and man-made lakes. *Anthropological Quarterly* 41:122–131.

Armelagos, G. J., G. H. Ewing, K. Greene, and D. L. Greene. 1965. Report of the Physical Anthropology Section, University of Colorado Nubian Expedition. *Kush* 13:24–27.

Armelagos, G. J., A. H. Goodman, K. N. Harper, and M. H. Blakey. 2009. Enamel hypoplasia and early mortality: Bioarcheological support for the Barker hypothesis. *Evol Anthropol Issues, News, and Reviews* 18:261–271.

Armelagos, G. J., K. Kolbacher, K. Collins, J. Cook, and M. Krafeld-Daugherty. 2001. Tetracycline consumption in prehistory. In *Tetracyclines in biology, chemistry and medicine*, ed. M. Nelson, W. Hillen, and R. A. Greenwald, 219–236. Verlag, Switzerland: Birkhäuser Basel.

Armelagos, G. J., and D. L. Martin. 1990. Advances in paleopathology: A biocultural approach to understanding osteoporosis in prehistoric populations. In *Para conocer al hombre: Homenaje Santiago Genoves*, ed. L. L. Tapia. Mexico D.F.: Universidad National Autonoma Mexico.

Armelagos, G. J., J. H. Mielke, K. H. Owen, D. P. Van Gerven, J. R. Dewey, and P. E. Mahler. 1972. Bone growth and development in prehistoric populations from Sudanese Nubia. *J Hum Evol* 1:89–119.

Armelagos, G. J., and D. P. Van Gerven. 1993. Paleopathologist as detective: Disease and death in prehistory. In *Ela'Qua: Essays in Honor of Richard Woodbury*, ed. R. B. Thomas and J. W. Cole. Amherst: University of Massachusetts, Department of Anthropology, Research Reports.

Arnold, J. S. 1960. Quantification of mineralization of bone as an organ and tissue in osteoporosis. *Clinical Orthopaedics* 49:7–38.

Arriaza, B. T., C. F. Merbs, and B. M. Rothschild. 1993. Diffuse idiopathic skeletal hyperostosis in Meroitic Nubians from Semna south, Sudan. *Am J Phys Anthrop* 92:243–248.

Bademci, G., T. Kendi, and F. Agalar. 2007. Persistent metopic suture can mimic the skull fractures in the emergency setting. *Neurocirugia* 18:238–240.

Baker, B., and G. J. Armelagos. 1988. Origin and antiquity of syphilis: A dilemma in paleopathological diagnosis and interpretation. *Current Anthropology* 29:703–737.

Barberini, F., E. Bruner, R. Cartolari, G. Franchitto, R. Heyn, F. Ricci, and G. Manzi. 2008. An unusually-wide human bregmatic Wormian bone: Anatomy, tomographic description, and possible significance. *Surgical and Radiologic Anatomy* 30:683–687.

Barker, D. J. P., and A. J. Hall. 1986. The epidemiology of Perthes' disease. *Clinical Orthopaedics and Related Research* 209:89–94.

Bassett, E. J., M. S. Keith, G. J. Armelagos, D. L. Martin, and A. R. Villanueva. 1980. Tetracycline-labeled human bone from ancient Sudanese Nubia (AD 350). *Science* 209:1532–1534.

Batrawi, A. M. 1935. Report on the human remains. *Mission archeologique de Nubie, 1929–1934*. Cairo: Government Press.

Batrawi, A. M. 1945. The racial history of Egypt and Nubia. Part I, The craniology of lower Nubia from Predynastic times to the sixth century A.D. *JR Anthrop Inst* 75:81–101.

Batrawi, A. M. 1946. The racial history of Egypt and Nubia. Part II, The racial relationship of the ancient and modern populations of Egypt and Nubia. *JR Anthrop Inst* 76:131–156.

Batrawi, A. M. 1947. Anatomical reports. *Annales du service des antiquities de l'Egypte* 47:97–109.

Becker, M., and F. Wendorf. 1993. A microwear study of a late Pleistocene Qadan assemblage from southern Egypt. *Journal of Field Archaeology* 20(4):389–398.

Beckett, S., and N. C. Lovell. 1994. Dental disease evidence for agricultural intensification in the Nubian C-Group. *Int J Osteoarch* 4(3):223–239.

Bennett, K. A. 1965. The etiology and genetics of wormian bones. *Am J Phys Anthrop* 23:255–260.

Blume, S. W., and J. R. Curtis. 2011. Medical costs of osteoporosis in the elderly Medicare population. *Osteoporosis International* 22:1835–1844.

Blumenbach, J. F. [1795] 1969. *On the Natural Varieties of Mankind*. 3rd ed. originally published in Gottinberg in 1795. New York: Bergmann.

Boas, F. 1911. *Changes in Bodily Form of Descendants of Immigrants*. Sixty-First Congress, 2nd Session, Washington, D.C.

Boas, F. 1940. *Race, Language, and Culture*. Chicago: University of Chicago Press.

Bocquet-Appel, J. P., and C. Masset. 1982. Farewell to paleodemography: Rumors of its death have been greatly exaggerated. *J Hum Evol* 11:321–333.

Bridges, P. S. 1991. Degenerative joint disease in hunter-gatherers and agriculturalists from the southeastern United States. *Am J Phys Anthrop* 85:379–391.

Bridges, P. S. 1994. Vertebral arthritis and physical activities in the prehistoric southeastern United States. *Am J Phys Anthrop* 93:83–93.

Bronowski, J. 1952. Statistics of discrimination in anthropology. *Am J Phys Anthrop* 10(4):385–394.

Bronowski, J. 1967. *The Common Sense of Science*. Cambridge, Mass.: Harvard University Press.

Bronowski, J., and W. M. Long. 1951. Statistical methods in anthropology. *Nature* 168(4279):794.

Brooks, S., and J. M. Suchey. 1990. Skeletal age determination based on the os pubis: A comparison of the Acsádi-Nemeskéri and Suchey-Brooks methods. *Hum Evol* 5:227–238.

Brothwell, D. R. 1959. Teeth in earlier human populations. *Proceedings of the Nutrition Society* 18:59–65.

Brothwell, D. R. 1963. The macroscopic dental pathology of earlier human populations. In *Dental Anthropology*, ed. D. R. Brothwell. New York: Pergamon.

Brune, M., L. Rossander-Hulter, L. Hallberg, and A. Gleerup. 1992. Iron absorption from bread in humans: Inhibiting effects of cereal fiber, phytate and inositol phosphates with different numbers of phosphate groups. *J Nutr* 122:442–449.

Bruzek, J. 2002. A method for visual determination of sex, using the human hip bone. *Am J Phys Anthrop* 117:157–168.

Burger, T. D., and E. Trinkhaus. 1995. Patterns of trauma among the Neandertals. *Journal of Archaeological Science* 22:841–852.

Burnor, D. R., and J. E. Harris. 1968. Racial continuity in Lower Nubia: 12,000 B.C. to the present. *Proceedings of the Indiana Academy of Science for 1967*, 73:113–121.

Burr, D. B. 1993. Remodeling and the repair of fatigue damage. *Calcified Tissue International* 53:S75–S81.

Burr, D. B., C. Ruff, and D. Thompson. 1990. Patterns of skeletal histological change through time: A comparison of archaic native American populations with modern populations. *Anatomical Record* 226(3):307–313.

Buzon, M. R., and R. Richman. 2007. Traumatic injuries and imperialism: The effects of Egyptian colonial strategies at Tombos in Upper Nubia. *Am J Phys Anthrop* 133:783–791.

Camper, P. 1791. *Report of the content of two lectures*. Utrecht: R. Wild & J. Altheer.

Cardoso, H. 2007. Environmental effects on skeletal versus dental development: Using a documented subadult skeletal sample to test a basic assumption in human osteological research. *Am J Phys Anthrop* 132:223–233.

Carlson, D. S., G. J. Armelagos, and D. P. Van Gerven. 1974. Factors influencing the etiology of cribra orbitalia in prehistoric Nubia. *J Hum Evol* 3:405–410.

Carlson, D. S., and D. P. Van Gerven. 1977. Masticatory function and post-Pleistocene evolution in Nubia. *Am J Phys Anthrop* 46:495–506.

Cauley, J. A. 2013. Public health impact of osteoporosis. *The Journals of Gerontology Series A: Biological Sciences and Medical Sciences* 68:1243–1251.

Chakravarthi, K., and N. Venumadhav. 2012. Morphological study of metopic suture in adult south Indian skulls. *International Journal of Medical and Health Sciences* 1:23–28.

Chhem, R. 2008. *Paleoradiology: History and New Developments in Paleoradiology*. New York: Springer.

Child, V. G. 1936. *Man Makes Himself*. London: Watts.

Christie, A. 1937. *Death on the Nile*. New York: Black Dog and Leventhal.

Clark, J. D., and S. A. Brandt. 1984. *From Hunters to Farmers: The Causes and Consequences of Food Production in Africa*. Berkeley: University of California Press.

Cohen, M. N., and G. J. Armelagos, eds. 1984. *Paleopathology at the Origins of Agriculture*. Cambridge: Academic Press.

Cohen, M. N., and G. J. Armelagos, eds. 2013. *Paleopathology at the Origins of Agriculture*. Gainesville: University Press of Florida.

Condon, K., and J. C. Rose. 1992. Intertooth and intratooth variability in the occurrence of developmental enamel defects. *J Palaeopathol Monogr Publ* 2:61–77.

Corondan, G., and W. L. Haworth. 1986. A fractographic study of human long bone. *J Biomechanics* 19:207–218.

Count, E. W. 1950. *This Is Race*. New York: Schuman.

Crichton, J. M. 1964. *A multiple discriminant analysis of Egyptian and African Negro crania.* Senior Honors Thesis, Peabody Museum Library.

Crossby, A. W. 2004. *Ecological Imperialism: The Biological Expansion of Europe, 900–1900.* Cambridge: Cambridge University Press.

Crubézy, E., and E. Trinkaus. 1992. Shanidar 1: A case of hyperostotic disease (DISH) in the middle Paleolithic. *Am J Phys Anthrop* 89:411–420.

Dahlin, D. C., and J. W. Beabout. 1971. Dedifferentiation of low-grade chondrosarcomas. *Cancer* 28:461–466.

Daly, M. W. 2004. *Empire on the Nile: The Anglo-Egyptian Sudan, 1898–1934.* Cambridge: Cambridge University Press.

Darby, W. J., P. Ghalioungui, and L. Grivett. 1977. *Food: The Gift of Osiris.* London: Academic Press.

Del Bigio, M. R. 1993. Neuropathological changes caused by hydrocephalus. *Acta Neuropathologica* 85:573–585.

Derry, D. E. 1913. A case of hydrocephalus in an Egyptian of the Roman period. *J Anat Phys* 48:436–458.

DeStefano, F., R. F. Anda, H. S. Kah, D. F. Williamson, and M. Russell. 1993. Dental disease and risk of coronary heart disease and mortality. *British Medical Journal* 306:688–691.

Dettwyler, K. A. 1991. Can paleopathology find evidence for "compassion"? *Am J Phys Anthrop* 84:375–378.

Dewey, J. R., M. H. Bartley, and G. J. Armelagos. 1969. 6 rates of femoral cortical bone loss in two Nubian populations: Utilizing normalized and non-normalized data. *Clinical Orthopaedics and Related Research* 65:61–66.

Dickens, C. 1843. *A Christmas Carol.* London: Chapman and Hall.

Dorfman, H. D., and B. Czerniak. 1995. Bone cancers. *Cancer* 75:203–210.

Dorit, R. L. 1997. A review of Darwin's Black Box: The biochemical challenge to evolution, by Michael J. Behe. *American Scientist* (September–October).

Doyle, A. C. 1891. The Boscombe Valley mystery. In *The Adventures of Sherlock Holmes.* London: Strand Magazine.

Edwards, D. N. 2004. *The Nubian Past.* London: Routledge.

Edwards, D. N. 2007. The archaeology of Sudan and Nubia. *Annual Reviews of Anthropology* 36:211–228.

Einstein, A., and L. Field. 1932. *The Evolution of Physics.* Cambridge: Cambridge University Press.

Ellis, W. M. 2004. *Ptolemy of Egypt.* London: Routledge.

El-Najjar, M. Y., B. Lozoff, and J. D. Ryan. 1975. The paleoepidemiology of porotic hyperostosis in the American Southwest: Radiological and ecological considerations. *Am J Roentgen* 125:918–924.

Emery, W. B. 1948. *Nubian Treasure: An Account of the Discoveries at Ballana and Qustul.* London: Methuen.

Emery, W. B. 1954. *Excavations at Saqqara: Great Tombs of the First Dynasty.* Cairo: Ministry of Finance, Cairo Government Press.

Eng, L. I. 1958. Chronic iron deficiency anemia with bone changes resembling Cooley's anemia. *Acta Haematologica* 19:253–268.

Errobidart, O. R. 2013. *Dental prosthesis for bovine animals with fully or partially worn down teeth.* U.S. Patent 8,573,970.

Eveleth, P. B., and J. J. M. Tanner. 1976. *World-wide Variation in Human Growth.* CUP Archive 8.

Facchini, F. E., E. Rastelli, and P. Brasili. 2004. Cribra orbitalia and cribra cranii in Roman skeletal remains from the Ravenna area and Rimini (I–IV century AD). *Int J Osteoarch* 14:126–136.

Fahrer, H., R. Barandun, N. J. Gerber, N. Friederich, B. Burkhardt, and M. H. Weisman. 1989. Pelvic manifestations of diffuse idiopathic skeletal hyperostosis (DISH): Are they clinically relevant? *Rheumatology International* 8(6):257–261.

Fairgrieve, S. I., and J. Molto. 2000. Cribra orbitalia in two temporally disjunct population samples from the Dakhleh Oasis, Egypt. *Am J Phys Anthrop* 3:319–331.

Featherstone, J. D. 1999. Prevention and reversal of dental caries: Role of low level fluoride. *Community Dentistry and Oral Epidemiology* 27:31–40.

Fernea, R. A., and J. G. Kennedy. 1966. Initial adaptations to resettlement: A new life for Egyptian Nubians. *Current Anthropology* 7:349–354.

Firth, C. M. 1912. *The Archaeological Survey of Nubia: Report for 1908–1909 Catalogue of Graves and their Contents.* Cairo: Cairo Government Press.

Firth, C. M. 1915. *The Archaeological Survey of Nubia: Report for 1909–1910.* Cairo: Cairo Government Press.

Firth, C. M. 1927. *The Archeological Survey of Nubia: Report for 1910–1911.* Cairo: Cairo Government Press.

Frost, H. M., A. R. Villanueva, H. F. Hospital, and H. Roth. 1960. Tetracycline staining of newly forming bone and mineralizing cartilage in vivo. *Stain Technology* 35:135–138.

Gabora, L. 2006. The fate of evolutionary archaeology: Survival or extinction? *World Archaeology* 38:690–696.

Garn, S. M. 1961. *Human Races.* Springfield, Ill.: C. C. Thomas.

Garn, S. M., and C. Coon. 1955. On the number of races of mankind. *Am Anthrop* 57:996–1001.

Garrod, D. A. E., D. M. A. Bate, T. D. McCown, and A. Keith. 1939. *The Stone Age of Mount Carmel.* Oxford: Clarendon Press.

Gatto, M. C. 2009. The Nubian pastoral culture as link between Egypt and Africa: Egypt in its African context. In *Proceedings of the Conference held at the Manchester Museum, University of Manchester, October 2–4.*

Gilberg, M. 1997. Alfred Lucas: Egypt's Sherlock Holmes. *J Am Instit for Conser* 36:31–48.

Goodman, A. H., and G. J. Armelagos. 1988. Childhood stress, cultural buffering, and decreased longevity in prehistoric populations. *Am Anthrop* 90:936–944.

Goodman, A. H., G. J. Armelagos, and J. C. Rose. 1980. Enamel hypoplasias as indicators of stress in three prehistoric populations from Illinois. *Hum Biol* 52:515–528.

Goodman, A. H., J. Lallo, G. J. Armelagos, and J. C. Rose. 2013. Health changes at Dickson Mounds, Illinois (AD 950–1300). In *Paleopathology at the Origins of Agriculture*, ed. M. N. Cohen and G. J. Armelagos. Gainesville: University of Florida Press.

Goodman, A. H., D. L. Martin, and G. J. Armelagos. 1984. Indications of stress from bone and teeth. In *Paleopathology at the Origins of Agriculture*, ed. M. N. Cohen and G. J. Armelagos. Cambridge: Academic Press.

Gorstein, J., K. Sullivan, R. Yip, M. De Onis, F. Trowbridge, P. Fajans, and G. Clugston. 1994. Issues in the assessment of nutritional status using anthropometry. *Bulletin of the World Health Organization* 72:273–283.

Gottfried, R. S. 1983. *Black Death*. London: Hale.

Gould, S. J. 1965. Is uniformitarianism necessary? *American Journal of Science* 263:223.

Gould, S. J. 2008. A biological homage to Mickey Mouse. *Ecotone* 4:333–340.

Granville, A. B. 1825. An essay on Egyptian mummies with observations on the art of embalming among the ancient Egyptians. *Phil Trans Royal Soc* 115:269–319.

Green, S. S., and G. J. Armelagos. 1974. Settlement and mortality of the Christian site (AD 1050–1300) of Meinarti (Sudan). *J Hum Evol* 3:297-316.

Greene, D. L. 1965. *Dentition and taxonomy of Meroitic, X-Group, and Christian populations from Wadi Halfa, Sudan*. Ph.D. diss., University of Colorado, Boulder.

Greene, D. L. 1966. Dentition and biological relationships of some Meroitic, X-Group, and Christian populations from Wadi Halfa, Sudan. *Kush* 14:285–288.

Greene, D. L. 1967a. Dentition of Meroitic, X-Group, and Christian populations from Wadi Halfa, Sudan. In *Anthropological Paper, Department of Anthropology*, Vol. 85. Salt Lake City: University of Utah Press.

Greene, D. L. 1967b. *Genetics, Dentition and Taxonomy*. Vol. 33. Laramie: University of Wyoming Publications.

Greene, D. L. 1972. Dental anthropology of early Egypt and Nubia. *J Hum Evol* 1:315–324.

Greene, D. L. 1973. Dental anthropology of Egypt and Nubia. In *Population Biology of the Ancient Egyptians*, ed. D. R. Brothwell and B. A. Chiarelli. New York: Academic Press.

Greene, D. L. 1982. Discrete dental variations and biological distances of Nubian populations. *Am J Phys Anthrop* 58:75–79.

Greene, D. L., and G. J. Armelagos. 1972. *The Wadi Halfa Mesolithic Population No. 11*. Department of Anthropology, University of Massachusetts.

Greene, D. L., G. H. Ewing, and G. J. Armelagos. 1967. Dentition of a Mesolithic population from Wadi Halfa, Sudan. *Am J Phys Anthrop* 27:41–55.

Greene, D. L., D. P. Van Gerven, and G. J. Armelagos. 1986. Life and death in ancient populations: Bones of contention in paleodemography. *J Hum Evol* 1:193–207.

Hafsaas-Tsakos, H. 2010. Between Kush and Egypt: The C-Group people of Lower Nubia during the Middle Kingdom and Second Intermediate Period. *Academia.edu PAM Supplement Series* 2.2/2.

Harper, K. N., and G. J. Armelagos. 2010. The changing disease-scape in the third epidemiological transition. *Internat J Environl Res Pub Heal* 7:675–697.

Harper, K. N., and G. J. Armelagos. 2013. Genomics, the origins of agriculture, and our changing microbe-scape: Time to revisit some old tales and tell some new ones. *Yearb Phys Anthrop* 57:135–152.

Harper, K. N., M. L. Zuckerman, J. D. Kingston, and G. J. Armelagos. 2011. The origin and antiquity of syphilis revisited: An appraisal of Old World pre-Columbian evidence for treponemal infection. *Am J Phys Anthrop* 146:99–133.

Harper, K. N., M. K. Zuckerman, B. L. Turner, and G. J. Armelagos. 2013. Primates, pathogens and evolution. In *Primates, Pathogens, and Evolution*, ed. J. Brinkworth and E. Pechenkina. New York: Springer Publishing.

Herlihy, D. 1997. *The Black Death and the Transformation of the West.* Cambridge, Mass.: Harvard University Press.

Hewes, G. W., H. Irwin, M. Papworth, and A. Saxe. 1964. A new fossil human population from the Wadi Halfa area, Sudan. *Nature* 203:341–343.

Hibbs, A. C., W. Secor, D. P. Van Gerven, and G. J. Armelagos. 2011. Irrigation and infection: The immunoepidemiology of schistosomiasis in ancient Nubia. *Am J Phys Anthrop* 145:290–298.

Hillson, S. W. 1979. Diet and dental disease. *World Archaeology* 11:147–162.

Hillson, S. W. 2007. *Dental Pathology: Biological Anthropology of the Human Skeleton.* Hoboken, N.J.: John Wiley & Sons.

Hooton, E. 1930. *The Indians of Pecos Pueblo: A Study of their Skeletal Remains.* New Haven, Conn.: Yale University Press.

Hujoel, P. P., M. Drangsholt, C. Spiekerman, and T. A. DeRouen. 2000. Periodontal disease and coronary heart disease risk. *JAMA* 284:1406–1410.

Hummert, J. R., and D. P. Van Gerven. 1982. Tetracycline-labeled human bone from a medieval population in Nubia's Batn el Hajar (550–1450 AD). *Hum Biol* 54:355–363.

Hummert, J. R., and D. P. Van Gerven. 1983. Skeletal growth in a medieval population from Sudanese Nubia. *Am J Phys Anthrop* 60:471–478.

Iheozor-Ejiofor, Z., H. V. Worthington, T. Walsh, L. O'Malley, J. E. Clarkson, R. Macey, R. Alam, P. Tugwell, V. Welch, and A. M. Glenny. 2013. Water fluoridation for the prevention of dental caries. *The Cochrane Library* 6.

Irish, J. D. 2005. Population continuity vs. discontinuity revisited: Dental affinities among late Paleolithic through Christian-era Nubians, 2005. *Am J Phys Anthrop* 128:520–535.

Jantz, R. L., and D. W. Owsley. 1984. Long bone growth among Arikara skeletal populations. *Am J Phys Anthrop* 63:13–20.

Jarcho, S. 1964. The Fielding H. Garrison lecture: Some observations on diseases in prehistoric North America. *Bulletin of the History of Medicine* 38:1.

Johnson, G. 2010. Unearthing prehistoric tumors, and debate. *New York Times*, December 28.

Johnston, F. E. 1962. Growth of the long bones of infants and young children at Indian Knoll. *Am J Phys Anthrop* 20:249–254.

Jones, F. W. 1908. The pathological report. In *Archaeological Survey of Nubia, Bulletin 1.*

Judd, M. A. 2000. *Trauma and interpersonal violence in ancient Nubia during the Kerma period (ca. 2500–1500 BC).* Ph.D. diss., University of Alberta.

Judd, M. A. 2002. Comparison of long bone trauma recording methods. *Journal of Archaeological Science* 29:1255–1265.

Judd, M. A., and S. Roberts. 1998. Fracture patterns in a medieval leper hospital in Chichester. *Am J Phys Anthrop* 105:43–55.

Karhu, S. L. 1991. *Childhood stress and dental histopathologies in a medieval Christian Nubian population.* Ph.D. diss., University of Colorado, Boulder.

Katzenberg, M. A., D. Herring, and S. R. Saunders. 1996. Weaning and infant mortality: Evaluating the skeletal evidence. *Am J Phys Anthrop* 101:177–199.

Keith, A. 1913. Abnormal crania—achondroplastic and acrocephalic. *J Anat Physio* 47:189–206.

Keith, M. S., and G. J. Armelagos. 1983. Naturally occurring dietary antibiotics and human health. In *The Anthropology of Medicine*. New York: Praeger Press.

Keith, M. S., and G. J. Armelagos. 1988. An example of in vivo tetracycline labelling: Reply to Piepenbrink. *Journal of Archaeological Science* 15:595–601.

Keller, E. T., and J. Brown. 2004. Prostate cancer bone metastases promote both osteolytic and osteoblastic activity. *Journal of Cellular Biochemistry* 91:718–729.

Kemp, B. J. 1989. *Ancient Egypt: Anatomy of a Civilization*. London: Routledge.

Kerley, E. 1965. The microscopic determination of age in human bone. *Am J Phys Anthrop* 23:149–164.

Kilgore, L. 1989. Possible case of rheumatoid arthritis from Sudanese Nubia. *Am J Phys Anthrop* 79:177–183.

Kilgore, L., R. Jurmain, and D. P. Van Gerven. 1997. Palaeoepidemiological patterns of trauma in a medieval Nubian skeletal population. *Int J Osteoarch* 7:103–114.

Kilgore, L., and D. P. Van Gerven. 2010. Congenital scoliosis: Possible causes and consequences in a skeleton from Nubia. *Int J Osteoarch* 20:630–644.

Kim, S. H., J. P. Meehan, T. Blumenfeld, and R. M. Szabo. 2012. Hip fractures in the United States: 2008 nationwide emergency department sample. *Arthritis Care and Research* 64:751–757.

Kirwan, L. P. 1937. A survey of Nubian origins. *Sudan Notes and Records* 20:47–62.

Kozlowski, K., D. Sillence, and F. Taylor. 1993. Short stature, mental retardation, craniosynostosis, Klippel-Feil syndrome, Scheuerman kyphosis, rib gaps and other distinctive skeletal and genital anomalies. *Pediatric Radiology* 23:442–445.

Kramer, M. S., and R. Kakuma. 2004. The optimal duration of exclusive breast feeding. *Protecting Infants through Human Milk* 554:63–77.

Kranzler G., J. Moursund, and J. Kranzler. 2006. *Statistics for the Terrified*. 4th ed. Upper Saddle River, N.J.: Prentice-Hall.

Kroeber, T. 1964. *Ishi: Last of His Tribe*. Berkeley, Calif.: Parnassus Press.

Krogman, W. M. 1951. The scars of human evolution. *Scientific American* 185:54–57.

Krogman, W. M. 1962. *The Human Skeleton in Forensic Medicine*. Springfield, Ill.: Charles C. Thomas.

Kuhn, T. S. 1962. *The Structure of Scientific Revolutions*. Chicago: University of Chicago Press.

Lafleur, M., M. Seamont, P. Sandberg, and D. P. Van Gerven. 2010. *The dish on DISH: A "severe" case of diffuse idiopathic skeletal hyperostosis from medieval Nubia with implications for etiology of DISH and the progression of knowledge on this disorder*. Paper presented at the annual meeting of the American Association of Physical Anthropologists, Albuquerque, N.M.

Lakatos I., and E. Zahar. 1975. Why did Copernicus' research program supersede Ptolemy's? In *The Copernican Achievement*, ed. R. S. Weisman. Berkeley: University of California Press.

Lallo, J., R. P. Mensforth, and G. J. Armelagos. 1977. The role of diet, disease and physiology in the origin of porotic hyperostosis. *Hum Biol* 49:471–483.

Larsen, C. S. 1994. In the wake of Columbus: Native population biology in the postcontact Americas. *Am J Phys Anthrop* 37:109–154.

Larsen, C. S. 2001. *Bioarchaeology of Spanish Florida: The Impact of Colonialism*. Ripley P. Bullen Series. Gainesville: University Press of Florida.

Larsen, C.S. and G. R. Milner, eds. 1993. *In the Wake of Contact: Biological Responses to Conquest*. Hoboken, N. J.: John Wiley and Sons.

Linden, S. V. D., H. A. Valkenburg, and A. Cats. 1984. Evaluation of diagnostic criteria for ankylosing spondylitis. *Arthritis and Rheumatism* 27:361–368.

Lips, P., P. Courpron, and P. J. Meunier. 1978. Mean wall thickness of trabecular bone packets in the human iliac crest: Changes with age. *Calcified Tissue Research* 26:13–17.

Livingstone, F. B. 1958. Anthropological implications of the sickle cell gene in West Africa. *Am Anthrop* 60:533–561.

Livingstone, F. B. 1962. Discussion and criticism: On the non-existence of human races. *Curr Anthrop* 3:279–281.

Livingstone, F. B., and T. Dobzhansky. 1962. On the non-existence of human races. *Curr Anthrop* 3:279–281.

Loesche, W. J. 1986. Role of *Streptococcus mutans* in human dental decay. *Microbiological Reviews* 50:353–380.

Logothetis, C. J., and S. H. Lin. 2005. Osteoblasts in prostate cancer metastasis to bone. *Nature Reviews Cancer*: 5:21–28.

Long, A. R. 1931. Cardiovascular renal disease: Report of a case of 3000 years ago. *Archaeol Path* 12:92.

Lortet, L. C. 1907. Crane syphilitique et necropoles prehistoriques de la Haute-Egypte. *Bulletin de la Société Antropologie* 26:211.

Lovejoy, C. O. 1981. The origin of man. *Science, New Series* 211(4480):341–350.

Lovejoy, C. O., A. H. Burnstein, and K. G. Heiple. 1976. The biomechanical analysis of bone strength: A method and its application to playcnemia. *Am J Phys Anthrop* 44:489–506.

Lovejoy, C. O., and K. G. Heiple. 1981. The analysis of fractures in skeletal populations with an example from the Libben site, Ottawa County, Ohio. *Am J Phys Anthrop* 55:529–541.

Lovell, N. C. 2008. Analysis and interpretation of skeletal trauma. In *Biological anthropology of the human skeleton*, ed. M. A. Katzenberg and S. R. Saunders. Hoboken, N.J.: John Wiley and Sons.

Magnus, S. P. M. 1968. *Kitchener: Portrait of an Imperialist*. London: Penguin.

Maresh, M. M. 1955. Linear growth of long bones of extremities from infancy through adolescence: Continuing studies. *Archives of Pediatrics and Adolescent Medicine* 89:725–742.

Marsh, P. D. 2004. Dental plaque as a microbial biofilm. *Caries Research* 38:204–211.

Martin, D. L., and G. J. Armelagos. 1979. Morphometrics of compact bone: An example from Sudanese Nubia. *Am J Phys Anthrop* 51:571–577.

Martin, D. L., and G. J. Armelagos. 1985. Skeletal remodeling and mineralization as indicators of health: An example from prehistoric Sudanese Nubia. *J Hum Evol* 4:527–537.

Martin, R. B., and P. J. Atkinson. 1977. Age and sex-related changes in the structure and strength of the human femoral shaft. *Journal of Biomechanics* 10:223–231.

Martin, R. B., and D. B. Burr. 1984. A non-invasive measurement of long bone cross-sectional moment of inertia by photon absorptiometry. *Journal of Biomechanics* 17:195–201.

May, J. M., and I. S. Jarcho. 1961. *The Ecology of Malnutrition in the Far and Near East (Food Resources, Habits, and Deficiencies)*. New York: Hafner.

McDade, T. W., and C. M. Worthman. 1998. The weanling's dilemma reconsidered: A biocultural analysis of breastfeeding ecology. *Journal of Developmental and Behavioral Pediatrics* 19:286–299.

Mendieta, C., J. Miranda, L. Brunet, J. Gargallo, and L. Berini. 2005. Alveolar bone necrosis and tooth exfoliation following *Herpes zoster* infection: A review of the literature and case report. *Journal of Periodontology* 76:148–153.

Mensforth, R. P., C. O. Lovejoy, J. W. Lallo, and G. J. Armelagos. 1978. Part Two: The role of constitutional factors, diet, and infectious disease in the etiology of porotic hyperostosis and periosteal reactions in prehistoric infants and children. *Med Anthrop* 2:1–59.

Mindell, J. A., and J. A. Owens. 2015. *A Clinical Guide to Pediatric Sleep: Diagnosis and Management of Sleep Problems*. Philadelphia: Lippincott Williams and Wilkins.

Mitchell, J. K. 1900. Study of a mummy affected with anterior poliomyelitis. *Trans Assoc Amer Physic* 15:134–136.

Mittler, D. M., and D. P. Van Gerven. 1994. Developmental, diachronic and demographic analysis of cribra orbitalia in the medieval Christian populations of Kulubnarti. *Am J Phys Anthrop* 93:287–297.

Molnar, P. 2011. Extramasticatory dental wear reflecting habitual behavior and health in past populations. *Clinical Oral Investigations* 15(5):681–689.

Moodie, R. L. 1931. *Studies in Palaeopathology of Egypt*. Chicago: University of Chicago Press.

Moore, K. P., S. Thorp, and D. P. Van Gerven. 1986. Patterns of dental eruption, skeletal maturation, and stress in a medieval population from Sudanese Nubia. *Hum Evol* 1:325–330.

Morton, S. G. 1844. Crania Aegyptica. *Journal of the American Philosophical Society*. Philadelphia: Penington.

Moseley, J. E. 1965. The paleopathologic riddle of symmetrical osteoporosis. *Am J Roentgen* 95:135–142.

Moss, M. L. 1972. Twenty years of functional cranial analysis. *Am J Orthodon* 61:479–485.

Moss, M. L., and R. W. Young. 1960. A functional approach to craniology. *Am J Phys Anthrop* 18:281–292.

Mulhern, D. M. 2000. Rib remodeling dynamics in a skeletal population from Kulubnarti, Nubia. *Am J Phys Anthrop* 111:519–530.

Mulhern, D. M., and D. P. Van Gerven. 1997. Patterns of femoral bone remodeling dynamics in a medieval Nubian population. *Am J Phys Anthrop* 104:133–146.

Myers, C. S. 1905. Contributions to Egyptian anthropology: II. The comparative anthropometry of the most ancient and modern inhabitants. *JR Anthrop Inst* 35:80–91.

Myers, C. S. 1908. Contributions to Egyptian anthropometry. V. General conclusions. *JR Anthrop Inst* 38:99–102.

Neel, J. V. 1949. The inheritance of sickle cell anemia. *Science* 110:64–66.

Nelson, M. L., A. Dinardo, J. Hochberg, and G. J. Armelagos. 2011. Brief communication: Mass spectroscopic characterization of tetracycline in the skeletal remains of an ancient population from Sudanese Nubia 350–550 CE. *Am J Phys Anthrop* 143:151–154.

Nordstrom, H. A. 1962. Excavation and survey in Faras, Argin, and Gezira Daborosa. *Kush* 10:34–61.

Ortner, D. J. 1998. *Male-Female Immune Reactivity and Its Implications for Interpreting Evidence in Human Skeletal Paleopathology: Sex and Gender in Paleopathological Perspective*. Cambridge: Cambridge University Press.

Owsley, D. W., and R. L. Jantz. 1985. Long bone lengths and gestational age distributions of post-contact period Arikara Indian perinatal infant skeletons. *Am J Phys Anthrop* 68:321–328.

Oxenham, M. F., and I. Cavill. 2010. Porotic hyperostosis and cribra orbitalia: The erythropoitic response to iron deficiency anemia. *Anthropological Sciences* 118:199–200.

Oxenham, M. F., H. Matsumura, and T. Nishimoto. 2006. Diffuse idiopathic skeletal hyperostosis in late Jomon Hokkaido, Japan. *Int J Osteoarch* 16:34–46.

Pauling L., H. A. Itano, S. J. Singer, and I. C. Wells. 1949. Sickle cell anemia: A molecular disease. *Science* 110:543–548.

Pettigrew, T. J. 1934. *A History of Egyptian Mummies*. London: Longmans.

Piel, F. B., S. I. Hay, S. Gupta, D. J. Weatherall, and T. N. Williams. 2013. Global burden of sickle cell anaemia in children under five, 2010–2050: Modelling based on demographics, excess mortality, and interventions. *PLoS Medicine* 10:e1001484.

Piepenbrink, D. B. H. 1986. Two examples of biogenous dead bone decomposition and their consequences for taphonomic interpretation. *Journal of Archaeological Science* 13:417–430.

Piepenbrink, D. B. H., B. Herrmann, and P. Hoffmann. 1983. Tetracyclintypische fluoreszenzen an bodngelagerten skeletteilen. *Zeitschrift für Rechtsmedizin* 91:71–74.

Pinhashi, R., P. Shaw, B. White, and A. R. Ogden. 2006. Morbidity, rickets, and long-bone growth in medieval Britain: A cross population analysis. *Annals of Human Biology* 33:372–389.

Pinhashi, R., A. Timpson, M. Thomas, and M. Slaus. 2013. Bone growth, limb proportion and non-specific stress in archaeological populations from Croatia. *Annals of Human Biology Online* 41:1–12.

Platt, J. R. 1964. Strong inference. *Science* 146:347–353.

Ponce, P., and P. Novellino. 2014. A palaeopathological example of Legg-Calvé-Perthes disease from Argentina. *Int J Paleopath* 6:30–33.

Prates, C., S. Sousa, C. Oliveira, and S. Ikram. 2011. Prostate metastatic bone cancer in an Egyptian Ptolemaic mummy: A proposed radiological diagnosis. *Int J Paleopath* 1:98–103.

Redfield, R. 1947. The folk society. *Am J Sociolo* 52:293–308.

Reisner, G. A. 1909. Archaeological survey of Nubia. *Egypt Survey Department* 3:5–20.

Relethford, J. H. 2004. Boas and beyond: Migration and craniometric variation. *Am J Hum Biol* 16(4):379–386.

Resnick, D., and G. Niwayama. 1976. Radiographic and pathologic features of spinal involvement in diffuse idiopathic skeletal hyperostosis (DISH). *Radiology* 119:559–568.

Rose, J. C. 1977. Defective enamel histology of prehistoric teeth from Illinois. *Am J Phys Anthrop* 46:439–446.

Rose, J. C., G. J. Armelagos, and J. W. Lallo. 1978. Histological enamel indicator of childhood stress in prehistoric skeletal samples. *Am J Phys Anthrop* 49:511–516.

Rosenberg, K. R. 1992. The evolution of modern human childbirth. *Am J Phys Anthrop* 35:89–124.

Rosenberg, K., and W. Trevathan. 1995. Bipedalism and human birth: The obstetrical dilemma revisited. *Evolutionary Anthropology: Issues, News, and Reviews* 4:161–168.

Rosenberg, K., and W. Trevathan. 2002. Birth, obstetrics and human evolution. *BJOG: An International Journal of Obstetrics and Gynaecology* 109:1199–1206.

Ruff, C. B., and W. C. Hayes. 1983a. Cross-sectional geometry of Pecos Pueblo femora and tibiae—a biomechanical investigation. I. Method and general patterns of variation. *Am J Phys Anthrop* 63:383–400.

Ruff, C. B., and W. C. Hayes. 1983b. Cross-sectional geometry of Pecos Pueblo femora and tibiae—a biomechanical investigation. II. Sex, age and size difference. *Am J Phys Anthrop* 63:383–400.

Ruffer, M. A. 1909. Preliminary note on the histology of Egyptian mummies. *British Medical Journal, London* 1:1005.

Sadig, A. M. 2013. *Reconsidering the Mesolithic and Neolithic of Sudan: Neolithisation of Northern Africa. Studies in Early Near Eastern Production, Subsistence, and Environment 16.* Berlin.

Sandberg, P. A., M. Sponheimer, J. Lee-Thorp, and D. P. Van Gerven. 2014. Intertooth analysis of dentine: A step toward addressing selective mortality in the reconstruction of life history in the archaeological record. *Am J Phys Anthrop* 155:281–293.

Sandison, A. T. 1967. Sir Marc Armand Ruffer (1859–1917) pioneer of palaeopathology. *Medical History* 11:150–156.

Sandison, A. T. 1972. Evidence of infective disease. *J Hum Evol* 1:213–224.

Sarzi-Puttini, P., and F. Atzeni. 2004. New developments in our understanding of DISH (diffuse idiopathic skeletal hyperostosis). *Current Opinion in Rheumatology* 16:287–292.

Save-Soderberg, T. 1987. *Temples and Tombs of Ancient Nubia: The International Rescue Campaign at Abu Simbel, Philae and Other Sites.* London: Thames and Hudson.

Savitt, T. L., and M. F. Goldberg. 1989. Herrick's 1910 case report of sickle cell anemia. *JAMA* 261:266–271.

Scarr, G. 2008. A model of the cranial vault as a tensegrity structure, and its significance to normal and abnormal cranial development. *International Journal of Osteopathic Medicine* 11:80–89.

Schillaci, M. A., D. Nikitovic, J. N. Akins, L. Tripp, and A. M. Palkovich. 2011. Infant and juvenile growth in ancestral Pueblo Indians. *Am J Phys Anthrop* 145:318–326.

Shapiro, H. L. 1959. The history and development of physical anthropology. *Amer Anthrop* 61:371–379.

Shattock, G. S. 1909. A report upon the pathological conditions of the aorta of King Merneptah. *Proceed Royal Soc Med (Pathological Section)* 2:122–127.

Sibley, L., G. J. Armelagos, and D. P. Van Gerven. 1992. Obstetric dimensions of the true pelvis in a medieval population from Sudanese Nubia. *Am J Phys Anthrop* 89:421–430.

Siqueira, J., and I. Rôças. 2009. The microbiota of acute apical abscesses. *Journal of Dental Research* 88:61–65.

Smith, G. E. 1909a. Anatomical remains. *Bulletin of the Archaeological Survey of Nubia* 3:21–28.

Smith, G. E. 1909b. *The Ancient Egyptians and Their Influence upon the Civilization of Europe*. New York: Harper and Bros.

Smith, G. E., and W. R. Dawson. 1924. *Egyptian Mummies*. New York: Dial Press.

Smith, G. E., and D. E. Derry. 1910. Anatomical report. In *Archaeological Survey of Nubia, Bulletin* 6.

Smith, G. E., and F. W. Jones. 1908. Anatomical report. In *Archaeological Survey of Nubia, Bulletin* 1.

Smith, H. S. 1962. *UNESCO's International Campaign to Save the Monuments of Nubia: Preliminary Reports of the Egypt Exploration Society's Nubian Survey*. Cairo: General Organisation for Government Printing Offices.

Smith, R. W., and R. R. Walker. 1964. Femoral expansion in aging women: Implications for osteoporosis and fractures. *Science* 145:156–157.

Smrcka, V., I. Marik, M. Svenssonova, and J. Likovsky. 2009. Case reports: Legg-Calvé-Perthes disease in Czech archaeological material. *Clinical Orthopaedics and Related Research* 467:293–297.

Sofaer, J. A. 1973. A model relating developmental interaction and differential evolutionary reduction in tooth size. *Evolution* 27:427–434.

Sofaer, J. A., H. L. Bailt, and C. J. MacLean. 1971. A developmental basis for differential tooth reduction during hominid evolution. *Evolution* 25:509–517.

Sponheimer, M., and J. A. Lee-Thorp. 1999. Isotopic evidence for the diet of an early hominid, *Australopithecus africanus*. *Science* 283:368–370.

Steckel, R., and J. Rose. 2002. *The Backbone of History: Health and Nutrition in the Western Hemisphere*. Cambridge: Cambridge University Press.

Stewart, T. 1957. Distortion of the pubic symphyseal surface in females and its effect on age determination. *Am J Phys Anthrop* 15:9–18.

Stini, W. A. 1979. Nutritional stress and growth: Sex difference in adaptive response. *Am J Phys Anthrop* 31:417–426.

Stodder, A. L. 1997. Subadult stress, morbidity, and longevity in Latte period populations on Guam, Mariana Islands. *Am J Phys Anthrop* 104:363–80.

Stoltzfus, R. J., M. Albonico, H. M. Chwaya, L. Savioli, J. Tielsch, K. Schulze, and R. Yip. 1996. Hemoquant determination of hookworm-related blood loss and its role in iron deficiency in African children. *Am J Trop Med Hyg* 5(4):399–404.

Stout, S. D. 1978. Histological structure and its preservation in ancient bone. *Current Anthropology* 19:601–604.

Strouhal, E. 1971. A contribution of the anthropology of the Nubian X-Group. In *Anthropological Congress Dedicated to Ales Hrdlicka*. Prague: Publishing House of the Czechoslovak Academy of Science.

Strouhal, E. 2015. Survey and analysis of malignant tumors of past populations in England and Scotland. *Journal of Paleopathology* 10:101–109.

Stuart-Macadam, P. 1991. Anaemia in Roman Britain: Poundbury Camp. In *Health in Past Societies: Biocultural Interpretations of Human Skeletal Remains in Archaeological Contexts*, ed. H. Bush and M. Zvelebil. Oxford: Tempvs Reparatvm Archaeological and Historical Associates.

Tabachnick, B. G., and L. S. Fidell. 2013. *Using Multivariate Statistics*. Boston: Pearson.

Tague, R. G., and C. O. Lovejoy. 1986. The obstetric pelvis of AL 288-1 (Lucy). *J Hum Evol* 15:237–255.

Thompson, D. W. 1942. On growth and form. In *On Growth and Form*. Cambridge: Cambridge University Press.

Todd, T. W. 1920. Age changes in the pubic bone. I. The male white pubis. *Am J Phys Anthrop* 3:285–334.

Trapper, M. 1995. Interrogating bodies: Medico-racial knowledge, politics and the study of a disease. *Comparative Study of Society and History* 1:76–93.

Trapper, M. 1998. *The Blood: Sickle Cell Anemia and the Politics of Race*. Philadelphia: University of Pennsylvania Press.

Trevathan, W. R. 1988. Fetal emergence patterns in evolutionary perspective. *Amer Anthrop* 90:674–681.

Turner, B. L., J. L. Edwards, E. A. Quinn, J. D. Kingston, and D. P. Van Gerven. 2007. Age-related variation in isotopic indicators of diet at medieval Kulubnarti, Sudanese Nubia. *Int J Osteoarch* 17:1–25.

Tylor, E. B. 1871. *Primitive Culture: Researches into the Development of Mythology and Philosophy*. London: J. Murray.

Ungar, P. 2004. Dental topography and diets of *Australopithecus afarensis* and early *Homo*. *J Hum Evol* 46:605–622.

Vagn Nielsen, O. 1970. *Human Remains. Metrical and Non-Metrical Anatomical Variations. The Scandinavian Joint Expedition to Sudanese Nubia*. Vol. 9. Munksgaard, Copenhagen: Scandinavian University Books.

Van Gerven, D. P. 1981. Nubia's last Christians: The cemetery of Kulubnarti. *Archaeology* 34:22–30.

Van Gerven, D. P. 1982. The contribution of time and local geography to craniofacial variation in Nubia's *Batn el Hajar*. *Am J Phys Anthrop* 60:471–478.

Van Gerven, D. P., and G. J. Armelagos. 1980. Sexual dimorphism and human evolution. *J Hum Evol* 9:437–446.

Van Gerven, D. P., and G. J. Armelagos. 1983. Farewell to paleodemography? Rumors of its death have been greatly exaggerated. *J Hum Evol* 12:353–360.

Van Gerven, D. P., R. Beck, and J. Hummert. 1990. Patterns of enamel hypoplasia in two medieval populations from Nubia's Batn-el Hajar. *Am J Phys Anthrop* 82:413–420.

Van Gerven, D. P., J. R. Hummert, and D. B. Burr. 1985. Cortical bone maintenance and geometry of the tibia in prehistoric children from Nubia's Batn el Hajar. *Am J Phys Anthrop* 66:275–280.

Van Gerven, D. P., J. Hummert, K. Pendergast-Moore, and M. K. Sandford. 1990. Nutrition, disease, and the human life cycle: A bioethnography of a medieval Nubian community. In *Primate Life History and Evolution*, ed. C. J. DeRousseau. New York: Wiley.

Van Gerven, D. P., S. G. Sheridan, and W. Y. Adams. 1995. The health and nutrition of a medieval Nubian population. *Am Anthrop* 97:468–480.

Van Gerven, D. P., M. K. Sandford, and J. R. Hummert. 1981. Mortality and culture change in Nubia's Batn el Hajar. *J Hum Evol* 10:395–408.

Verwers, G. J. 1962. The survey from Faras to Gezira Dabarosa. *Kush* 10:19–33.

Wakely, J., T. Anderson, and A. Carter. 1995. A multidisciplinarian case study of prostatic carcinoma from mediaeval Canterbury. *Journal of Archaeological Science* 22:469–477.

Wallace, D. C. 1992. Mitochondrial genetics: A paradigm for aging and degenerative diseases. *Science* 256:628–632.

Walker, G. F. 1972. A new approach to the analysis of craniofacial morphology and growth. *Am J Orthod* 61:221–232.

Walker, P. L. 1985. Anemia among prehistoric Indians of the American Southwest. *Health and Disease in the Prehistoric Southwest* 34:137.

Walker, P. L., R. R. Bathurst, R. Richman, T. Gjerdrum, and V. A. Andrushko. 2009. The causes of porotic hyperostosis and cribra orbitalia: A reappraisal of the iron-deficiency anemia hypothesis. *Am J Phys Anthrop* 139:109–125.

Washburn, S. L. 1951. The new physical anthropology. *Transactions of the New York Academy of Sciences* 13:258–304.

Washburn, T. C., D. Medearis, and B. Child. 1965. Sex differences in susceptibility to infections. *Pediatrics* 35:57–64.

Webb, S. 1982. Cribra orbitalia: A possible sign of anaemia in pre- and post-contact crania from Australia and Papua New Guinea. *Archaeology in Oceania* 17:148–156.

Wells, C. 1964. *Bones, Bodies, and Disease: Evidence of Disease and Abnormality in Early Man. Ancient Peoples and Places Series*. New York: Frederick A. Praeger.

Wendorf, F., and W. Chmielewski. 1965. *Contributions to the Prehistory of Nubia*. Dallas: Southern Methodist University.

Wendorf, F., R. Schild, N. El Hadidi, A. E. Close, M. Kobusiewicz, H. Wieckowska, B. Issawi, and H. Haas. 1979. Use of barley in the Egyptian late paleolithic. *Science* 205(4413):1341–1347.

White, C. D., and H. P. Schwartz. 1994. Temporal trends in stable isotopes for Nubian mummy tissues. *Am J Phys Anthrop* 93:165–187.

White, L. A. 1945. History, evolutionism, and functionalism: Three types of interpretation of culture. *Southwestern Journal of Anthropology* 1(2): 221–248.

White, T. D., M. T. Black, and P. A. Folkens. 2011. *Human Osteology*. Cambridge: Academic Press.

White, T. D., and P. A. Folkens. 2005. *The Human Bone Manual*. Cambridge: Academic Press.

Wiener, P. 1996. Experimental studies on the ecological role of antibiotic production in bacteria. *Evolutionary Ecology* 10:405–421.

Wilkie, A. O. 1997. Craniosynostosis: Genes and mechanisms. *Human Molecular Genetics* 6:1647–1656.

Wolpoff, M. H. 1976. Evolutionary aspects of hominid tooth reduction and early hominid dental variation. In *Les Plus Anciens Hominides*, ed. P. Tobias and Y. Coppens. Paris: Nat de la Res Scientifique.

Wood, J. W., et al. 1992. The osteological paradox. *Current Anthropology* 3:343–370.

Yakovlev, P. I. 1947. Paraplegias of hydrocephalics. *American Journal of Mental Deficiency* 51:561–576.

Yokochi, K. 1996. Tongue thrust swallowing in severely physically disabled children. *Brain Development* 18:242–244.

Zaino, E. C. 1967. Symmetrical osteoporosis: A sign of severe anemia in the prehistoric Pueblo Indians of the Southwest. In *Miscellaneous Papers in Paleopathology, Museum of Northern Arizona*. Flagstaff: Northern Arizona Society of Science and Art.

ABOUT THE AUTHORS

George J. Armelagos

George Armelagos (1936–2014) received his B.A. degree at the University of Michigan in 1958. He earned his master's degree in anthropology in 1963 and his Ph.D. in anthropology in 1968, both at the University of Colorado, Boulder. He was a professor of anthropology at the University of Massachusetts, Amherst, from 1968 to 1990, and then chair of the department of anthropology at the University of Florida from 1990 to 1993. He was the Goodrich C. White Professor of Anthropology at Emory University from 1993 until his retirement in 2014.

His research career in skeletal biology began in 1963 with his position as a research assistant for the University of Colorado Nubian Expedition to Wadi Halfa in Sudanese Nubia. His analysis of the skeletal remains excavated by the expedition focused on the interaction between patterns of mortality and disease and the cultural circumstances of the populations. The Nubia research and his biocultural approach contributed importantly to what is known today as bioarchaeology.

Armelagos's research extended far beyond his Nubia research. He did pioneering work on skeletal remains from the Dickson Mound in Illinois, and was a career-long critic of the race concept both in ancient and contemporary human populations. He also did groundbreaking work on the evolution of human infectious diseases. In addition to his many accomplishments as a researcher, he was an extraordinary award-winning teacher and mentor of both undergraduate and graduate students. He also liked to tell people that he was an avid outdoors person with a particular love for hang gliding and white-water rafting.

Dennis P. Van Gerven

Dennis Van Gerven received his B.A. in anthropology from the University of Utah in 1968. He did his graduate work at the University of Massachusetts, Amherst, and received his M.A. in 1969 and his Ph.D. in 1971. He became an assistant professor of anthropology at the University of Kentucky, Lexington, in 1971 and subsequently joined the faculty in the department of anthropology at the University of Colorado, Boulder, in 1974. He achieved the rank of associate professor in 1975, professor in 1983, and professor emeritus in 2013.

His research career has focused primarily on the analysis of human remains from Wadi Halfa and Kulubnarti in northern Sudanese Nubia. He codirected, with David Greene (University of Colorado) and W. Y. Adams (University of Kentucky), a December 1978–May 1979 joint University of Colorado/Kentucky expedition to Kulubnarti in support of that research. The Kulubnarti collection consisting of over 400 human remains resides at the University of Colorado. He also conducted research on Hohokam remains from Arizona as well as the Dickson Mound site in Illinois.

Van Gerven taught in areas of human origins, human adaptability, skeletal biology, and quantitative methods. He directed the University of Colorado Honors Program from 1996 to 2006. He is a two-time winner of the Boulder Faculty Assembly Teaching Award and three-time winner of the Student Alumni Association Teaching Award. He was named a University of Colorado President's Teaching Scholar in 1995 and was the 1998–1999 Carnegie Foundation Colorado Teacher of the Year.

INDEX

Page numbers in *italics* refer to illustrations.

www.ingramcontent.com/pod-product-compliance
Lightning Source LLC
LaVergne TN
LVHW091533200926
848483LV00002B/391
* 9 7 8 0 8 1 3 0 5 4 4 5 2 *